After the Wrath of God

After the Wrath of God

AIDS, Sexuality, and American Religion

ANTHONY M. PETRO

OXFORD
UNIVERSITY PRESS

OXFORD
UNIVERSITY PRESS

Oxford University Press is a department of the University of Oxford.
It furthers the University's objective of excellence in research, scholarship,
and education by publishing worldwide.

Oxford   New York
Auckland   Cape Town   Dar es Salaam   Hong Kong   Karachi
Kuala Lumpur   Madrid   Melbourne   Mexico City   Nairobi
New Delhi   Shanghai   Taipei   Toronto

With offices in
Argentina   Austria   Brazil   Chile   Czech Republic   France   Greece
Guatemala   Hungary   Italy   Japan   Poland   Portugal   Singapore
South Korea   Switzerland   Thailand   Turkey   Ukraine   Vietnam

Oxford is a registered trade mark of Oxford University Press
in the UK and certain other countries.

Published in the United States of America by
Oxford University Press
198 Madison Avenue, New York, NY 10016

Library of Congress Cataloging-in-Publication Data
Petro, Anthony Michael, 1981–
After the wrath of God : AIDS, sexuality, and American religion / Anthony M. Petro.
p.   cm.
Includes bibliographical references and index.
ISBN 978–0–19–939128–8 (cloth : alk. paper) 1. AIDS (Disease)—Religious aspects—
Christianity. 2. Sex—Religious aspects—Christianity. 3. AIDS (Disease)—Patients—
Religious life—UnitedStates. I. Title.
BX2347.8.A52.P48 2015
261.8'321969792—dc23
2014036658

1 3 5 7 9 8 6 4 2

Printed in the United States of America on acid-free paper

Contents

List of Illustrations	vi
Acknowledgments	vii
Introduction: AIDS, Sexuality, and Moral Citizenship	1
1. *Emerging Moralities:* American Christians, Sexuality, and AIDS	18
2. *Governing Authority:* The Surgeon General and the Moral Politics of Public Health	53
3. *Ecclesiastical Authority:* AIDS, Sexuality, and the American Catholic Church	91
4. *Protest Religion!* ACT UP, Religious Freedom, and the Ethics of Sex	137
Afterword	186
Notes	199
Selected Bibliography	257
Index	279

List of Illustrations

2.1 Gary Brookins, "I take it the Surgeon General's 'AIDS' pamphlet came today!" 56

2.2 Portrait of C. Everett Koop in Public Health Service uniform. 62

2.3 Cover of *Understanding AIDS*. 75

2.4 Ralph Dunagin, "If anything comes in the mail from the Surgeon General, don't open it!" 77

4.1 ACT UP New York's, "Silence = Death" poster. 142

4.2 ACT UP New York's, "Safe sex is hot sex" poster. 145

4.3 ACT UP New York's, "Stop the Church" flier for demonstration at St. Patrick's. 156

4.4 ACT Up New York's, "Stop the Pope: John Paul is a drag" poster. 163

4.5 ACT UP New York's, "Criminales de SIDA" poster. 169

4.6 ACT UP New York's, "Let me demonstrate," poster 1. 182

4.7 ACT UP New York's, "Let me demonstrate," poster 2. 183

Acknowledgments

I HAVE BENEFITED from the kindness, insight, and patience of more people than I can properly thank in a few pages. Though the shortcomings of this work remain mine, any successes arise from the wonderful colleagues and friends who have nurtured my research and writing over the last several years.

Marie Griffith supported this project from the start. Her scholarly insight, and her vision for what academic work can be, inspired this project throughout. Anyone who has worked with Judith Weisenfeld knows how lucky I have been to have her as a mentor, reader, and intellectual guide. Her advice and encouragement strengthened this project at every turn. Leigh Schmidt, Albert Raboteau, and especially Wallace Best (who always knows just what to say) generously provided their time, counsel, and critical feedback. Buzzy Teiser, Jeffrey Stout, Robert Wuthnow, Eddie Glaude, and Eric Gregory were excellent mentors and interlocutors. This book would not exist without Mark Jordan and his commitment to helping the rest of us try to say something about religion and sexuality that even approaches the incisiveness of his own work. Whether miracle-worker, angel, or saint I know not, but Kathryn Lofton read, critiqued, and championed this project at every step along the way. I could not have made it this far without mentors as wonderful as Tim Renick, Kathryn McClymond, Duane Corpis, and Amy Hollywood. Joyce Stavick and the late Diane Nix introduced me to critical thinking—I hope to have learned their lessons well.

I received helpful feedback on proposals and chapter drafts during a number of workshops and presentations at Princeton University, including the Religion and Public Life and the Religion and Culture workshops at the Center for the Study of Religion; the Women and Gender Studies Colloquium; and the American Religious History Workshop. I would particularly like to thank Patty Bogdziewicz, Jenny Wiley Legath, and Anita Kline for their support. I also received excellent feedback at the Religion and Sexuality Initiative at Emory University; the Politics of Religion conference at CUNY; various meetings of the American Society of Church History, the American Historical Association, and the American Academy of Religion; the American Religious History workshop at Yale University; the Center for Religion and Media at NYU; the GLBT Historical Society in San Francisco; and the departments of religion at Georgia State University and Boston University. My thanks to Levi McLaughlin and the Department of Religion at North Carolina State University for inviting me to present my work. Students in my seminar on "American Religion in the Age of AIDS" at Eugene Lang College of the New School pushed me to think anew about much of this material. I thank them and Mark Larrimore for that opportunity. I have benefited from generous funding and other material support from the Center for the Study of Religion, the Program in Women and Gender Studies, the Department of Religion, and the Program in American Studies at Princeton. My thanks go to the Boston University Center for the Humanities for providing generous funding to include the images in this book.

Archivists and librarians (and perhaps also baristas), as every historian knows, are the backbone of our scholarship. I thank the archival staff at the National Library of Medicine at the NIH in Bethesda; the AIDS History Project at UCSF Library; the National Archive of Lesbian, Gay, Bisexual, and Transgender History in New York City; the History Project in Boston; and the Billy Graham Center Archives at Wheaton College as well as the amazing ILL staff at Princeton University, NYU, and Boston University, who tracked down the many documents that eluded me. Though I have not met them in person, I remain indebted to the amazing work of Sarah Schulman and Jim Hubbard, who coordinate and make publicly available the very rich collection of interviews held in the ACT UP Oral History Project.

I was lucky to spend two years in the Religious Studies program at NYU, where Angela Zito, Adam Becker, Ann Pellegrini, and Jeremy Walton graciously taught me what it means to be a good colleague and interlocutor. Since then, my colleagues at Boston University have provided a most welcoming environment. My thanks go especially to Stephen Prothero, David Frankfurter, Deeana Klepper, and Adam Seligman for their support as chairs and mentors, and to Wendy Czik and the tireless Karen Nardella for their guidance and good cheer. My YSAR cohort at the Center for the Study of Religion and American Culture provided rich discussion and a critical eye on my introduction: my thanks to Courtney Bender and Bob Orsi for leading us; to Philip Goff, Art Farnsely, and Becky Vasko for bringing us together; and to Shelby Balik, Omri Elisha, Allison Greene, Rosemary Corbett, Katie Holscher, Hillary Kaell, David King, John Seitz, and Josef Sorett for their conversation.

I thank Laura Davulis for seeing potential in this project and Diane Winston for providing feedback on a draft of the proposal. At Oxford University Press, Theo Calderara provided support and critical feedback, making my work sharper. Marcela Maxfield graciously answered my many questions and ushered this project to completion. I am most grateful for the anonymous reviewers of this manuscript. I have no doubt fallen short of their suggestions, but I hope they will see how I have wrestled with their insightful, critical engagements with my work. My thanks to Cathy Hannabach for help with the index and to Jerry Altobelli for his keen eye in copyediting.

Fellow colleagues and friends often provided the best encouragement to keep thinking and to keep writing. For conversation, debate, references, and all the other little things, I offer abundant thanks to April Armstrong, Emily Mace, Josh Dubler, Kathleen Holscher, Briallen Hopper, Rachel Lindsey, Levi McLaughlin, Molly Farneth, Ryan Harper, Nicole Kirk, Elizabeth Jemison, Caleb Maskell, Harvey Stark, Beth Stroud, Joe Moshenska, Leah Hunt Hendrix, Lindsay Reckson, Allison Schnable, Megan Goodwin, Kristy Smolinski, Leslie Ribovich, Will Smith, Gina Cogan, Chris Lehrich, and Ricky Martin. Kathryn Gin Lum, Tisa Wenger, Rebecca Davis, Dan Williams, Amy Kittlestrom, Jon Pahl, Lauren Winner, Monique Moultrie, and Debra Levine offered references, suggestions, and critical advice that have stuck with me. Heather White, who paved the way, Jessica Delgado, Phillip Haberkern, Kathi Kern, Gayle Salamon, and Ann Neumann pushed my thinking, asked amazing questions, and offered their support, as have Kent Brintnall and the incomparable Lynne Gerber. Christienna Fryar, Samira Mehta, Russell Cambron, Tonie Boykin, Michael Melton, Zachary Herz, Freddie Lai, Paulo Natenzon, Moulie Vidas, Carey Seal, Mark Robinson, Andy Ferguson, and Adrienne Brown offered homes away from home, family away from family, and many laughs. Talia Dan-Cohen has, for almost a decade now, proven to be a great phone companion on walks from here to there and always knows how to make my thinking more precise. Nathan Ha read, discussed, and improved just about every word of this book—a friendship-defining feat if ever there was one.

My parents, Barbara and George, and brothers, George and Ryan, have blessed me with their love and support. They always encouraged my plans to go to college, then to study for a master's, and then to go on for a doctorate—even if they didn't quite understand why I was *still* in school. I cannot imagine better fortune in life than happening upon Patrick McKelvey. He went beyond the call of duty in reading drafts of every chapter, several times, talking through problems, and cheerleading me through the final stages. Along with our whippet Shelby, he reminded me why this work matters, but also when it was time to stop and go for a walk. Better interlocutors I could neither imagine nor love more.

*   *   *

I dedicate this work to my fellow traveler and thinker, Renata Hicks—she stays with me always—and to the many people who have been affected by the HIV/AIDS crisis. I wasn't certain why I started researching the history of religion and AIDS until I read the final pages of Paul Monette's *Borrowed Time*. The memoir recounts the death of Monette's lover, Roger, from AIDS. I was sitting in a coffee shop in Princeton when I came to the end—of the memoir and of his lover's life. As the meningitis reached Roger's brain, "the battle," Monette wrote, "was over." I couldn't hold back tears, couldn't stop reading. But I don't think I cried simply because Roger had died. I was moved, as well, by the love his partner had for him—not a romantic love, but a down in the trenches, dirty, unwavering, hard-fought love grounded in companionship, care, and respect. I was moved by what he'd lost, and for his strength in the midst of it. Also for what I'd lost, we'd lost: a generation of mentors, friends, neighbors, enemies, lovers, family. And for those we continue to lose.

After the Wrath of God

Introduction

AIDS, SEXUALITY, AND MORAL CITIZENSHIP

"The contemporary culture war is ultimately a struggle over national identity—over the meaning of America, who we have been in the past, who we are now, and perhaps most important, who we, as a nation, will aspire to become in the new millennium."

—JAMES DAVISON HUNTER, *Culture Wars*

"Medicine is at the core of our soteriological vision."

—BYRON GOOD, *Medicine, Rationality, and Experience*

"A good discipline tells you what you must do at every moment."

—MICHEL FOUCAULT, *Security, Territory, Population*

IN THE FALL of 1993, the Reverend Billy Graham—"America's pastor," as he had been known for decades—stood before an audience of more than forty thousand people in Columbus, Ohio. Over the years, Graham had been transformed from religious leader to celebrity to national icon. He had become, in the words of historian Grant Wacker, the "Great Legitimator," whose very presence "conferred sanctity on events, authority on presidents, acceptability on wars, desirability on decency, shame on indecency, and prestige on dessert recipes."[1] Standing before his audience in Columbus, Graham asked, "Is AIDS a judgment of God?" "I could not say for sure," he answered, "but I think so." Graham later apologized for his remarks, but his hesitance mirrored other Christian responses to AIDS.[2]

In 1986, the weekly Jesuit magazine *America* dedicated an issue to pastoral responses to the AIDS epidemic. The introduction was written by

Fr. Thomas Stahel, who had recently returned to the United States after a two-year stint mentoring young priests in Paraguay to take up his post as executive editor of the magazine. By that time, AIDS had become national news, and leaders of the Christian Right were quick to assert that it was a punishment from God. Stahel pushed back: "AIDS is not God's wrath poured out on homosexuals." Such a "vicious idea," he charged, "overlooks the fact that people who are not gay, even children, get AIDS." Even more, this condemnation "demeans God, attributing to Him the specifically vengeful intent characteristic of us, but not God. AIDS is not their problem, but ours."[3] Yet Catholics still faced an obstacle, he asserted: "How to promote a validly Christian attitude to the gay community, without saying that homogenital behavior is acceptable."[4]

These two examples capture a central tension that faced American Christians—and often Americans more broadly—in the first decade and a half of the AIDS epidemic. AIDS may not have been God's wrath, but neither, it seemed, were members of the gay community hapless victims of a strange new biomedical disease. Rather, from its start, AIDS was also a moral epidemic, complete with a hierarchy of victimhood that placed innocent children above implicitly guilty homosexuals. If AIDS was not God's wrath, many believed it was still in some sense a clear indication of God's morality for individuals and for the nation.

After the Wrath of God examines how religious leaders, organizations, and activists constructed AIDS as a *moral* epidemic, which has not only shaped cultural and political responses to the disease in the United States and abroad, but has helped draw the battle lines for the wider war over religion and sex. While recent accounts of religion and the AIDS epidemic have foregrounded the role of the Christian Right, this book examines the much broader—and more influential—range of American Christians who shaped public discussions of AIDS, sexuality, and public health.[5] Mainstream religious groups almost uniformly called for care and compassion for those afflicted with the disease, but the epidemic also prompted Protestants and Catholics alike to enter public debates about homosexuality and sex education, with far-reaching social and political ramifications for the trajectory of HIV prevention and care. American Christians responded to the epidemic, both at home and abroad, through means both medical and moral.

This book tracks the emergence of this moral and religious rhetoric in the first decade and a half of the epidemic. I focus on this period, which we might think of as the "long 1980s," for two reasons. First, it marks the introduction of AIDS itself into the public sphere, and consequently the advent of Christian reaction. AIDS became national news only gradually and unevenly over this period. But most Christians, and indeed most Americans, began to grapple with the epidemic between the mid-1980s and early 1990s.[6] Second, the introduction of the AIDS cocktail in the mid-1990s marked a sharp break in the history of AIDS in the United States.[7] This medical breakthrough largely redefined the idea that AIDS was a necessarily fatal disease into the notion that it was a chronic condition for those with access to good medical care.[8]

By the mid-1990s, in the popular imagination, AIDS was no longer just a gay disease, but was becoming a heterosexual—and eventually African—epidemic. Public health workers and AIDS activists in the United States increasingly targeted their efforts toward racial minorities, who were often overlooked in national media and by Christian AIDS workers. As the AIDS cocktail made the disease manageable in the United States, at least among those with sufficient means, Africa became the new focus of attention. By the early 2000s, American evangelicals made African AIDS into a major cause, one helped along the way by the decoupling of AIDS from homosexuality. Still, we should not divide the period this neatly. The rhetoric declaring AIDS a disease of sexual immorality did not disappear after the mid-90s; rather, it shifted the sin from homosexuality to promiscuity. Christian responses that have come after the wrath of God did not so much move beyond this rhetoric as layer upon it. Changes across the years should be considered not ruptures but laminations.

After the Wrath of God also reinterprets the last thirty years of American religious history through the AIDS crisis. Histories of American Christianity since the Second World War have ably, and often rightfully, underscored religious and political division and the rise of the Christian Right. But this emphasis has come at the expense of mainstream forms of American religion, often described as being in decline—a kind of demographic reductionism.[9] The religious history of the AIDS epidemic disrupts this narrative, since the crisis cannot easily be parsed along the lines of conservative and progressive or even religious and secular. This book employs a wider lens to make room for liberal and evangelical Protestants, Catholic bishops and lay parishioners, public health workers, AIDS activists, and gay and lesbian community leaders. It dwells upon the particularities of their religious and moral visions to demonstrate their differing responses to the disease, the diversity of American Christianity, and the form that Christian influence takes in the modern, secular age.

This book places the history of religious reactions to AIDS within the broader cultural and political history of the United States since the 1980s.[10] I seek to demonstrate how religious actors have shaped moral language surrounding AIDS, as well as to broaden scholarly interpretations of religion in America, especially since the 1980s. While focusing on Christian responses, I also attempt to elucidate the broader cultural and political influence that religious constructions of disease, sex, and morality have exerted. To that end, *After the Wrath of God* surveys the many books, pamphlets, pastoral guides, and major denominational statements about sexuality and AIDS published by religious writers in this period. It also draws from the archival records and oral and documentary histories of religious figures, political and public health leaders, and AIDS activists and organizations. I examine these sources alongside religious and secular media, including national magazines like *Christianity Today*, *Christian Century*, and *America* and newspapers like the *New York Times*, as well as local news sources such as the archdiocesan paper *Catholic New York* and the gay and lesbian magazine *OutWeek*.

Each chapter in this book identifies a particular site of religious and moral engagement—the emergence of moral approaches to HIV/AIDS and sexuality, the moral governing of public health, ecclesiastical authority, and grassroots protest against the Catholic hierarchy. Taken together, they demonstrate the pervasive moral and religious rhetoric that has gained purchase not merely by declaring AIDS a divine punishment, but by promoting moral prescriptions for sexuality. Saying yes to sex has proven far more persuasive than saying no, and religious Americans have learned this lesson. The ability to shape notions of morality in American discussions of AIDS, sexuality, and public health has grown into a source of religious power in modern America.[11] This form of power is perhaps most visible in cases where it has been translated into a conventionally secular vocabulary, in both the moral language of health and medicine and in rhetoric about American citizenship and its limits.[12] Before moving forward, it will be helpful to clarify two of the key terms that frame this study: morality and citizenship.

Morality, AIDS, and Biomedicine

Religious actors have reframed political approaches to AIDS, sexuality, and public health by amplifying the moral dimensions of this epidemic. But how have moral languages become attached to HIV/AIDS, and what are the form and content of this morality? Few words have the potential to carry as much authority or to be as rhetorically flexible as *morality*. In modern America, especially among political conservatives, invocations of morality have become a useful tool for public debate precisely because the term is unwieldy and shifting: morality doubles as both a religious and secular concept, often becoming the site of translation between the two. This is particularly true for moral claims about health. "Health," writes Lynne Gerber in her study of modern evangelicals, is "often used as a way to talk about moral concerns in language more broadly accessible than that of sin, giving an ostensibly secular category theological meaning."[13] Moral claims can translate ideas about sinfulness into statements about health because morality cuts across modern American religious and secular vocabularies. Morality is what's "good" about modern religion; it is also what leaves room to debate how people ought to act—and what their actions say about their humanity—in the seemingly disenchanted world of modern medicine.[14]

In this book, I use *morality* and *moral languages* to describe correct behavior, especially in regard to codes of sexual conduct or norms, and the ways that people talk about these norms.[15] Moral languages about health and sexuality deem some practices to be right (or moral) and others wrong. Sometimes they do so in ways that are explicit, but they can also be implicit, even to the speaker or writer. At times, I use the term *ethics* to mark a slight departure—from codes or ideas of proper behavior to practices or techniques that contribute to the formation of an ethical or moral person.[16] While this book emphasizes how religious actors in particular employed moral languages, morality need not be tied to any specific religious tradition. Indeed, one of my key arguments is that through the AIDS crisis, Christian moral assumptions regarding sexuality were elaborated by, attached to, and translated into broader political and public health discourses, which in turn often reappeared in theological and religious rhetoric.[17] The convergence of scientific, theological, and religious rhetoric proved powerful in the moral languages about sexuality that developed in the wake of—and through—the epidemic.

But not all forms of morality work in the same way. Michel Foucault suggests the different forms that morality can take when he distinguishes between two approaches to the creation and enforcement of norms.[18] In one, a standard is defined in advance and people are measured against it—they are either normal or abnormal. In the other approach, the standard for what is normal is deduced from the population itself, and people are encouraged to move toward the center of the curve. The former is grounded in discipline, the latter in regulation.[19]

Mainline Christian models for pastoral care, like most public health models, largely followed this latter approach. Evangelical and official Catholic models, on the other hand, focused on discipline. Those approaches, in turn, relied on two distinct conceptions of the disease. Most public health workers and mainline Christians described AIDS as a biomedical issue: that is, as a virus. They believed prevention should focus on changing behavior to the extent that these changes in behavior blocked the spread of HIV. Evangelical and Catholic leaders, on the other hand, held a different view, one that did not displace but worked alongside this biomedical explanation. For them, AIDS was both a viral and a moral crisis. Their efforts to fight the epidemic concentrated not merely on preventing the spread of a virus but also on changing human moral behavior precisely in order to realign such behavior with a specific, predetermined moral code. This moral approach has included specific norms governing where and how sex should take place—at the very least, that sex should occur only within the bounds of monogamous, heterosexual marriage.

I do not mean to say, however, that biomedical approaches were not moral, or that Christians simply joined a moral argument to a biomedical one. On the contrary, biomedicine is itself a moral enterprise, though it does not embrace this notion.[20] As we will see, the language of medical objectivity often obscures the moral claims that medicine makes, while other moral arguments, usually Christian or biblical, become fused with biomedical knowledge. What I hope to demonstrate is that some Christians moved beyond targeting the *virus* to prevent its spread because the disease, in this view, was not fundamentally biomedical. Their tactics aimed to shape individual and social moral values. Their aim was not merely to stop the flow of microbes but to spread religious and moral conduct. The treatment of AIDS, in other words, could not be limited to the prevention of HIV: condoms might *slow* the spread of the epidemic, evangelical leaders Rick and Kay Warren would argue, but they cannot *stop* it. Only moral behavior could do that. This is the morality that I attempt to trace.[21]

Moral Citizenship

The content of this modern Christian morality—the focus on abstinence and (heterosexual) monogamy—both emerged through and became a defining feature of local and national political debates. Particular languages of Christian sexual morality were further expressed through attempts to define what I call "moral citizenship." This raises a series of questions. What forms did American sexual morality take in this period, and of what did it consist? How has it been advanced through religious discussions of the AIDS epidemic and prevention? And how does it draw the boundaries of national citizenship around questions of legitimate and illegitimate sexual practice and identity?

In using the term *moral citizenship*, I draw upon historical and sociological descriptions of citizenship as a culturally and legally defined *status*. They emphasize citizenship as an identity rather than something people exercise.[22] Recent scholarship on *sexual citizenship*, in particular, has examined the historical struggles of sexual and gender minorities to gain legal rights.[23] During the 1980s, gays, lesbians, and people with HIV/AIDS made a number of claims on local, state, and federal governments. These included requests for legal protection against discrimination based on sexual orientation and HIV status. They also called for larger-scale and faster federal responses to HIV/AIDS, especially in the first few years when activists accused the government of sidestepping an issue that was imagined only to affect a small, marginal population. Government agencies have the authority to bestow or withhold the status of legal citizenship or to bestow it partially, as is often the case for those at the margins of society. For instance, gays and lesbians have struggled to gain full citizenship status through the decriminalization of sodomy (achieved in the 2003 Supreme Court case *Lawrence v. Texas*, which overturned the 1986 case *Bowers v. Hardwick*), through local, state, and federal anti-discrimination protections (which have been successful in some cities and states), and most recently through state and federal recognition of same-sex marriages. Here, citizenship status provides access to various state resources.

But citizenship has also long functioned as a site for cultural identity and recognition. For instance, in addition to demanding legal protections and funding, AIDS activists often expressed their frustration that President Ronald Reagan did not speak publicly about AIDS until 1986. Beyond material and legal recognition, these activists also sought public recognition. To be a citizen, in this sense, is to become a recognized part of a national community. I use *moral citizenship* here to emphasize the history of competing visions of sexual morality for this idea of the imagined nation.[24] To be sure, sexual morality has enjoyed a long career in the business of defining not just citizenship, but even personhood.[25] I use this term to highlight the struggle for sexual citizenship among sexual and gender minorities, but also to name the pervasive, if sometimes ethereal, rhetoric of Christian and secular sexual morality that continues to shape notions of personhood and ideas of who constitutes a "real" American. This book examines how arguments about proper sexual morality have framed the boundaries of the American nation and the definition of moral citizenship. To address this, however, we must also understand the shifting historical contours of citizenship itself, especially the ways that Reagan-era conservatism reshaped American citizenship and political practice.[26]

In *The Queen of America Goes to Washington City*, Lauren Berlant describes the reemergence and intensification in the 1980s of what she calls the "intimate public sphere . . . a rhetorical shift from a state-based and thus political identification with nationality to a culture-based concept of the nation as a site of integrated social membership."[27] The shift stretches back at least to the 1960s, a moment in American history before the organizing mantra of "equal rights" gave way to the dominant refrain of "family values" in the 1980s and 1990s. Americans intensely debated issues of gender and sexuality over this period. These battles led to what Robert Self calls a "transformation of the national polity itself," which included "how Americans conceived of the nation and the possibility of improving society."[28] The family became a key site of intervention, especially for members of the embryonic Christian Right. By the late 1970s, conservative evangelicals and Catholics set new sights on national politics as they fought against what they perceived to be moral threats to the "traditional family"—key among them were feminism (particularly efforts to pass the Equal Rights Amendment), abortion, and gay rights.[29]

Conservative Christian rhetoric quickly gained traction, as groups like Jerry Falwell's Moral Majority and James Dobson's Focus on the Family put the traditional family in the national spotlight. More and more we would see what Berlant calls "the marketing of nostalgic images of a normal, familial America."[30] This marketing corresponded to a new form of politics. Berlant tracks this shift—from the kinds of claims activists made upon the state in the 1960s and 1970s (such as for civil rights) toward an increasingly sentimentalized notion of citizenship defined not through one's relation to the state, but in terms of one's sense of national belonging. Note the important distinction here between the *state*, which was receding as the site for the provision of civil rights and social goods, and the imagined *nation*, which was becoming the privileged site for making claims to American citizenship. The AIDS crisis has played a critical role in this transformation.

To the extent that the sexual revolution of the 1960s and 1970s focused on securing rights to birth control, abortion, and divorce, it was a revolution, Berlant argues, "largely, in heterosexuality."[31] The modern gay and lesbian rights movement advanced alongside this revolution, but it would not come fully into the national spotlight until the 1980s, when AIDS brought the sexual lives of gay men—and, to a lesser extent, lesbians—into public discussion, including among American Christians. The introduction of gay sexuality into national debates about AIDS thus converged with new ways of imagining citizenship as a mode of national belonging. In the context of AIDS hysteria, political and cultural conservatives, including those within the Christian Right, could declare gay men and lesbians not fully American. As Thomas Yingling describes it: "conservatives may thus not only ignore the need for the nation-state to respond to population groups not visible within 'America' (predominantly gays and IV drug users in the early years of the AIDS epidemic) but may even cast those needs as anti-American, as a danger *to* rather than *within* the state."[32]

This political and cultural realignment transformed both the idea of the "American nation" and the meanings of American citizenship, including moral citizenship.[33] By linking sexual discipline to the idea of the America nation, religious leaders promulgated no less than a national sexuality. This national sexuality has proclaimed some forms of sex—namely, abstinence until marriage and monogamy in marriage—not merely respectable, but fundamental to the health of the American public.

Sexuality and the Moral Narratives of AIDS

After the Wrath of God builds upon a rich body of historical and cultural studies that have illuminated AIDS not only as a medical event but as a social and political one as well.[34] I take this proposition a step further: AIDS has been since its emergence both a religious and moral event. The particular religious and moral languages surrounding the epidemic in the United States cannot be separated from narratives of sexuality, especially those of gay sex.

While medical authorities identified Haitian immigrants, intravenous drug users, and female sex workers among the earliest cases of AIDS, media portrayals of a new "gay plague" largely defined popular and political opinions of the epidemic. Medical researchers and the media associated the disease not only with sexuality, but with the gay (and quickly gay male) population and with practices of sexual "promiscuity." The gay and

lesbian community—lesbians were not immune to the social stereotyp-
ing—was increasingly defined by sexual practices that many scientists and
members of the general public considered immoral, if not bizarre. The
mainstream media sensationalized stories of gay men claiming hundreds,
if not thousands, of sexual partners and participating in a range of sexual
practices largely unknown outside of urban gay populations, including
BDSM, fisting, and frequenting bathhouses.[35]

The question of how to talk about gay sex has haunted discussions
of the AIDS epidemic and reveals the power of moral and moralizing
narratives. To be sure, some practices, including anal sex and sex with
multiple partners, contributed to the rapid spread of HIV through the
gay community. Yet popular and scholarly narratives of this fact have
varied in the extent to which they have morally faulted the gay community itself for spreading AIDS. Here I discuss two examples. In his
groundbreaking 1987 account *And the Band Played On,* gay journalist
Randy Shilts emphasized sexual promiscuity as a leading cause of the
spread of AIDS, a position echoed in historian Jonathan Engel's more
recent *The Epidemic: A Global History of AIDS.* Public health officials,
religious leaders, and some gay activists used this rhetoric of promiscuity to support state-led efforts to encourage gay men to decrease
their sexual contacts (if not to stop having sex altogether) and to close
bathhouses.

The moral narrative of *And the Band Played On* centered on the character of Gaëtan Dugas, the infamous French Canadian flight attendant,
whom Shilts labeled "Patient Zero." In the first years of the epidemic,
Shilts explains, CDC researchers traced a number of men diagnosed with
AIDS back to sexual encounters with Dugas, an attractive and "sexually
voracious" gay man who flew from coast to coast expanding his list of
sexual exploits. "Quite pleased with himself," Shilts writes, Dugas "rattled
off" his list of conquests (already in the hundreds) to the health researchers. In these early years of the epidemic, anti-gay and anti-sex hysteria
outpaced scientific evidence. The flight attendant ignored doctors' claims
that he had what was then called "gay cancer" and refused to limit his
sexual activity. In Shilts' account, after having sex with a new partner the
airline steward would announce, "I've got gay cancer. I'm going to die and
so are you." Shilts morally indicted Dugas for continuing to have sex with
men and consequently spreading disease to a number of new victims.
Indeed, as Douglas Crimp puts it, Dugas served as the villainous center of
this AIDS exposé.[36]

Timothy Murphy contends that Dugas represents for Shilts "the sexual ethos of gay life itself" and even "an occasion for lamentation about the evils of (gay) men." He continues:

> To the extent that Shilts uses Dugas as a figure for gay men—no other gay man in *And the Band Played On* is said to represent what every man wanted from gay life; not an activist, not a politician, not a journalist—the very defining properties of gay life provide the conditions for the epidemic's possibility.[37]

Murphy questions why a tragic figure like Dugas is presented as a greater social evil than educational failures that continue to leave many people confused about how HIV/AIDS is transmitted. Moving into the late 1980s and 1990s, we might add to Murphy's list of social problems conservative opposition to the dissemination of safe sex information, the narrowing of sex education to abstinence instruction, or advertising the scientifically inaccurate claim that condoms are ineffective in preventing the transmission of HIV (often translated into the language of "failure rates").[38]

Engel also foregrounds the "sexual promiscuity" of gay men, whose reluctance to stop having sex and resistance to closing bathhouses are deemed moral failures that abetted the rapid spread of AIDS. He elevates the rhetoric of sexual perversity glimpsed in Shilts' account, detailing for his readers the range of sex practices in which gay men indulged during the heyday of sexual liberation. "In some bathhouses," Engel gushes, "customers could have oral sex through a hole cut between plywood partitions, nullifying even the need for eye contact." A page later, his repugnance erupts:

> It wasn't just the quantity of sex that raises hackles; it was the increasing perversity of it. Many young gay men in San Francisco, New York, and Los Angeles in the 1970s relentlessly pursued increasingly bizarre and extreme sexual experiences, ranging from urination, to bondage, to beatings. Men had themselves tied up and bullwhipped, chained to a cross, urinated on while crouching in a bath-tub, suspended in slings to be masturbated, and penetrated in every way imaginable.[39]

Caught up in the "perverse" sexual practices "relentlessly pursued" by voracious gay men who wanted it "in every way imaginable," Engel's moralizing (and salacious) narrative proved irresistible. But it ignores the fact that most of the sex practices listed here, including those perhaps considered most perverse by a general audience—glory holes, sadomasochism, golden showers—were relatively unlikely to transmit HIV. The latter two do not necessarily involve swapping semen or blood, the bodily fluids in which the virus lives, thus making them—despite their shock value—safer practices than unprotected anal or vaginal intercourse, even if it were monogamous. In fact, Engel's portrait of gay sex has less to do with relaying the history of AIDS than with advancing a view of history tethered to moral consequence rather than medical accuracy. In his account, the unrestrained hedonism of gay men would eventually square off against the punishing truth of nature's will, which would descend upon them in the form of AIDS.

Engel's discussion of gay sexuality reflects a broader conservative approach to public health decision-making. This position trivializes political resistance by gay and AIDS activists to public health initiatives proposed in the 1980s, such as those to close bathhouses and to limit or abstain from sexual encounters.[40] While presenting public health measures as being of the utmost importance, Engel sidesteps the need to weigh potentially invasive public health measures against individual liberties, such as the political and social ramifications that mandatory testing would have had in an atmosphere in which people who tested positive risked losing their health insurance, housing, and jobs. By contrast, Engel upholds the U.S. military as a model for dealing with the AIDS epidemic. The military instituted mandatory testing for all soldiers and "faced few of the limits on civil discourse or *politically correct stigmatization* that undermined public health efforts."[41] Engel thus privileges the public health model for dealing with epidemics, without considering the cultural and political factors underlying the lived reality of those affected by AIDS or the formation of scientific knowledge itself. Though Engel would surely maintain that AIDS was caused by a virus, not by God's punishment, his narrative nonetheless implicates the "sexual promiscuity" of gay men in the spread of AIDS. Consequently, the failure to curb such practices—by closing bathhouses and limiting sex to monogamous relationships—was, in his view, a moral failure on the part of the gay community.

What have been the rhetorical effects of focusing upon sexual identity or invoking "sexual promiscuity"? What difference does it make when drawing upon the loaded connotations of "promiscuity" in particular, a term historically reserved for that other class of sexual deviants, female prostitutes?[42] My point here is not that there is a correct way to represent

AIDS or sexuality, but that our rhetorical choices nonetheless bear discernable moral and political consequences. The Reagan administration's long silence regarding AIDS, for example, had much to do with the idea that it was a "gay disease" and that gay lives were of limited value to an imagined "American public."

There are alternative renderings. In separate studies published in the 1980s, journalist Cindy Patton and political scientist Dennis Altman explicitly resisted labeling the sexual practices of gay men as *moral* failings.[43] They demonstrated how scientific and media reports of the epidemic quickly slipped from descriptions of specific sexual *practices* that could transmit disease to forms of sexual *identity* associated with AIDS. Homosexual identity and homosexuality in general, not just specific sexual practices, were subject to both epidemiological concern and moral blame. As a result, the medical model employed to stem the spread of the disease itself promoted the moral and health benefits of monogamy, if not heterosexuality, rather than focus on safe sexual practices.[44]

A form of sexual conservatism arose when medical authorities and the media increasingly faulted "sexual promiscuity" for the spread of AIDS. Both Altman and Patton insisted that it was not sexual promiscuity that was the problem, but rather specific sexual acts: that is, not the volume of sexual partners, as Engel would later claim, but what people were doing. Some practices such as mutual masturbation (and to a lesser extent oral sex) posed lower or even virutally no risk of infection, regardless of the number of sexual partners. The real culprit was unprotected anal and vaginal intercourse, which did put people at risk—and which put them at greater risk as their partners multiplied. Patton and Altman offered what has been called a "sex-positive" narrative of the epidemic. They avoided stigmatizing "sexual promiscuity" (and by extension the ostensible perversity of homosexuals) by focusing instead on the types of sexual practices that proved capable of spreading this disease.[45] In this view, calls for monogamy betrayed a conservative sexual moralism that has subsequently been written into the history of AIDS.[46] Their writings emphasized how a growing culture of conservatism shaped medical, political, and popular responses to the epidemic—an ideology that they located within the Christian heritage of American sexual mores.

All too quickly, however, such accounts begin and end their discussions of religion and AIDS with the Christian Right. Altman first published his book on the American AIDS epidemic in Great Britain under the title *AIDS and the New Puritanism*. Invocations of "Puritanism" cast a long shadow over the history of AIDS (and of sexuality) in the United States, particularly for gay and lesbian authors who were part of a political tradition that has often perceived—and reproduced—a historical opposition between Christianity and gay liberation.[47] This perception has fueled narratives of gay and lesbian history that overlook the long record of religious entanglement with homosexuality, including at times support for gay and lesbian rights.[48]

Most accounts of the AIDS epidemic repeat this pattern by depicting the relationship between religious practitioners and AIDS activists primarily as one of conflicting beliefs and interests, a pattern that stems partly from the overrepresentation of conservative religious figures, who are made to stand in for religion in general.[49] The specter of the Christian Right has thus preoccupied popular and historical representations of AIDS. By reducing religious responses to the statements of the Christian Right, we risk understating both the range of conservative, mainstream, and progressive religious engagements with AIDS as well as their influence upon popular constructions of the epidemic and health care policy. *After the Wrath of God* addresses the wider spectrum of public religious discourse both to enlarge historical narratives of AIDS and to provide a new lens through which to assess the moral and religious constructions of this epidemic.

Moving Forward

Given this book's attention to Christian engagements with AIDS, readers may wonder how "religion"—highlighted in its title—figures into the analysis. My intention is not to read Christianity as American religion writ large. Nor is it to suggest that other religious traditions did not figure prominently into the history of AIDS, which could be told with greater attention to Jewish, Buddhist, Native American, and New Age viewpoints in particular.[50] I use the term "religion" to distinguish certain kinds of language considered religious from ostensibly nonreligious AIDS discourses, including those of biomedicine, public health, and state policy. In this sense, the term operates descriptively, following the historical separation of religious and secular spheres. Analytically, however, *After the Wrath of God* ultimately unsettles the historical presumptions of this separation, not least by showing how easily Christian speech traveled into or even constituted purportedly secular rhetoric through morality.[51] The term *religion* itself comes under scrutiny in my final chapter, where I describe how

AIDS activists, Catholic leaders, and lay members of the church drew upon the category of "religion" more often than "Catholic" to articulate their concerns about sexual protest and religious freedom.

I do not want to insist upon sharp delineations in the terminology used to describe various kinds of Christians, in part because the moral rhetoric that this book examines does not cleave to common divisions. But some clarifications are in order. They are meant to offer a roadmap, not a final definition. I employ *evangelical* in this work to designate a specific subset of Protestant Christians who take the Bible as an authoritative message from God that is not only applicable to, but normative in, their daily lives, and who understand spiritual rebirth—or being born again—as a moment of personal conversion marking their Christian identity. Most of the people I label evangelicals would likely recognize themselves in this term, but might prefer "Bible-believing Christians." Evangelicals tend to be more theologically conservative than "liberal" or "mainline" Protestants, who stress reading the Bible within its cultural and historical context and the need to re-interpret its meaning for today's world. While many of the evangelicals I describe in this book are also political and social conservatives, there are of course moderate and progressive evangelicals, too.[52] When I refer to "conservative" Christians, whether Protestant or Catholic, I aim to highlight their political positions, especially in regard to issues of gender and sexuality, in the context of American politics since the 1960s.[53] When I speak of members of the Christian Right, I have in mind historian George Marsden's definition of fundamentalists as evangelicals who are militantly opposed to shifts from what they consider biblical or traditional values toward those aligned with "secular humanism." Or, as he put it more playfully (though no less accurately), a fundamentalist is an "evangelical who is angry about something."[54] Emotions, like these religious identities, shift over time and are often inflected through other feelings— of urgency, disgust, love, compassion, worry. In this regard, I am interested in examining moments of speech that could be aligned with the Christian Right, or with evangelicals, or with mainline Protestants or Catholics, with the understanding that such moments may not be definitive of their particular religious identities or political alignments. This point should become clear moving forward.

Within this book, I alternate between using the terms *gay* or *lesbian* and *homosexual*. The former terms have become preferable in recent years among both historians and members of these communities to refer to personal and political identities. Since the 1990s, public health and medical researchers have also used "MSM" (men who have sex with men) to include men—especially racial and ethnic minorities and men outside of the United States—who do not identify as gay or bisexual, identities sometimes associated with being white or American. Since this book emphasizes the cultural and religious power of representation, I prefer to use *gay* to mark this history. I often use *homosexual* to connote how this term has been used in specific contexts, especially religious and medical writing, to reproduce "homosexuals" as objects of medical and moral attention.[55]

I employ *AIDS epidemic* in this work to signify the cultural history and effects of HIV and AIDS. Strictly speaking, AIDS (acquired immune deficiency syndrome) is a syndrome, which according to the vast majority of medical experts is caused by HIV (the human immunodeficiency virus), a retrovirus that harms the immune system by attacking white blood cells.[56] Not all people who test positive for HIV develop AIDS. Advances in drug treatment since the 1990s have made this especially true for people who have access to quality medical care. It has become common popular and scholarly parlance to use *HIV/AIDS* or simply *AIDS* to capture the broader cultural complex of this epidemic, including the specific medical conditions and social and political responses to it since the 1980s. Following the lead of members of this community who have found empowerment in denying their status as "victims," it has become preferable to refer to people diagnosed with HIV or AIDS as people with AIDS (PWAs) or people with HIV.[57]

Finally, I must note that by emphasizing public debates about AIDS and sexual morality, and especially homosexuality, I focus selectively on some aspects of this history at the expense of others. This emphasis skews my analysis towards the words and actions of religious and political actors and organizations that exerted national influence. This book is far less concerned with internal religious experience or celebrations of religious agency than with the powerful intellectual, political, and cultural effects of religious engagements with AIDS in the public sphere.[58] It places grassroots AIDS ministry work, lay parishioners, and AIDS activists alongside religious and political elites in order to discern the national implications of their encounters. I thus favor some debates and historical contexts over others. For instance, the morality of drug use and of other forms of sexual practice, such as female prostitution, enter this discussion, but a rigorous account of these perspectives falls outside my scope. Other renderings of this history could foreground different geographical, historical, or ideological contexts. In this manner, studies of gender and race in the moral and religious history of AIDS appear especially pressing. There is a clear need for further studies to account for these and countless other complexities. My aim is merely to contribute to the larger history of American religion, AIDS, and sexuality.

***

This book elucidates the central role that American Christianity has played in the AIDS epidemic, especially in its first decade. Even more, it demonstrates how religious actors and activists constructed AIDS as a moral epidemic. This construction has left an indelible mark not only on understandings of the disease itself, but also upon efforts to provide care for people with AIDS, upon political debates over AIDS prevention, and, not least, upon far-reaching battles over the link between sex and disease, morality and consequence, and the ethics of sexuality in America.

Chapter One

Emerging Moralities

AMERICAN CHRISTIANS, SEXUALITY, AND AIDS

> *"[T]he notion that certain sexual activities especially or uniquely violate nature is a theological claim constructed over centuries of Christian exegesis and argument."*
> —MARK JORDAN, *The Ethics of Sex*

> *"Communicable disease compels attention—for scientists and the lay public alike—not only because of the devastation it can cause but also because the circulation of microbes materializes the transmission of ideas."*
> —PRISCILLA WALD, *Contagious: Cultures, Carriers, and the Outbreak Narrative*

ON DECEMBER 1, 2008, the twentieth anniversary of World AIDS Day, Southern Baptist pastor Rick Warren presented President George W. Bush with the first "International Medal of PEACE" on behalf of the Global PEACE Coalition. The award recognized Bush's "unprecedented contribution to the fight against HIV/AIDS and other diseases," particularly through the President's Emergency Plan for AIDS Relief, or PEPFAR, which had provided over $18 billion to combat HIV/AIDS globally since 2003.[1] Bush received the award during the Saddleback Civil Forum on Global Health held in Washington, D.C.'s Newseum, a museum predictably dedicated to the history of news.

Bush reciprocated the praise. He lauded Warren's international PEACE plan for bringing government agencies together with faith and business leaders to solve global problems. "Government is justice, and love comes from a higher government, higher calling—from God," Bush explained. "People from across America, motivated by faith," he continued, "are already involved in the process" of bringing faith and government together:

"so why not bring some order and focus. That is a proper role of the government in this case, and it's working."[2] Bush's praise suggests he was not the only winner on this newsworthy occasion. His very presence signaled the arrival of American evangelicals as leaders in the international fight against AIDS.

While evangelicals have been involved in fighting AIDS since the early 1980s, their work received little national attention until the early twenty-first century, when prominent leaders like Rick Warren made the crisis a key priority. Author of the best-selling guide to Christian living *The Purpose Driven Life*, Warren founded Saddleback Church in 1980, and it has since grown into one of the largest congregations in the United States. Along with his wife Kay, he has championed a "biblically based" approach to AIDS work, one that places an evangelical notion of sexual morality at its center. That moral proposition includes abstinence before marriage and fidelity within a monogamous union. Since the early 2000s, this approach to HIV/AIDS prevention has gained prominence not only within the voluntary sector of AIDS relief, but also at the level of national policy, evidenced by the success of evangelical lobbying for abstinence education funding in Bush's PEPFAR.

Bush's presidency marshaled into the American mainstream a new constellation of conservative and religious politics that championed faith-based activism as a tool for national policy and social reform. Conservatives had been gaining influence in the United States as far back as the 1970s, and proponents of the Christian Right held sway within Ronald Reagan's administration. But George W. Bush elevated to a new level faith-based approaches to humanitarian concerns. Few measures advocated under his administration were more significant to politically conservative Christians and Jews than PEPFAR.[3] The president's global fight against AIDS marked a significant battleground for conservative religious leaders who opposed comprehensive sex education in favor of programs that promoted abstinence as the best, if not the only, way to prevent the spread of HIV. Under pressure from evangelicals—and under fire from most public health professionals—PEPFAR earmarked a significant percentage of its prevention funding for abstinence-based education.[4] In doing so, it signaled Bush's commitment to faith-based approaches to AIDS activism that focused on the moral training of abstinence and marital fidelity. Warren's bestowal of an award on Bush for his fight against AIDS thus advanced the moral platform of evangelical AIDS activism as well, including Warren's own HIV/AIDS Initiative, which was launched in 2004 and has since become one of the biggest players in the global fight against AIDS.

But support for faith-based AIDS prevention has not been limited to conservatives like Bush and his fellow Republicans. Appearing on *The To-night Show with Jay Leno* in 2006, Senator Barack Obama also called upon the church to become a central ally in the fight against AIDS. "Let me say this: I don't think we can deny that there is a moral and spiritual compo-nent to prevention," Obama explained: "that in too many places all over the world where AIDS is prevalent—including our own country, by the way—the relationship between men and women, between sexuality and spirituality, has broken down, and needs to be repaired."[5] Obama thus di-agnosed one of the key factors hindering efforts to win the fight against HIV/AIDS, both in the United States and abroad: the failure of men and women to maintain healthy relationships with one another, relationships that combined sexual intimacy with spirituality.

Obama's point reflected a shift over the previous decade and a half in how many Americans thought about AIDS: no longer a "gay disease," it also affected heterosexuals, often those living in Africa. Obama resisted characterizing AIDS solely as an "African" problem, noting its presence in the United States, where it has disproportionately affected African Ameri-can and Latino communities and is spread through both intravenous drug use and sexual intercourse. For Obama, the epidemic nonetheless re-mained sexual, even heterosexual—its continued spread stemming from the failures of male-female relationships. The salve for this breakdown was no less than the reunion of "sexuality and spirituality," the return to a moral foundation for sexual relationships between men and women. This moral foundation was also a medical foundation, one in which spirituality and health mutually constituted one another. If we didn't know better, we might think Obama an evangelical.

Indeed, Obama's call to enlist a moral and spiritual component in AIDS relief work followed only days after his participation in the 2006 Global Summit on AIDS and the Church, hosted by Rick and Kay Warren. Held annually since 2005, this conference brought together politicians, religious leaders, and health experts to discuss the place of the church in the AIDS epidemic. The 2006 Summit witnessed Obama praying hand-in-hand with Rick Warren and Republican Senator Sam Brown-back before he affirmed the need for the participation of churches in the fight against AIDS. Obama's participation drew criticism from Chris-tians on the Far Right, who denounced Warren for inviting leaders who dissented from the hardline evangelical stance regarding abstinence, fidelity, and abortion.[6]

Obama supported comprehensive sex education and called upon evangelical leaders and health professionals to move past debates over condoms versus abstinence. Indeed, this has remained a key difference between Obama and evangelical AIDS activists like Warren. Nonetheless, Obama's presence, along with other international leaders and celebrities who have attended in the past—including former British Prime Minister Tony Blair, President of Rwanda Paul Kagame, Hillary Clinton, Bill and Melinda Gates, and even Bono—helped legitimate Warren's cause. In 2009, Obama would invite Warren to deliver the invocation at his first Presidential Inauguration. This decision drew an outcry from many on the Left, including prominent lesbian and gay leaders who pointed to Warren's comparison of gay marriage to incest. But it also placed the evangelical pastor one step closer to inheriting Reverend Billy Graham's decades-long role as "America's Pastor."[7]

In the last decade, evangelicals have emerged as perhaps the best-known, or at least most newsworthy, religious leaders providing AIDS relief in the twenty-first century—with figures like Rick and Kay Warren heading up efforts to help women, men, and children around the globe through their Saddleback Church HIV/AIDS Initiative. I open with this example to foreground evangelicals' success in shaping how many American Christians have come to understand the HIV/AIDS crisis in the United States and especially in sub-Saharan Africa and Southeast Asia. It also reveals something they share with nonevangelical American leaders and with Americans more broadly—the idea that AIDS remains a sexual epidemic and that some combination of moral and spiritual healing will be crucial to ending it.

Needless to say, this cooperation on the topic of AIDS between national political figures like Hillary Clinton and Barack Obama and religious figures like the Warrens demonstrates how very far evangelicals have come from Christian Right fulminations against homosexuals for causing AIDS. It also suggests how much closer leading Democrats have come to conservative evangelicals in their attempt to forge an American mainstream in the wake of political division. They may not agree on the preferred methods of HIV prevention, but both camps see religious and moral reform as central to the future of AIDS work. This chapter examines how we have come to this point. It excavates the history of American Christian responses to AIDS in order to demonstrate how this rhetoric has shifted from condemnation to compassion, from claims that AIDS was God's wrath to calls for pastoral care for people with HIV or AIDS and for religious support to end the crisis.

To narrate this history requires stepping into the thick of what sociologist James Davison Hunter has called America's "culture war," a pitched battle for the control of moral authority in public life. Hunter describes two polarizing impulses at the heart of this struggle: the impulse toward orthodoxy, characterized by a commitment to external or transcendent authority; and the impulse toward progressivism, in which moral authority derives from "the spirit of the modern age, a spirit of rationalism and subjectivism."[8] For Hunter, this clash between two opposing moral visions was ultimately a battle to define American national identity. Within this struggle, confronting the AIDS crisis, and especially its lamination upon homosexuality, would become a key way to elaborate diverse visions of the nation. Rather than narrating this history through the binary rhetoric of the culture wars, however, this chapter emphasizes the shifting moral, theological, and affective registers of (mostly Protestant) Christian speech about AIDS, particularly during its emergence in the 1980s.[9]

Staging AIDS in America: The Long Eighties

On a frosty February morning in 1987, a handful of conservative protesters stood outside the Unitarian Universalist Church of Amherst in Massachusetts. As driving winds and freezing rain battered them from all sides, they began to recite the Rosary. Some carried signs reading, "A Wolf in Sheep's Clothing" and "Promotion of Condoms Will Procure the Rath [sic] of God."[10] They assembled outside the church that Sunday morning to protest the Reverend Carl F. Titchener, who planned to hand out condoms during a sermon about AIDS. The married father of four felt moved to discuss the epidemic in his church after learning that a fellow minister had contracted HIV. He hoped this largely symbolic act of passing out condoms would draw attention to the need for the church and for society to confront the quickened pace of the disease, which was surging through communities of gay men and drug users and which was, by the late 1980s, headed toward white, middle-class heterosexuals as well.

About twenty minutes into his sermon, the minister and six ushers handed out nearly four hundred condoms to the members of his congregation. "It should not be necessary for me to do what we are doing this morning," Titchener pronounced. "But the only ways we have to stop the spread of this dread disease is [*sic*] to abstain, or, if we do not abstain," he continued, "to use a condom."[11] The audience exploded into applause several times throughout the morning, building to a standing ovation at the service's close. But Titchener could not hang around to enjoy it. Worried from death threats he had received earlier, the minister dashed out of the church once the service ended.

Titchener's AIDS service came six years into the epidemic, which first became known to the medical community in 1981. That June, the United States Centers for Disease Control (CDC) reported the diagnosis of five relatively healthy young men living in Los Angeles with a rare form of pneumonia, called *Pneumocystis carinii* (PCP). The one factor all the men shared was that they were homosexual.[12] By the fall, medical researchers had diagnosed dozens more gay men with either PCP or Kaposi's sarcoma, a rare cancer usually afflicting older men of Mediterranean descent. While the cause remained unknown, public health officials conjectured that a common factor was at work in cases of what gay and mainstream presses alike dubbed "gay pneumonia" and "gay cancer."[13] Despite reports of Haitians, intravenous drug users, and female sex workers also contracting these rare infections, in the first months of the epidemic, researchers with the CDC associated the new disease with homosexuality. The high incidence of infection among homosexual men led the condition to be called GRID, or gay-related immune deficiency, and later acquired community immune deficiency, before the CDC officially adopted the name AIDS, for acquired immune deficiency syndrome, late in 1982.[14]

The early association of AIDS with homosexuality has had lasting effects. It marked the epidemic from its very beginning not simply as a biological catastrophe, but as a political, religious, and moral epidemic as well. Debates about the distribution of condoms, no less than arguments about the sinfulness of homosexuality, played into the rising culture wars—the rhetorical polarization of American public life through a division of cultural and political ideals. Cultural-values conservatives balked at government-funded (or church-sponsored) condom distribution while social progressives pushed for publicly funded safe sex programs. Political scientist Dennis Altman and communications scholar Cindy Patton have argued that "traditional" sexual mores—which they attributed to a new "American Puritanism" or "Calvinism" resurging in the 1970s and 1980s—shaped how people thought about and responded to the epidemic. Public health officials and later the media often cited "sexual promiscuity," as opposed to a viral agent, as the cause of AIDS: the implication being that heterosexual monogamy was the clear remedy. The conflation of sexual promiscuity, homosexuality, and AIDS led many Americans to infer that the purportedly immoral lifestyle of homosexuals was a central reason for the outbreak and spread of the disease.[15]

Media attention increased through the early 1980s, when it first became clear that hemophiliacs and other patients who had received blood transfusions had contracted the new disease. AIDS finally appeared in the national spotlight in 1985, when actor Rock Hudson died from AIDS-related complications. As the 1980s wore on, Americans began to view AIDS as a threat not only to homosexuals, but also to the broader (ostensibly heterosexual and non-drug-using) public as well. Mainstream media suggested with sensationalist rhetoric that the disease would likely spread from marginalized populations of gay men, drug users, and sex workers to the general heterosexual population. The 1985 cover for *LIFE* magazine's first story about the epidemic captured the sentiment, warning, "Now No One Is Safe from AIDS."[16] As people across the United States began to fear that AIDS would spread from urban gay ghettos to their own communities, gay men in particular were blamed for the crisis and became the focus of moral reprobation.

These mainstream media accounts emerged alongside and by means of the rhetoric of conservative Christians, who gained national recognition in this period.[17] The AIDS epidemic offered leaders of the Christian Right a new site to elaborate their political positions, as the appearance of a virus afflicting mostly gay men provided the proof needed to trumpet the moral superiority of "traditional values" and to warn Americans to scale back the freedoms granted through the "sexual revolution." Fundamentalist Jerry Falwell, founder of the Moral Majority, thus declared: "AIDS is not just God's punishment for homosexuals. It is God's punishment for the society that tolerates homosexuals."[18] Here, gay men threatened the nation itself—AIDS was not simply their punishment, but America's, too. Perhaps because their voices were the loudest, or the most vitriolic, leaders within the emerging Christian Right largely defined the religious reaction to the AIDS epidemic among gay and AIDS activists and in national media.

In its 1985 "Report on Sexual Orientation Discrimination," the Human Rights Commission of San Francisco identified the rise of AIDS discrimination as one of four major problem areas. The report cited "individuals going so far as to state that they see this disease as a punishment for the gay population" as one of the "unreasonable fears" that led to increased homophobia. "The rise of this illness," the statement proceeded,

> [A]lso happened to coincide with a rise of homophobia seen in the 'Moral Majority' and 'Fundamentalist' right-wing backlash. The timing acted to increase vitriolic attacks against Gay persons that became increasingly vocal in the last year, in media as well as in the streets.[19]

The San Francisco AIDS Foundation even organized a brochure campaign that targeted the Religious Right. Titled the "Right to Life Campaign," it co-opted the language of religious conservatives. It equated the "Moral Majority" with safe sex, noting "Safe sex *is* the norm of gay men today." "Family Values" highlighted the validity of gay men's relationships, explaining that "no matter how they are defined or configured," they are "as valid as those of any 'traditional' family." And finally, the brochure usurped the "Right to Life" motif itself, contending: "The Right to Life is ours—when we make a *lifetime* commitment to safe sex."[20] For many gay rights groups, it seemed, the Religious Right was public enemy number one.[21]

National secular media also homed in on conservative Christian speech when covering AIDS. News outlets capitalized on the occasion to cite media-savvy religious leaders like Falwell or televangelist Pat Robertson, who offered nationally recognized names attached to punchy statements fit for print. As a result, in the first decade of the epidemic, stories often repeated the trope that AIDS was God's punishment.[22] This religious speech proved powerful—and persistent—in large measure because it drew upon and extended public emotions of fear, a conservative evangelical tactic dating back to the 1960s.[23] Christian books and leaflets published in the 1980s exploited the dangers of AIDS—which turned out to be the dangers of homosexuality—by warning Americans not only that they missed the "facts" about AIDS, but even worse that the nation itself was under siege.

AIDS, Homosexuality, and the Wrath of God

Fitting for the postmodern context in which AIDS came to public attention, the epidemic raised competing concerns over the "truth" about the disease, from the Left and the Right, and spurred theories of conspiracy.[24] Some conservative Christians capitalized on public fear, combined with gaps in medical knowledge, to advance alternative theories about HIV and

S and its connection to homosexuality. Two works by the discredited chologist and sex researcher Paul Cameron—*AIDS: A Special Report* 86), co-written with David A. Noebel and Wayne C. Lutton and published by Summit Ministries, and *Exposing the AIDS Scandal* (1988)— along with Gene Antonio's *The AIDS Cover-Up? The Real and Alarming Facts about AIDS* (1986), published by the Catholic Ignatius Press, exemplify this mode of writing.[25] They constructed a pastiche of paranoid claims about the AIDS epidemic by drawing from an assortment of published writings, including established medical and public health journals, discredited scientific studies (many authored by Cameron himself), writings by social scientists (gay political scientist Dennis Altman is cited three times in *Special Report*), and articles from gay presses describing the sexual practices of gay men.[26] These authors sought to alarm readers, to incite anger against the gay community for causing AIDS, and to raise doubts for Americans about the facts they were getting from mainstream media and public health experts (even though they cited such studies approvingly when they support claims about the devastations wrought by AIDS). They accomplished this through common rhetorical devices. Mark Jordan describes how Cameron creates authority in *Exposing the AIDS Scandal* by modeling his presentation on forms of scriptural exegesis that evangelical readers would find familiar, including those used in the popular *Scofield Reference Bible*. Moreover, Cameron's writing echoes the technique of proof-texting, in which "quotations taken out of context and identified only by brief citation are expected to produce conviction in the reader."[27]

These works emerged within what Didi Herman has called a new Christian Right cultural genre "consisting of books, videos, and special reports, specifically dedicated to identifying the gay threat, and calling Christian believers to arms."[28] AIDS offered a new way through which to advance this political and theological point. In *AIDS, Gays, and You*, Enrique Rueda, a Cuban native who founded the Catholic Center at the Free Congress Research and Education Foundation, and Michael Schwartz, who directed its Child and Family Policy Division, explained that the "AIDS plague in America is a result of promiscuous homosexual behavior." They wrote this book "to show you what you need to know to protect [your children], and by doing so protect yourselves, your community, your country."[29] In *The Power in the Blood: A Christian Response to AIDS*, Christian reconstructionist David Chilton hesitated to declare AIDS a "homosexual disease." He listed counterpoints, noting means of transmission that are not through homosexual sex, including drug use. But his main example of nonhomosexual transmission was the prevalence of hetero-sexually transmitted HIV in Africa.[30]

First, he argued, sexual promiscuity "is rampant among Africans to an extent much greater than in the United States" (except, presumably, among gay men). This was true as well in the case of Haitians, he explained, another major risk group mentioned in early reports about AIDS. In addition to naming promiscuity, Chilton added the *kind* of sex that people were having. Anal sex, "even between heterosexuals," he continued, "is a hazardous and destructive practice" which "could account for the higher incidence of AIDS among Africans and Haitians." The United States has largely been spared from the prevalence of "this brutal and unhygienic practice" of anal sex by "the restraining effects of Christian ethics." Finally, Chilton explained, African heterosexuals might really be homosexuals in disguise: "Another factor in the African situation, often ignored, is that homosexuality is common, and is widespread even among those listed as 'heterosexuals.'" Thus, Chilton concluded, "[w]hile it is clear that AIDS is not precisely and universally a 'homosexual disease,' it is also clear that it is an '*immorality disease*,' and most of those 'really nice' but immoral people contracting and spreading it are homosexuals."[31]

Why go to such lengths to depict AIDS as a homosexual disease? First, as should be obvious by now, conservative Christian writers coupled AIDS with homosexuality in order to demonstrate the folly of this sexual practice, considered not merely sinful but also medically dangerous. But even more, they tethered homosexuality and AIDS to theological warnings about the dangers of accepting homosexuality and, for some, the meaning AIDS carries as divine punishment not only for homosexuals but for all Americans. Almost synonymous, homosexuality and AIDS together threatened to destroy the American nation. Thus, Chilton cautioned, "[w]e must not miss the *eschatology* of AIDS," its status as a divine signal about what has gone wrong and how to change it.[32] To miss these warnings would be dire, as Rueda and Schwartz explained in a passage warning readers about the dangers of churches embracing homosexuals:

> Churches, once they have been infiltrated by the homosexual movement, constitute one of its most important allies . . . Thus readers are reminded that if they belong to a religious body—whether parish, congregation, or temple—their organization is of great interest to, indeed is a target of, the homosexual movement, which works relentlessly to take over its structures for its own purposes.[33]

Note the resonance here between AIDS invading human bodies and the homosexual movement, like a virus, infiltrating religious bodies, after which it "takes over its structure for its own purposes." The language of this passage also looks back toward older rhetorical devices for thinking about homosexuals. For the initiated reader, it conjures the image of homosexuals as communists, bent on infiltrating America.[34] The resonance is not uncanny once we understand that conservative Christians writing about AIDS in the 1980s drew upon older scripts for talking about sexuality, disease, and the nation. They could align AIDS with homosexuals not only because the first reported cases of this disease included gay men, but also because Christians already had languages for talking about homosexuality as an epidemic, the nations it had infiltrated, and the cities it destroyed.

Feeling God's Wrath: AIDS, Sodomy, and the Threatened Nation

The association of AIDS with God's wrath for sexual immorality proved pervasive in the early years of the epidemic. While leaders of the Christian Right most infamously declared that God was serving out just punishments for sexual sin, less militant, big-tent evangelical leaders also leaned on this rhetoric. Billy Graham worried in a 1986 sermon in Tallahassee that AIDS "may be a judgment of God on the nation," or if not a judgment, "it may be a warning from God."[35] Outside of the pulpit and the public spotlight, everyday people, even many gay men with AIDS, also worried that this disease—their disease—could be some form of divine retribution. In the first decade and a half of the epidemic, before an effective cocktail of medications transformed AIDS into a chronic condition rather than a death sentence, sometimes the best answers a patient could hear were reassurances that AIDS was not God's punishment and that God loved them. This was the line that noted progressive William Sloane Coffin, senior minister of Riverside Church in Manhattan, repeated to the numerous gay men he counseled and that other religious caregivers like Sister Patrice Murphy of St. Vincent's Hospital in Greenwich Village shared daily with AIDS patients.[36] This fear that AIDS could be God's punishment proved ubiquitous partly because it was, in many ways, not a new argument, but an older one recast.

Take for instance Billy Graham's 1983 speech in Orlando, called "Herpes, Sex and the Bible." Before AIDS emerged in epidemiological sights, public health experts worried about an outbreak of herpes, which in 1982 *Time* dubbed "The New Scarlet Letter" threatening to reverse the sexual revolution.[37] In his speech, Graham described it as a "raging plague" that was already curbing promiscuous sexual behavior. "It may be a judgment of God on the country," he continued: "or it may be a warning from God."[38] That Graham could use nearly identical language in describing AIDS and herpes suggests not only that arguments about God's wrath well exceeded the scourge of AIDS, but also that these arguments have much longer histories. Conservative Christians were not inventing a new theological or political rhetoric when they labeled AIDS "the wrath of God," when they collapsed AIDS into homosexuality, or when they saw in this epidemic a central threat to the American nation. They encountered AIDS through older conventions for speaking about sexuality and society, including jeremiads (a form of religious lamentation) against moral declension, tropes for understanding homosexuality itself as an epidemic, and reading practices that tied homosexuality to the older biblical category of sodomy.[39]

Conservative Christians published a number of books during the 1970s and 1980s warning Americans about the bleak future of their nation.[40] These works depict revolutionary shifts in American cultural values—especially regarding sexuality, gender, and the family—since the 1960s. In earlier, more idyllic times, most Americans lived in conformity to the "biblical sexual ethic," writes Baptist pastor Randy Alcorn, who would later found and direct an evangelical nonprofit called Eternal Perspective Ministries. He defines this ethic in his 1985 book *Christians in the Wake of Sexual Revolution* as "affirming personal chastity, modesty, fidelity, and marriage as the only proper context for sexual intimacy." The few Americans who did not share these standards, he continued, at least kept their vices out of public view. But this was no longer the case.[41]

Alcorn and Tim LaHaye, in his 1978 *Unhappy Gays*, trace similar genealogies of the sexual revolution that stretch back to Renaissance humanism and the European Enlightenment—that is, to what conservative Christians often lament as the rise of secular humanism. Two years earlier, LaHaye coauthored with his wife Beverly a self-help sex manual for Christians, *The Act of Marriage: The Beauty of Sexual Love*. He would become even more famous in the 1990s, both within Christian communities and in the secular reading public, for the best-selling apocalyptic fiction series *Left Behind*, which he co-wrote with Jerry B. Jenkins.[42] Like other conservative Christian tracts about the sexual revolution, homosexuality, and AIDS, these books by Alcorn and LaHaye often reference one another, usually implicitly and without citation. This repetition has the rhetorical effect of producing a sense of truth when these books are read together— the creation of and support for an alternative worldview. Depending on who tells the story, their history of the sexual revolution winds through some assortment of Sigmund Freud (who turned the sin of homosexuality into mental illness), Havelock Ellis (who made homosexuality not only an innate quality, but something good), Bertrand Russell, Margaret Sanger, and finally Alfred Kinsey (the "most harmful" for American morality, be- cause he led people to believe a large number of Americans engaged in sexually immoral behavior).[43]

The 1960s became a turning point in such accounts for two reasons. This decade witnessed the development of what these writers described as a new sexual morality. This emerging morality, which was rooted in secu- lar humanism but had remained just below the surface, finally achieved public expression. They worried that public recognition increasingly bent toward toleration and acceptance. In the first few pages of *Unhappy Gays*, LaHaye narrates his impression of America after returning from a trip to Europe in the late 1970s. "Everywhere I turned," he laments, "newspa- pers, television, and many individuals bombarded me with the realization that America is experiencing a homosexual epidemic." A few pages later: "What was once a secret sin, rarely mentioned, has become an epidemic sweeping the land."[44] Conservative evangelical authors aligned this epi- demic with the fate of America. In his 1977 screed *The Homosexual Revo- lution*, David Noebel asked: "Will America maintain a Biblical value system and move toward moral health and restoration, or will She follow other civilizations on the road to paganism and decay?"[45]

This language suggests that in order to make sense of claims that AIDS was the wrath of God—against both homosexuals and the American nation—we ought to consider how Christians have approached homosex- uality not only as a modern category of identity, but also through the much older theological category of sodomy.[46] Allow me to clarify: conservative Christians writing in the late twentieth century also understood "homo- sexuality" through the modern, therapeutic lenses of psychology and med- icine, even as many would resist modernist claims that homosexuality was a fixed category of identity.[47] Since the late nineteenth century, according to Michel Foucault's well-known history, medical and psychiatric disci- plines have redefined sexuality as a component of one's inner psychologi- cal state and thus as part of one's true self. As this understanding gained traction, it led to the formation of classes of people aligned with various sexual identities, the most salient today being heterosexual and homosexual.[48] My point here is that this modern medical understanding of "the homosexual" (and later political and legal ones too) did not wholly replace the earlier theological category of "the sodomite."[49]

Mark Jordan traces the naming of the theological category of *sodomia*, "Sodomy," to the eleventh-century theologian Peter Damian. The naming came in two acts. First, Damian simplified readings of Genesis 19 into the story of punishment for just one sin, that of the Sodomites. Then, he assembled together several sins "under the old Roman category *luxuria*," which "came to be seen as the source of sinfulness in diverse acts, many of them having to do with the genitals."[50] Damian drew upon an older "misreading or overreading" of Paul's First Letter to the Romans, where he vaguely described sexual or homoerotic relations between women (1:26) and then men (1:27) as beyond nature. The exact acts remained vague, Jordan notes, because this genre of moral speech operated more effectively when its listeners discerned for themselves what was being condemned. Christian writers, including Augustine, yoked this reading of Paul's description of acts against nature to their reading of the story of Sodom (though, as Jordan clarifies, Paul never explicitly mentions Sodom in his letter). The connection suggested that specific acts must be avoided to prevent God's wrath. "The lesson of Sodom is not so much about sex as about the urgency of avoiding whatever (sexual) acts will provoke divine wrath," Jordan writes: "In this way, the story encourages Christians to draw up a sexual code backed by severe punishments."[51]

Damian's first innovation, then, was to combine four kinds of same-sex acts (between men)—masturbation, mutual masturbation, copulation between the thighs, and copulation "in the rear"—and to designate these acts under the term "sodomy." His second was to connect "his synthetic definition of sins with a sin-identity," to explain that these sins are what sodomites do and, once named, to designate the sins of the sodomite as "the most outrageous violation of nature." The formation of the sodomite as a kind of person is crucial here, as Jordan argues: in this new understanding, sexual acts do not form the sodomite but rather reveal who he already is.[52]

Medieval Christian writers would come to characterize the sodomite as a "rebellious sinner" or "universal traitor." In the fifteenth-century writings of Archbishop Dominican Antoninus of Florence, sodomites—or even contact with sodomites, who could expose a society to contagion—threatened whole communities with divine retribution, just as earlier sodomites led to the destruction of the city of Sodom. The Protestant Reformation intensified the moral depravity of the sodomite, as Protestant polemicists associated sodomy with the celibate Catholic clergy. In the context of religious and political warfare, this link between sodomy and Catholics allowed Protestants to elevate the sin of sodomy to the charge of treason. The sodomite no longer threatened only Christian communities, but political states as well. Thus, Jordan demonstrates, the sin of sodomy "became now more than ever a triple threat—an accusation of personal filthiness, of shared heresy, and of high treason."[53]

Conservative Christians reproduced these theological tropes in their descriptions of the growing "homosexual subculture," in their understandings of "the epidemic of homosexuality," and in their worry that AIDS could be a sign of divine retribution, not only for gay men, but for the American nation. David Noebel was not merely imitating the heightened rhetoric of the Cold War—or the emerging culture wars—when he claimed that the "homosexual sub-culture . . . destroys lives, families, institutions, and nations,"[54] or that homosexuals threatened national security because of "the fact that homosexuals in sensitive positions have a tendency to place their own sexuality above national security and end up giving government secrets to the enemy."[55] Noebel and LaHaye even suggested that, at the end of the world, the anti-Christ could be a homosexual. They cite the final phrase from the King James translation of Daniel 11:37, which comments on the rule of the anti-Christ just before Christ's return: "Neither shall he regard the God of his fathers, *nor the desire of women.*"[56]

Putting the jeremiad form in the service of American nationalism, these writers warned that the United States would face a fate all too familiar to their Christian readers. The historical signs pointed in a clear direction. LaHaye, for instance, attributed the "rapid decline" of Great Britain as a world power to the legalization of homosexuality there in 1957. America was next. In language recalling the great flood in the age of Noah, he feared the "tidal wave of homosexuality that will drown our children in a polluted sea of sexual perversion—and will eventually destroy America as it did Rome, Greece, Pompeii, and Sodom."[57] Alcorn and Noebel both invoked Ruth Graham, the wife of the famous evangelical crusader: "If God doesn't judge America, He'll owe Sodom and Gomorrah an apology."[58]

I place conservative Christian writing about homosexuality and AIDS within this longer theological genealogy to suggest a different reading of their rhetorical and religious affects. They tie together homosexuality and AIDS with biblical accounts about sodomy as a special category of sin (against nature) that already resonates with long-standing theological and political notions of identity, community, contagion, national threat, and destruction. In doing so, they speak both a modern language and a much older theological one. The non-initiated reader sees where these texts fail. One could pinpoint a number of ways in which the "facts" presented in such accounts are easily refuted by the competing "facts" of history or of medical science read correctly (that is, in secular fashion).[59] One could likewise counter these authors' theological or biblical claims with others, as many mainstream and progressive Christians have (as I will soon describe). Both operations are no doubt important and valuable for anyone interested in combatting misinformation or reconsidering theological resources for responding to the AIDS crisis. But the recitation of these "failures" should not blind us to the work these texts have done and the force they continue to exert.

While many of these books draw upon the languages of medicine and public health, alongside those of the Bible and of history, they do not take the form of these secular languages. They speak in a different rhetorical tongue, one that Susan Harding captures brilliantly in her reading of evangelical witnessing.[60] The secular reader is interested in the facts; the conservative Christian reader is interested in the message and how it is conveyed. The message here is clear: homosexual activity is a biblical sin, a flaunting of God's law; this sin threatens to infect the nation; AIDS is the just recompense for America's failure to stamp it out; and things will only worsen if we (Christians, Americans) do not act quickly. This conservative Christian reading posits homosexuals in opposition to Christianity, to biblical morals, and to American citizenship. It holds out hope that, if forewarned—through these books and sermons, and through the AIDS epidemic and its "alarming facts"—Americans may return to their Christian past and biblical destiny.

The older history of this rhetoric of God's wrath and its repetition through religious and national media combined to make it a powerful force in the moral construction of the AIDS epidemic: one that figured Christian speech about AIDS that came after it. I mean *after* in two senses here. In terms of chronology, Christian responses necessarily came after the rhetoric of the wrath of God, not because they came later than Christian Right speech about AIDS (though this largely was the case) but because this rhetoric prefigured Christian (and secular) responses to AIDS. Or, to put this another way, AIDS emerged within and through the theological and political framework of the sodomitical community—what would later be called the homosexual community—a point captured in earlier namings: the "gay plague" and gay-related immune deficiency (GRID). To the extent that medical researchers discovered AIDS through its connection to a homosexual community or a homosexual lifestyle, this epidemic was already cast in the shadow of the sodomite.

Second, outside of the Right, many Christians went after the rhetoric of the wrath of God—whether by refuting, sidestepping, or repressing it—to emphasize other theological and political resources for encountering AIDS. But however they ultimately responded, they found that when they tried to speak about AIDS, their language had to struggle against this history of the homosexual and the longer history of the sodomite.

After the Wrath of God: Calls for Compassion, Calls to Action

Many of the first organized religious responses that sought to help people with AIDS and those in danger of contracting the new disease arose in the urban communities where the crisis was most visible—especially San Francisco, New York, Los Angeles, and Chicago. Congregations that focused on gay and lesbian concerns often initiated such efforts, such as when the predominantly gay Congregation Beth Simchat Torah (CBST) in Manhattan organized a forum to discuss the new "gay plague" in February 1982. The meeting drew a bustling crowd of over three hundred and fifty people who came to hear medical professionals present the latest information about the mysterious epidemic affecting gay men and to learn how they could avoid it.[61]

The Universal Fellowship of Metropolitan Community Churches, founded in 1968 by defrocked Pentecostal Troy Perry to serve gay men and lesbians, has played an important role in the struggle for gay rights and in early AIDS activism. Metropolitan Community Church (MCC) congregations in Los Angeles, San Francisco, and New York quickly joined CBST to inform members of their congregations and the broader gay communities in their areas about AIDS. In 1983, MCC issued one of the first religious resolutions from any denomination about the epidemic, calling for further religious and medical resources to be devoted to fighting AIDS. Individual congregations followed with more hands-on measures. The Metropolitan Community Church of the Valley in North Hollywood has been engaged in activism since the early 1980s, when several members of the congregation developed AIDS. In 1985, one of the church's ministers, Stephen Pieters, learned of his own diagnosis. Asked to preach that year's Easter sermon, the 33-year-old gay activist broke out into dance in front of the congregation, with the tune of "Singing in the Rain" buzzing in his head, exhibiting his hope for life and his positive spirit in the face of the epidemic. Under his direction, the congregation produced a videotape ministry project to address issues of concern to the religious gay population. The first tape "AIDS: A Present Crisis, A Present Grace" featured four people with AIDS discussing their experiences with the disease and its effect on their faith. A second addressed the topic of "Safe Sex."[62] A long-term AIDS survivor, Pieters has continued his work with the MCC AIDS Ministry, publishing several articles and pamphlets about the spiritual aspects of AIDS, including "Spiritual Strength for Survival" and "HIV/AIDS: Is It God's Judgments? A Christian View of Faith, Hope and Love," which are available at the widely used online resource center *The Body*. Much of Pieters' work has been collected in his 1991 memoir, *"I'm Still Dancing!" A Gay Man's Health Experience.*[63]

In the mid-1980s, a number of congregations—both gay-oriented and gay-friendly, Protestant, Catholic, and Jewish—became active in AIDS ministry. One author, writing for *The Christian Century*, the flagship publication of mainline Protestant Christianity, even lauded how in San Francisco "the AIDS epidemic has actually brought religious groups and the gay community together as nothing has before."[64] As a theological crisis, AIDS forced religious individuals to confront their stances on issues such as homosexuality, leading some to revise theologies that considered it sinful. Rather than condemning homosexual behavior, for instance, Episcopal leaders in the city encouraged churches to fight AIDS by advocating that their gay parishioners form monogamous relationships. Other groups did not go quite so far, but even "once-hostile fundamentalists and evangelical groups have become compassionate toward gays," noted the article.[65]

Evangelical pastor Jim Lowder of the Dolores Street Southern Baptist Church in San Francisco spoke out against the president of his denomination—Charles Stanley—who declared in January 1986 that "AIDS is God indicating his displeasure." "That was one of the most disgusting statements I'd ever heard," Lowder remarked: "To use human suffering as an excuse to condemn people is absolutely intolerable and unchristian." Because of his stance, Lowder's church lost $15,000 in annual funds from his denomination, and he was removed from his teaching position at Southern Baptist Golden Gate Seminary.[66] Even as the AIDS crisis brought San Franciscans together, Lowder's story signaled the emotional intensity surrounding the epidemic and the factures it created even within his own denomination.

In Los Angeles, the Reverend Carl Bean established the Minority AIDS Program (MAP) as an outreach effort of the Unity Fellowship Church, a ministry program for the city's black gay and lesbian community founded in 1985. Bean described how his call to found MAP grew out of the realization, borrowed from other AIDS activists, that "Silence = Death." "I realized one day that as a black gay man who was aware of the virus, who had lost friends to it, who had to live daily with the fear of it possibly showing up in my own system some day," Bean explained, "that if I didn't spread my knowledge then I was the silence that would spell death for others." He thus concluded, "I HAD to do something." MAP focused its efforts in Los Angeles' black and Latino communities, as these populations witnessed increasing rates of infection in the second half of the 1980s. But the organization had a difficult start. Attempts to advertise MAP through predominantly black radio stations met with resistance. "Most slammed their doors right in my face," Bean complained, since they saw AIDS not as a black issue, but as "a white gay thing." MAP finally broke through to one station, KJLH with Jackie Stevens, and citywide coverage in the *Los Angeles Times* soon followed. After word got out, Bean noted, MAP's phones "rang off the hook; the brothers began to call."[67]

Bean joined other African American religious leaders in combating an epidemic that more and more affected racial minorities. Though there was little denomination-wide organization in the first two decades, the A.M.E. Church and the A.M.E. Zion Church issued public statements on AIDS calling for compassion for those living with the disease. More often, this ministry work was left to individuals, such as Bean, public health worker Pernessa Seele, and the Reverend Dr. Yvette Flunder. In 1989, Seele founded The Balm in Gilead (first started as the Harlem Week of Prayer for the Healing of AIDS), which offered one of the first efforts to confront AIDS in the black community in New York. Seele's organization convened the First African American Religious Leaders Summit on HIV/AIDS at the White House in 1994, at which time members adopted "The African American Clergy's Declaration of War on HIV/AIDS." Flunder, a noted gospel singer, became involved with AIDS work and opened a hospice facility while working at the Love Center Church in Oakland, California. She left her position there in 1991 to form City of Refuge Church, which opened an ancillary non-profit agency called Ark of Refuge, Inc., to provide services and care for people with HIV/AIDS across the Bay area. [68]

By the middle of the decade, a small number of religious leaders across the United States began to address the epidemic among congregations that were mostly heterosexual, and some leaders started to take action to combat social discrimination against people with AIDS. The Rev. Nancy Radclyffe led the first mass for people with AIDS at St. Paul's Episcopal Church in conservative Orange County in 1986, while California's twenty Catholic bishops issued a statement denouncing Proposition 64. Also known as the LaRouche Initiative, the proposition called for sweeping controls on people diagnosed with AIDS, even raising the possibility of quarantine, and threatened the confidentiality of people tested for HIV. The bishops joined the Interfaith Council of the AIDS Project in Los Angeles in opposing the proposition, which they referred to as "an irrational, inappropriate and misguided approach to a serious public health problem."[69] As AIDS became more familiar to the American public through the 1980s, the need for accurate information and education to stem the spread of the disease became a key issue for church leaders addressing their constituencies. Largely quiet up to this point, religious leaders outside of cities like San Francisco, Los Angeles, and New York started to realize, as one *Chicago Tribune* headline put it, that "AIDS May Be [the] Church's Ministry of the '80s."[70]

Mainline denominations, moderate and progressive evangelicals, and individual authors writing from within these traditions began discussing AIDS more publicly in the second half of the 1980s. By the end of that decade, most denominations and many ecumenical organizations had issued statements about the epidemic.[71] At least at the denominational level, most Christian and Jewish clergy in the United States steadfastly called for care and compassion for people with AIDS. The major differences among these leaders concerned their opinion of homosexuality with regard to the cause of AIDS and their position on the best methods to curb the spread of HIV.

While mainline Protestant denominations denied that homosexuality was the cause of AIDS, most withheld formal comment about the acceptability or sinfulness of homosexual behavior itself. The National Council of Churches of Christ, an ecumenical organization composed of a number of Christian faith groups, issued a resolution in 1986 "to address the churches directly." It cited increased discrimination against risk groups, including homosexuals, and called for governmental legislation that would protect the civil rights of gays and lesbians. In its 1986 resolution, the Presbyterian Church (U.S.A.) recognized that "many lesbians and gay men have felt that the church's teaching on homosexuality excluded them from the church's care." It called for Presbyterians "to condemn the potential threat of AIDS as an excuse for discrimination and oppression."[72] Other mainline denominations passed similar resolutions calling for an end to discrimination against people with AIDS because of their sexual identities, but likewise stopped short of affirming or castigating gay men's sexual behavior from the perspective of the church.

Apart from denominational statements, in the late 1980s and early 1990s many Christian writers began publishing articles and books about AIDS and organizing AIDS ministry programs. Readers could find New Age and spiritual approaches in works like Nick Bamforth's *AIDS and the Healer Within* and Louise L. Hay's *The AIDS Book: Creating a Positive Approach.*[73] John Fortunato, a gay psychotherapist, penned *AIDS: The Spiritual Dilemma* in 1987 to address the spiritual aspects of the AIDS crisis, drawing heavily from Christian traditions. Mainline and progressive responses—including those arising within lesbian and gay, AIDS, and queer theology—also began filling bookshelves.[74] Taken together, they demonstrate both the array of religious and spiritual responses and the effort to combat the vitriolic rhetoric issuing from the Christian Right. We can see this approach developed by two Southern Baptists—Earl Shelp and Ronald Sunderland—who together published a number of the earliest articles and books about the AIDS crisis and developed in 1985 one of the first and largest Christian AIDS ministry programs, which was based in Houston, Texas. Shelp and Sunderland served as Research Fellows at Texas Medical Center's Institute of Religion in Houston and later as the ethicist (Shelp) and the chaplain (Sunderland) for the Institute for Immunological Disorders, the nation's first research and treatment center devoted to AIDS.[75] Shelp and Sunderland have garnered national recognition for their AIDS work, including the Rosalyn Carter Caregiving Award, which they received in 1987, and the President's Community Award, which Bill Clinton presented to them in 1998.

Forging Christian AIDS Ministry

Shelp and Sunderland first called "the Church's attention" to AIDS in an essay published in *Christian Century* in 1985. One of the first statements on AIDS to appear in a national religious periodical, their article decried the slow pace with which Christian churches were responding to the epidemic. More than twelve thousand Americans had been diagnosed with

AIDS by that time, yet the church "was noticeably silent," Shelp and Sunderland lamented. "The personal tragedies and social failures associated with the disease," they continued, "appear to have been largely ignored by the church—except for those strident segments that view AIDS as God's retribution on a sinful people."[76] In contrast to this notable silence, willful ignorance, or cruel accusation, as they characterized the Christian response up to that point, Shelp and Sunderland sought to marshal the church's resources to combat the crisis. They called on pastors to offer spiritual guidance for people with AIDS and their loved ones. They further challenged the corporate church to "join—if not lead—the chorus of voices calling on government at every level to commit funds for research, personnel and facilities for treatment and for a hospice in which patients would be able to die in dignity."[77]

Shelp and Sunderland outlined their Christian response to AIDS in three books published in the 1980s. *AIDS: Personal Stories in Pastoral Perspective*, co-authored with Dr. Peter Mansell and published in 1986, presented the personal stories of people affected by AIDS and focused on the lives of gay men in particular. The goal of this volume was to introduce readers to real people with AIDS, personalizing their stories, in order to suggest the types of situations pastoral caregivers might encounter should they begin their own AIDS ministry work. Two more volumes followed the next year: *AIDS: A Manual for Pastoral Care* and *AIDS and the Church*, which was updated and released in its second edition in 1992.[78] Unlike those published by more conservative Christians or members of the Christian Right, these books presented accurate and current medical facts regarding AIDS, including information about how HIV could be transmitted, along with advice on providing pastoral care for people with the disease and their families. Shelp and Sunderland advocated a non-proselytizing approach to AIDS ministry that focused on understanding the needs of people with AIDS and advocating for them at local and national political levels. Such care, they claimed, might include material, emotional, and spiritual or religious support, but should not be conditioned upon the conversion to Christianity of the people receiving help. They also warned about the difficulty religious caregivers might face if they had limited experience working with gay men and drug users.

Growing out of this work, Shelp and Sunderland soon developed a comprehensive AIDS ministry program: an AIDS "care model" designed for replication by other congregations and lay caregivers. Emerging in the 1980s, this program originally focused on how to care for gay men. But it soon adapted to the needs of other populations, as the epidemic progressed among (or became more visible within) black and Latino communities, a shift that would also include the need to provide care more often for heterosexual women and intravenous drug users. To highlight the understanding of sexuality foundational to their ministry work, I focus here on their writing about gay men.[79]

Shelp and Sunderland denounced the claim that homosexual behavior caused the AIDS epidemic and called for comprehensive sex education to combat the spread of the disease. In their pastoral manual, they describe the difficult religious environment with which gay men with AIDS had to wrestle. They called the church to engage gay men on their own terms, without "moralizing." Shelp and Sunderland did not go so far as to claim that pastoral caregivers should "ignore their own value systems" in working with gay men—and their books did not condone homosexual practice. But they warned readers that not all clergy would be suited for this type of ministry, which required commitment to and patience with populations with whom many (ostensibly heterosexual) clergy remained unfamiliar in the mid-1980s. Indeed, this epidemic presented the church with an unusual opportunity: to draw the gay population into its embrace.[80]

Shelp and Sunderland rejected the condemnation of homosexuals, a position they shared with most leaders of mainline denominations. They called instead for the church to take on prophetic and pastoral roles in fighting AIDS. In doing so, they challenged the Christian Right's claim to moral authority and offered an alternative vision of the "true church." Following the example of Jesus, they insisted, the church ought to recommit itself to Christianity's central mission: the biblical imperative to help the "stranger," the "outcast," and the "poor."[81] "The true question for the church," they explained, "has nothing to do with the morality of certain conduct or the status before God of certain people associated with AIDS." These issues proved at best secondary. The main issue concerned "the integrity and credibility of the people who bear Christ's name." Their mandate as Christians was to love the "the outcast," and in this moment that figure was the person with AIDS. "This is the only acceptable attitude," they maintained, "and it ought to produce appropriate reconciling and compassionate ministries."[82]

Shelp and Sunderland thereby founded their pastoral AIDS ministry on Jesus' commitment to the poor, even devoting a chapter of *AIDS and the Church* to develop this idea. At several turns in their writing, they compared work with AIDS patients to Jesus' interactions with sinners, tax collectors, the impoverished, publicans, prostitutes, and the sick. The tax collector and the publican provided particularly relevant examples for how Jesus might have regarded people with AIDS. "Despite the moral condemnation and ostracism directed toward publicans and others similarly situated," they explained, "Jesus had fellowship with them, undeterred by their conduct or the societally mandated judgment of their actions."[83] In modern times, they insisted, people with AIDS filled the criteria for being included among the biblical category of the poor. If the person is gay or bisexual, they explained, then "these labels are cited as an additional justification for relegating him or her to the edges of society." In their reading, gay and bisexual people, and people with HIV/AIDS, represented modern-day "manifestations of the poor who, despite society's judgments to the contrary, are loved by God and deserve to be treated compassionately by God's people."[84]

Through their published works and their ministry program, Shelp and Sunderland provided a vocal counterargument to religious condemnations of gay and bisexual men with HIV/AIDS. Taking the Christian traditions of healing and social justice as their starting point, they led the way in developing an effective AIDS ministry program. As their program grew, and as they also began to include Jewish congregations within their fold, it was renamed an "interfaith" AIDS ministry. The program quickly became the largest in the United States, and Shelp and Sunderland, along with other lay caregivers, helped thousands of people living with the disease. They did so without condemning—or condoning—the sexual practices of the people they served.

By casting people with AIDS as exemplars of Jesus' poor, as the privileged outcast, Shelp and Sunderland countered claims that AIDS was God's wrath and reinterpreted the epidemic in a manner that invited many mainstream Christians into the pastoral care project. But in doing so, they also (if perhaps unwittingly) called for the care of people with AIDS not despite their ostracized position, but precisely because of it. Without offering a theological affirmation of homosexuality, mainline Christian positions left no way out of the marginal position of this identity. In short, gay men with AIDS remained perpetually other—always the stranger or the outcast. This approach ran counter to the goals of many secular and pro-gay religious AIDS activists in the 1980s, who sought to render both gay life and living with AIDS into acceptable lifestyles rather than exceptional forms of otherness. For instance, a group of people with AIDS formed an early movement to empower those grappling with the epidemic. "We

condemn attempts to label us as 'victims,' a term which implies defeat,"
they argued in a statement drafted during a meeting in Denver in 1983:
"and we are only occasionally 'patients,' a term which implies passivity,
helplessness, and dependence upon the care of others. We are 'People
With AIDS.'"[85] In contrast, by modeling people with AIDS after marginalized figures in the Bible, Shelp and Sunderland recast the rhetoric of the
AIDS "victim" in theological terms. This formuation no doubt offered a
more pragmatic way to reach the Christian communities they hoped to
bring into AIDS care, but it also limited theological and political efforts to
validate the health status of the person with AIDS and, if gay, the moral
status of his or her sexual identity.

In discussing the stigmas attached to homosexuals, bisexuals, and
drug users, Shelp and Sunderland followed modern medical and political
trends in positing sexuality as a fixed part of one's identity. Thus, they
maintained, "in the cases of homosexual and bisexual men, the stigma
applies to who they are—a matter about which they have no choice—
rather than (or in addition to) what they do—a matter about which they do
have a choice."[86] Sexuality was a natural part of one's identity, a secular
component independent of free will or religious faith. In articulating sexuality this way, they echoed a modern understanding of the relationship
between the individual and his or her sexuality.

While agnostic about the morality of homosexuality and bisexuality,
Shelp and Sunderland did not contest the idea that sexuality was central to
people's identities or, further, that sexual identity formed part of a person's
essential and natural self. And though they drew attention to the disjunc-
tion between identity and practice—that is, between being homosexual
versus practicing same-sex sex—Shelp and Sunderland nonetheless premised the prevention component of their AIDS ministry work on education that included reduction of partners, long-term monogamy, and
condom use, rather than conversion to Christian heterosexuality. In doing
so, they bracketed off the specific moral status of sexual identity or sexual
practice. Of course, to bracket something off is also to take a kind of position, and this bracketing put them at odds both with gay AIDS activists
and with a number of other Christians.

Given its formation in the 1980s, their ministry program has emphasized providing pastoral and everyday care for people with AIDS more than
advocating prevention strategies for at-risk populations, though both activities have been significant to their work. This marks a key difference between the work of many mainline and progressive Christians and that of

evangelicals, who since the 1980s have emphasized prevention to a far greater degree, even making it into tool of moral pedagogy. The importance of prevention for many evangelical AIDS workers suggests a stronger connection to missionary forms of activism, which center on helping those who have not yet contracted HIV/AIDS.[87] This focus on prevention has also meant that most evangelical writing about AIDS—rather than sidestepping issues of sexual morality, as Shelp and Sunderland tried to do—has foregrounded the importance of conservative Christian sexual morality in the fight against the epidemic.

Getting Evangelical about AIDS

Since the start of the epidemic, most evangelicals have considered AIDS a moral problem that requires a moral solution. In 1988, the National Association of Evangelicals (NAE), a collection of several denominations and churches dedicated to engaging public life, released a "Statement on AIDS" that drew attention to the moral issues surrounding transmission. "The nexus between immoral behavior and the spread of AIDS," it noted, "is self-evident."[88] The statement discouraged conferring "special 'civil rights' on persons afflicted with AIDS." It also called for mandatory testing for high-risk groups and that test results be reported to public health officials—measures that more liberal Christian bodies and nearly all AIDS activists rejected. Many evangelical leaders upheld what they considered "a Biblical approach" for dealing with the epidemic. The NAE called for "chastity before marriage and fidelity within marriage" to stem the spread of HIV.[89] The Southern Baptist Convention, the International Pentecostal Church of Christ, and the Independent Fundamental Churches of America issued similar statements in the late 1980s and pushed to limit any form of sex education that went beyond advocating abstinence and monogamous heterosexual marriage.[90]

Once people considered AIDS a threat not only for homosexuals, sex workers, and drug users, but for middle-class (and ostensibly non-drug-using) white, heterosexual Americans as well, sex education took on a renewed political relevance as one way to protect teens and adults from this life-threatening disease. But health professionals, AIDS activists, and religious leaders disagreed about what sex education should look like. At the start of the epidemic, gay and lesbian activists led debates about safe sex, which focused on promoting the use of condoms in addition to teaching about specific sexual practices less likely to transmit HIV. Gay and lesbian AIDS activists debated both among themselves and with health professionals over the public health risks of bathhouses, the practice of anonymous sex, and the value of monogamy, but most agreed on one point: that people at risk of contracting HIV would continue having sex, so the best way to curb the spread of the virus was to promote safer sexual practices and the use of condoms.[91] In large measure, mainline Protestant denominations involved in AIDS work acceded to this position. Even Surgeon General C. Everett Koop, an evangelical Presbyterian, took what he called a pragmatic stance on sex education and the distribution of condoms. He considered comprehensive sex education—including the promotion of condoms—absolutely necessary.[92] But throughout the 1980s and into the 1990s, Koop's position proved unpopular among fellow evangelicals and drew criticism from religious conservatives, many of whom were his former colleagues and friends.[93]

Most American evangelicals situated AIDS prevention in the context of a broader push for traditional family values and upheld the idea that the Christian faith had specific moral lessons to offer in this regard. As part of its annual Washington Insight Briefing, the NAE hosted a conference in 1988 that brought together church leaders, health professionals, and government officials to address the role of American Christians in the AIDS epidemic. At the meeting, conservative Illinois State Representative Penny Pullen, who also served on the Presidential Commission on HIV, called upon Christian leaders to promote "behavior modification as an important prevention tool." She clarified, "The church is the institution that civilizes society . . . so the church must comment, persuade, lead, and be involved in these issues."[94] Evangelicals such as Pullen and members of the NAE called for moral training to stem the spread of infectious diseases such as AIDS both within American high schools and, by the first decade of the twenty-first century, around the globe. Thus, while comprehensive sex education proved common (even common-sense) for most public health experts and activists in the 1980s and early 1990s, evangelical leaders steadfastly promoted an abstinence movement that would gain national prominence by the late 1990s and the early twenty-first century.[95]

Even politically progressive evangelicals shared this view. A leader in the Christian social justice movement, Ron Sider, penned "AIDS: An Evangelical Perspective" for *Christian Century* in 1988. Like most writing on AIDS in the 1980s, his article depicted the epidemic almost solely in terms of sexual morality. He begins by declaring that people with AIDS, including gays, are "indelibly stamped in the divine image" and should be provided with care and support. He also counters the charge that "AIDS is God's punishment for gays," pointing out that there is no biblical precedent for the argument that specific sins could be linked to specific illnesses.[96] But then the line between God's wrath and God's consequences begins to blur.

Sider devoted several lines to defending the public stance of evangelicals to the mainline audience of *Christian Century*. "To the extent that there is a link between AIDS and homosexuality," he claimed, "the major point that must be made is that it is homosexual promiscuity that stands in condemnation, not evangelical belief that homosexual practice is wrong."[97] Sider argued that it would be "dishonest" and "unwise" to deny that most cases of AIDS resulted from sexual (especially homosexual) promiscuity: "the facts are that the only true safe intercourse is that within a lifelong monogamous relationship, and that AIDS is closely linked with homosexual promiscuity." According to Sider, God established a moral order, one "structured into nature": ignoring this order "has consequences." He goes further: "If the Bible teaches that homosexual practice is wrong, as I think it does, then it is right to suppose that violating God's law in this area will have negative consequences."[98] One major difference between Sider's position and that of the Christian Right was his insistence that homosexuality be placed alongside other sins, including environmental pollution, racism, and economic oppression.

Sider concluded by suggesting a compromise between Surgeon General Koop's call for sex education, which included discussions about condoms on television and in print media, and worries articulated by many conservative Christians that safe-sex advertisements would incite promiscuity. He imagines an ad that could please both sides. It would include a picture of actor Rock Hudson, who died from AIDS in 1985. He would be depicted with advanced physical symptoms of the disease, "where its ravages are unmistakable." A caption would parrot Hudson:

The only safe sex is within a lifelong monogamous relationship. I wish I had lived that way before I got AIDS. But if, in spite of today's harsh facts, you want to play Russian roulette with your life, then please use condoms. They are not fail-proof, but they do improve your chances.[99]

Sider's article joined the broader deployment of fear and disgust as techniques for teaching sexual morality and fighting AIDS. But it also evinces the grip that Christian rhetoric of homosexuality had on AIDS in the 1980s, as it crossed the lines of conservative and progressive evangelicalism.

Though most evangelical organizations had issued resolutions on AIDS by the late 1980s, by and large their participation in AIDS activism was limited to a handful of congregations in cities overwhelmed by the epidemic. In Orange Country, California, Bruce Sonnenberg founded He Intends Victory in 1990 to assist people with HIV/AIDS. It began as a small support group for local people in his community but has since grown into a global AIDS ministry program. It also operates a small publishing house. Dan Wooding's *He Intends Victory* (1994) and Joan Yorba-Gray's *In His Shadow: A Devotional for Christians Living with AIDS* (2001), two books the program has released, tell the stories of American Christians living (or helping others) with HIV/AIDS. The message of these books, and of the ministry as whole, has emphasized Christian compassion, and Sonnenberg has refuted the claim that AIDS is God's punishment for homosexuals.[100]

Before the twenty-first century, however, evangelical AIDS ministries like He Intends Victory proved exceptional. Uneasy discussing the unseemly matters of sexuality that AIDS brought to the fore, most evangelicals—like Americans generally—considered this disease somebody else's problem, one limited to homosexuals and drug users in urban enclaves.[101] This is how former Southern Baptist president (1978–1979) Jimmy Allen understood AIDS until it started to impact his own family. Allen reveals his encounter with AIDS in the 1995 memoir *Burden of a Secret*. His daughter-in-law contracted HIV through a blood transfusion and later unknowingly passed it along to her two children. His gay son also contracted HIV, this time sexually. All four family members would die from AIDS complications. Allen hoped that by telling his story, he would make the epidemic more familiar for his evangelical readers and help to destigmatize AIDS.[102]

But AIDS would not become a priority for evangelicals until it could be dislodged from its representation as a homosexual disease. In the late 1980s and throughout the 1990s, public health workers and media accounts increasingly addressed the heterosexual, racial, and global dimensions of the AIDS epidemic. In 1991, NBA star Earvin "Magic" Johnson made national headlines when he announced that he had contracted HIV. Johnson's revelation publicized heterosexual transmission, the idea, as he noted, that "anybody, even me" could get AIDS. He also drew attention to the acceleration of HIV/AIDS infection among racial minorities, who were disproportionately at risk compared to whites. By the late 1990s, advances in the treatment of HIV/AIDS, especially the release of the AIDS cocktail, rendered it a far more treatable condition for those with access to medical care. Attention then turned to marginal populations without access to medicine, often because of poverty or lack of information. This shift took some of the pressure off the "gay community," often imagined as white and well-connected. Though the link between AIDS and homosexuality would not disappear in public discourse, representations of AIDS as an epidemic of poverty and as heterosexual, especially in Africa, opened the crisis to new kinds of intervention.[103]

It was not until the turn of the twenty-first century that AIDS appeared on the radar for many evangelicals, who often first encountered the epidemic either during missionary work or upon hearing about mission trips to sub-Saharan Africa, rather than among gay men and drug users in the United States. In 1999, for instance, the epidemic failed to make the list of urgent concerns for the Christian humanitarian organization World Vision. It was not until a couple years later, according to Ken Casey of their AIDS ministry program, that World Vision "woke up" to realize that "[t]he AIDS pandemic is the greatest humanitarian crisis."[104] Once awoken to the AIDS crisis in Africa, a number of American evangelicals were quick to mobilize their vast financial, cultural, and moral resources.[105]

Evangelical leaders underscored how the past two decades of prevention efforts had failed to end the crisis. They promoted an alternative approach to AIDS relief, which they advanced through private organizations and by lobbying the government to redirect international AIDS relief. A 2002 editorial from the national evangelical magazine *Christianity Today* made the case for why churches proved best equipped to fight HIV/AIDS. After reciting statistics on the epidemic in Africa, the editorial condemned the "20 years of failed attempts to fight HIV/AIDS, mostly with billions upon billions of low-cost condoms (rarely used consistently) and costly drug cocktails (hard to administer and distribute fairly)." In place of these failed efforts, the editors cited the "sea change" taking place in the public health community regarding HIV/AIDS prevention, one that focused on abstinence and fidelity, methods that promoted "primary behavior change" far more effectively than condoms and drugs.[106] As this editorial suggests, evangelical AIDS workers set themselves the much grander task of moral education among their mostly African subjects, teaching them about abstinence and fidelity from a Christian perspective and remaking them in their own Christian image. One of the leading efforts in this regard has been the HIV/AIDS Initiative at Saddleback Church.

Evangelical AIDS Work and the Saddleback Initiative

The HIV/AIDS Initiative began in 2004 at Saddleback, the Southern Baptist mega-church co-founded by Rick Warren and his wife Kay in Lake Forest, California. While Rick Warren has headed up Saddleback Church, his wife Kay was the first to draw attention to the AIDS epidemic and the need for a church response. Since 2004, she has served as the executive director for Saddleback's HIV/AIDS Initiative. She describes becoming involved with AIDS relief work in her 2007 memoir *Dangerous Surrender: What Happens When You Say Yes to God.*

Warren's journey began with a photograph. One spring morning in 2002, sitting on her couch with a cup of tea, she began flipping through a newsmagazine. She turned to a story about AIDS in Africa, although not because she particularly cared about AIDS in Africa; as she confesses to her readers, she "didn't care about AIDS anywhere." But she was drawn in by "horrific" photographs—pictures of "skeletal men and women, children so weak they couldn't brush the flies away from their faces." Warren asked herself, "How could there be more than 30 million people infected with a lethal virus and I not know even one of them?" In the following days she remained "haunted by the thought of 12 million boys and girls left alone, their parents victims of AIDS." Confronted with this devastation, Warren became "a seriously disturbed woman." And "once I became disturbed," she continued, "I became passionate about ending AIDS in Rick's and my lifetime."[107]

With its personalized accounts of innocent victims, poor women, and motherless African children in need of help, Warren's narrative of her journey to AIDS work could be read as a product of the devolution of American religion into the sentimental terrain of emotion, manipulation, individualism, and ineffectiveness. Sentimentality has had a long, if sullied, career in the history of American Christianity. In *The Feminization of American Culture*, Ann Douglas lamented the erosion of Calvinist orthodoxy and literary refinement in the nineteenth century into the feminized spirituality and mass-marketed consumer fiction perhaps most famously—or infamously—evidenced in the work of Harriet Beecher Stowe. For generations, literary scholar Jane Tompkins has noted, twentieth-century critics of this sentimentalist history have taught us "to equate popularity with debasement, emotionality with ineffectiveness, religiosity with fakery, domesticity with triviality, and all of these, implicitly, with womanly inferiority."[108] The same holds true for more recent forms of Christian sentimentality. Perhaps because her work is seen as ineffective or superficial, Kay Warren barely enters journalistic and academic accounts of evangelical AIDS work, which tend to highlight male leaders like Rick Warren or Franklin Graham.[109] Less attention has been devoted to women leaders or to the particular religious understandings of health, disease, and morality informing evangelical AIDS work, including the politics of sentimentality. Building upon feminist and queer scholarship on the political work of affect, Melani McAlister has suggested that we understand American evangelicals as one kind of "intimate public" and that we examine the cultivation of religious feeling in their writing as a form of public practice, one that brings together accounts of the interiority of faith with social and political behavior.[110]

Read in this way, Kay and Rick Warren join a number of other evangelical leaders in the fight against AIDS, including several women, such as Deborah Dortzbach, who has served as the International Director for World Relief's HIV/AIDS program, and Lynne Hybels, who founded Willow Creek Community Church with her husband Bill and has been a leading advocate for AIDS relief in Africa. Many of their writings about AIDS evince the sentimental register recalled in Warren's narrative. McAlister adds to this roster the sentimental appeal of Franklin Graham, who has called for support from people who "have a heart" for HIV/AIDS work.[111] Together, these figures form an evangelical intimate public sustained through conferences, lectures, handbooks, and branded start-up kits instructing local congregations on how to join the fight against AIDS, as well as through the circulation of mass-marketed literature such as Kay Warren's *Dangerous Surrender* or Lynne Hybels' *Nice Girls Don't Change the World*, memoirs detailing the power of serving Christ through serving others. To appeal to fellow Christians, they recount stories about suffering in Africa and especially the need to help the "innocent victims" of this disease—usually women and children. They remind readers that Christ calls them to love and to help the less fortunate. This sentimental reasoning has, by most accounts, become quite effective in mobilizing evangelical Christians in the United States, who have quickly established one of the most influential platforms in global AIDS relief.[112]

Evangelical leaders contend that AIDS will not be stopped without the participation of the faith community. As Kay Warren explained in an interview with *Christianity Today*, "The church has the moral authority to ask people to make behavior changes. Governments and private sectors cannot do that."[113] The HIV/AIDS Initiative follows a two-part method in the fight against AIDS. At the broadest level, Kay and Rick Warren advocate the "P.E.A.C.E. Plan," an effort to enlist one billion Christians around the world to fight against what they consider "the five global, evil giants of our day," which include "spiritual emptiness," "egocentric leadership," "extreme poverty," "pandemic disease," and "rampant illiteracy."[114] To mobilize against these evils, they advocate following the same five activities that Jesus supported during his lifetime. These include "Planting churches," "Equipping servant leaders," "Assisting the poor," "Caring for the sick," and "Educating the next generation."[115] According to Rick Warren, this "mission effort" proves unique because it is based on God's biblical teaching, which he locates in five main purposes for Christians found in the Great Commandment and the Great Commission from the gospel of Matthew. Warren glosses these purposes as worship, service, evangelism, fellowship, and discipleship. The mission effort further gains power by drawing upon every member of the Christian church, pooling individuals together into a team effort that connects various congregations, and tackling global problems in a holistic manner. Even more, according to Warren's plan, this approach "makes local congregations the heroes. Not governments or other organizations."[116]

Saddleback's HIV/AIDS Initiative then describes two more specific strategies that have been used to fight the epidemic. The first recasts in new language the ABC approach (abstinence, be faithful, use a condom), which became popular in the 1990s but remained controversial among conservative evangelicals and Catholics. They explain in a care team training package that, since the 1980s, activists have been working to slow the spread of HIV. The techniques used to "S.L.O.W." the epidemic have included: "Supply condoms and eventually microbicides for everyone," "Limit the number of partners," "Offer needle exchange," and "Wait for sexual debut." While these techniques can be helpful for managing HIV, Kay Warren explains, they will not stop AIDS. In order to end the global crisis, the church must draw upon "its moral authority to S.T.O.P. the spread of HIV/AIDS by encouraging and supporting these four strategies": "Save sex for marriage," "Teach men and boys to respect women and children," "Open the door for the Church," and "Pledge fidelity to one partner for life." "When we reframe it like that," Kay Warren reasons, "barriers go down. We want to do the best for people, which is to stop it."[117]

Indeed, with these simple, copyrighted acrostics, the Saddleback Initiative has reshaped the global movement to fight HIV/AIDS.

Like other evangelical approaches, the Saddleback Initiative has emphasized the moral authority of the Christian community to promote behavior changes. According to Kay Warren, "Churches have *the moral credibility* to challenge high-risk lifestyles and to offer moral imperatives for the family and teach the moral motivation for abstinence and faithfulness."[118] To be sure, the initiatives that Shelp and Sunderland advocated also called for forms of "behavior modification." They promoted reduction in the number of sexual partners, settling into monogamous relationships, and using condoms when having sex, while the Warrens promote abstinence and fidelity, which they place above the use of condoms in their hierarchy of effective HIV prevention strategies. The difference between these two models arises not in their promotion of "behavior modification"—a coinage that sounds uncomfortable to the ears of most political liberals but one that evangelical activists use regularly. Rather, they differ in the languages and techniques each has employed to justify such changes.

Both models evince religious—and particularly Protestant Christian—approaches to helping others and caring for the sick. Shelp and Sunderland argued on biblical grounds for caring for people with AIDS, but the specific type of care and information they offered drew from medical and health professional guidelines: faith provided the impetus and the vehicle, but not necessarily the content of care. Their goal was to promote non-proselytizing means to care for people with HIV/AIDS and to prevent the further spread of the disease. The Warrens, on the other hand, have premised success upon the promotion of traditional Christian values among at-risk populations. Their model promotes changing not only sexual behavior, but the moral grounds upon which people engage in sex. Here, faith provides the impetus, the vehicle, and much of the content. Moreover, this approach to AIDS prevention cannot be severed from current-day evangelicals' stance on sexuality more generally and on homosexuality in particular.

Since the 1970s, a number of evangelicals have contended that although one's sexual orientation might be natural, sexual behavior must be guided biblically.[119] They have attached a powerful normative argument to debates about the social construction of sexual identities—if homosexuality is constructed, then homosexuals should be reconstructed, or reborn, as celibate Christians or (less often and with far less success) as heterosexual Christians.[120] For conservative evangelicals such as Rick and Kay Warren, proper moral education has the potential to promote behavior modification for homosexuals, who can—and for biblical reasons ought to—become sexually born again. In their sexual malleability, homosexuals in this approach resemble African men and women who, instead of being given condoms, should be given the proper moral training to practice abstinence and monogamous heterosexuality. Placing evangelical attitudes regarding sexual behavior modification among homosexual (Americans) and (heterosexual) Africans side by side reveals the common notion of sexuality undergirding this evangelical position. Rather than a natural component of one's identity, sexuality becomes a divine gift that can and ought to conform to biblical standards.

I emphasize this contemporary example for two reasons. First, the prominence of evangelical AIDS work today, which promotes a culturally conservative and increasingly common approach to sexual morality premised on abstinence and fidelity, disrupts any simple narrative of progression from negative to positive religious attitudes. It also shifts away from any simple dichotomy between religious conservatives and progressives by demonstrating instead the continuities and divergences in the theological and affective arguments that American Christians have drawn upon to understand and to confront the AIDS epidemic. Evangelicals working to end the AIDS crisis today extend earlier conservative Christian rhetoric about sexual immorality, though they focus less upon the wrath of God against sinners than upon promoting God's plan for sexuality. Likewise, they extend mainline Christian calls for care and compassion, for taking up the gospel of love. But in doing so they place biblical morality and biomedicine on nearly equal footing, and they merge pastoral care and evangelizing into a common goal. As President Obama might put it, they call for the reunification of "sexuality and spirituality" in the fight against AIDS.[121] They have been successful in this endeavor not by fulminating against sexual immorality, but by promoting a positive vision of sexual ethics that marries biblical morality to the language of public health. But they would not be the first to promote such a union.

Chapter Two

Governing Authority

THE SURGEON GENERAL AND THE MORAL POLITICS
OF PUBLIC HEALTH

"We would stop the spread of AIDS today if these high-risk people, these typhoid Marys, would stop spreading the disease. As a physician and a scientist, I'm appalled at their wildly having sex and spreading AIDS."

—HELEN SINGER KAPLAN, Human Sexuality Program, New York Hospital-Cornell Medical Center

"I am the surgeon general of the heterosexuals and the homosexuals, of the young and the old, of the moral [and] the immoral."

—C. EVERETT KOOP, United States Surgeon General

"God bless you, Dr. Koop."

—EUGENE L. STOWE, General Superintendent, Church of the Nazarene

IN A 1984 editorial in *Southern Medical Journal*, Dr. James Fletcher of the Department of Family Medicine at the Medical College of Georgia lamented, "a single disease syndrome, a true media rage, has brought gays a tremendous national outpouring of attention and sympathy." Fletcher acknowledged the social support and legal protections offered to gays and lesbians but encouraged readers to consider another approach. The Bible has served as a source of wisdom, even among "physicians," Fletcher explained, "who have consulted its pages and acknowledged its dictates."[1]

"But what of science?" the doctor asked. Fletcher surveyed the history of gay men's infection with sexually transmitted diseases since the

heyday of the gay sexual revolution of the 1970s. By the 1980s, the repercussions of this revolution had come into full view with the onset of
AIDS—and the convergence, he maintained, was no coincidence.[2] Given
the predominance of gay men with AIDS, Fletcher suggested looking
for a causal link between their actions and illness. "Might we be witnessing, in fact, in the form of a modern communicable disorder," he wondered, "a fulfillment of St. Paul's pronouncement: 'the due penalty of
error'?" For Fletcher, it appeared so, as "we see homosexual men reap-
ing not only expected consequences of sexual promiscuity, suffering
even as promiscuous heterosexuals the usual venereal diseases, but
other unusual consequences as well." Fletcher combined medical empir-
icism with Christian logic, noting that "the wisdom of the Bible" anticipated the medical conclusion that homosexuality was not merely an
alternative lifestyle, but "most certainly pathological." The only solution,
he concluded, was for healthcare providers "to seek reversal treatment
for their homosexual patients just as vigorously as they would for alco-
holics or heavy cigarette smokers, for what may not be treated might
well be avoided."[3]

Moral pronouncements against homosexuality come as no surprise.
They have existed nearly as long as the modern construction of homosexuality itself, dating back to the late nineteenth century.[4] Fletcher cast this
moral reproach in theological and medical terms, such that the empirical
reality of AIDS illustrated the divine rule laid out in his reading of the
Bible. He at once legitimates scientifically the "traditional" wisdom of the
Bible while illustrating the moral and scientific depravity of homosexual
behavior. Even more than heterosexuals, homosexuals in his view are
bound morally and medically to the "unusual consequences" of their
sinful acts, and their only cure is conversion. Medicine and morality speak
in one tongue, and it says no to gay sex.

To be sure, Fletcher was not representative of most physicians, just as
leaders of the Christian Right railing that AIDS was God's punishment for
homosexuality hardly represented most Christians. But neither was his
diagnosis far-flung. His position proved plausible enough to appear as an
editorial in a medical journal, which granted it not only visibility, but also
legitimacy. Most members of the medical community were less conspicuous in their moral condemnation. Though confusion and judgment were
commonplace, most doctors stopped shy of citing biblical injunctions
against gay sex. Medical injunctions proved sufficient, allowing religiously
based moral arguments to fade to the background or to be voiced by other

sectors of society. But moral and religious arguments did not disappear altogether in public health discussions of AIDS.[5]

Though Reagan did not speak publicly about AIDS until years after its emergence, members of Congress, the White House, and the Public Health Office debated strategies for confronting the epidemic and how to frame their responses. One leading voice belonged to United States Surgeon General C. Everett Koop, an evangelical and pro-life conservative appointed by Reagan. Initially shut out of conversations about the new epidemic, by the mid-1980s Koop took an active role in shaping a national HIV/AIDS education campaign. By emphasizing sex education and condom use, he surprised his conservative friends and liberal opponents alike, turning many of the former against him while garnering praise from the latter.

Throughout the 1980s, debates over sex education and condoms pitted religious morality against secular permissiveness, dividing conservatives and liberals largely on these grounds. In this battlefield of rhetoric, Koop seemed to be crossing the lines.[6] In 1986, he published a report on AIDS that detailed how HIV was transmitted and candidly discussed drug use and sexuality, including practices of oral and anal sex. The report drew the most attention, however, for its call for sex education in public schools to start at the earliest age possible. While public health experts and AIDS activists applauded Koop's bold approach, religious conservatives quickly spun Koop's position into a call to teach elementary schoolers about sodomy.

By 1988, Koop hadn't just crossed the line; he had redrawn it. That year his pamphlet *Understanding AIDS* brought straight talk about sex into nearly every American home. AIDS provided a learning experience, as media coverage of the epidemic introduced the lives of gay men and lesbians to mainstream America. Descriptions of gay sexual practices, often sensationalized, had never before reached so large an audience. And now the surgeon general pressed Americans to learn even more about sex through his education campaign, which included promoting abstinence and monogamy but also maintained the importance of using condoms. If the sexual revolution of the 1960s and 1970s had not yet reached every small town and rural outpost in the heartland, Koop's pamphlet did (Figure 2.1).

This chapter turns to Koop's national HIV/AIDS education campaign, and the political struggles leading up to it, to underscore how a particular moral politics of public health developed around AIDS in the

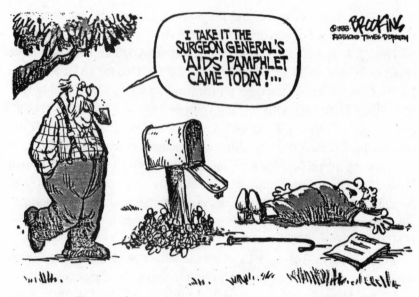

FIGURE 2.1 Gary Brookins' political cartoon, titled "I take it the Surgeon General's 'AIDS' pamphlet came today!" ran in the *Richmond Times-Dispatch* in 1988, shortly after the release of the pamphlet *Understanding AIDS*. (Gary Brookins: ©1988. Distributed by King Features Syndicate. Courtesy of the National Library of Medicine.)

second half of the 1980s.[7] To locate a moral politics of public health is to assert that medicine and public health became intertwined with religion and politics—a point that goes against common sense for most Americans, including medical professionals. Most of us think medical science is, or at least should be, free from the taint of religious or political bias. Religious and moral thought may have informed, if not dominated, public health campaigns in the nineteenth century, but, according to historians of medicine, these approaches gave way throughout the twentieth century to instrumental ones. Medical science, in short, became secular.[8] As least it should have. The federal government's public health campaign to educate Americans about AIDS invites us to revisit this narrative and to examine how religion shaped public health and medical responses to the AIDS crisis. White House staff and public health leaders not only debated conservative Christian approaches to public health and sexual morality: through Koop's AIDS campaign, they advanced a moral politics of public health and sexuality that touched more Americans than perhaps any previous discussion of sexuality.

Koop's Crusade

Charles Everett Koop—his friends called him Chick, a play on "Chicken Coop" from his student days at Dartmouth College—began his term as surgeon general in 1982. At the time, few could have guessed he would become the government's primary spokesperson for one of the most devastating diseases of the twentieth century. Even fewer could have predicted that he would become one of the most outspoken leaders in the call for sex education in public schools to combat the spread of HIV and other STDs. After completing his medical education at the University of Pennsylvania in 1947, Koop made a name for himself serving as surgeon-in-chief at the Children's Hospital of Philadelphia, where he established the first neonatal unit in the United States in 1956. He remained there until 1981. During those years, Koop attended Tenth Presbyterian Church, where he came under the influence of its pastor and renowned radio preacher Donald Barnhouse. For most of the twentieth century, Tenth Presbyterian was a member of the mainline Presbyterian denomination. In the 1970s, however, the mainline denominations witnessed a major push to expand roles for women and for gays and lesbians in church leadership. This movement reanimated long-standing rifts between theological conservatives and liberals in the larger denominational body. In 1979, Tenth Presbyterian left the mainline denomination to align with the theologically conservative Reformed Presbyterian Church, Evangelical Synod, which would merge with the Presbyterian Church in America (PCA) a few years later. This history shaped Koop's religious and public life.[9]

Koop did not experience the overwhelming emotional conversion typical of many American evangelicals—the often-sudden change that some would call being born again. He described, instead, coming to the "intellectual aspects of understanding" the gospel when he was 29, after hearing Barnhouse preach over a period of several months. During that time, Koop explained, "the Spirit of God made me realize [the Word] applied to me, and I accepted Christ into my heart and life."[10] This kind of conversion, hastened through learning, was not unusual in the history of American evangelicalism, especially among the headier denominations like the Reformed Presbyterians. Koop's exposure to the more intellectual side of the evangelical tradition, and to the demands of living in an urban setting like Philadelphia, would shape his participation in key culture wars issues, such as abortion, homosexuality, and AIDS, especially during his tenure as surgeon general.[11]

Koop gained notice in the broader evangelical community when he published *The Right to Live: The Right to Die* in 1976, in which he presented his case against abortion and euthanasia. Aimed at Christian readers, the book sold over one hundred thousand copies in its first year.[12] Seeking to awaken fellow evangelicals, Koop later explained, "I wrote as a physician, and also as a Christian, about the inexorable progression from abortion to infanticide to euthanasia." For Koop, life began at conception. It was his duty, both as a Christian and as a medical doctor, to preserve that life. Koop delivered the commencement address at the evangelical Wheaton College in Illinois six months after the Supreme Court decided *Roe v. Wade*, where he forecasted the dangerous effects of the case. He feared that it would devolve life-and-death ethics and medicine, leading not only to higher numbers of abortions, but also to an increase in "mercy killings" demanded by patients or their families. Legalized abortion, he warned, would hasten the loosening of American sexual morality. Finally, Koop worried the ruling would lead to the disabled newborn becoming the next victim considered incapable of having a "meaningful life."[13] As a pediatric surgeon, and as a Christian, he stood against this turn in *The Right to Live*.

But it was Koop's collaboration with well-known evangelical writer and philosopher Francis Schaeffer that brought him to the center of the Christian pro-life movement. Schaeffer, an intellectual forerunner of the Christian Right, founded L'Abri, an evangelical study center housed in Switzerland. In 1981, he published *Christian Manifesto*, which called for greater evangelical participation in political matters like abortion.[14] Koop and Schaeffer were longtime friends—the pediatric surgeon had treated Schaeffer's children, including his son Frankie, who had polio. They had not communicated in almost fifteen years when they happened to be lecturing at York University in Toronto around the same time. Though Koop and Schaeffer had worked separately to organize Christians against abortion, they decided now was the time to address the issue together. As Koop would later recall, "[T]he Schaeffers—father and son—and I determined to awaken the evangelical world—and anyone else who would listen—to the Christian imperative to do something to reverse the perilous realignment of American values on these life-and-death issues."[15]

Their collaboration over the next year and a half resulted in a book called *Whatever Happened to the Human Race?* First published in 1979, it sold fifty thousand copies. Thousands more people heard Koop and Schaeffer speak through a series of seminars or viewed one of the five films based on their work together.[16] By the end of the decade, Koop, now in his late sixties, had made a name for himself among conservative evangelicals through his work opposing abortion and euthanasia. He would soon come to the attention of Reagan's staff as well, through a tip from the offices of Billy Graham that came weeks before the presidential election in 1980.[17] For Reagan, who was about to sail into the White House largely through the support of evangelicals disappointed with born-again president Jimmy Carter, the pro-life pediatric surgeon seemed a fitting choice. But Koop's work on abortion also turned out to be one of the most controversial topics during his long and tumultuous confirmation process on the road to becoming the surgeon general.

A *Culture Wars Confirmation*

The 1980 presidential election marked a turning point in American politics. While the Republican Party had been courting southern and midwestern votes for decades, it was Ronald Reagan who shored up the alliance between the GOP and Bible Belt Christians that would endure to the present day. The topography of American Christianity had shifted dramatically since World War II. Up to that point, most Americans aligned with specific denominations, usually those in which they were reared, such as Catholic or Episcopalian, Methodist or Baptist. This denominational approach began to break down after the war for a number of reasons, including the expansion of higher education, greater geographic mobility, and the changing role of women in American society. More and more, Americans organized around moral and political sensibilities: conservatives gravitated toward other conservatives, and liberals to other liberals. This political and cultural realignment even helped melt divisions among Protestants, Catholics, and Jews, as religious identity came to matter less than one's moral and political positions regarding a host of key issues, including abortion, premarital sex, birth control, divorce, and homosexuality. These divisions began to calcify following the racial and sexual revolutions of the 1960s. By the late 1970s, conservative white evangelicals and Catholics had grown impatient with the Southern Baptist Jimmy Carter, who toed a fine line between this emerging conservative morality and the Democratic Party's more liberal platform. While not as fluent in evangelical rhetoric as Carter, Reagan voiced his support for the pro-life movement, which helped him court conservative Christian leaders and their ever-expanding audience. Upon assuming office, the new

president began to fill his administration with like-minded political conservatives, many of them religious.[18]

Pro-lifers hoped the new president would rein in the mistakes of *Roe v. Wade,* and the buzz about nominating Koop as the next surgeon general only confirmed their wishes. Even before his official nomination, the national evangelical magazine *Christianity Today* lauded Reagan's choice. "Koop is widely admired among evangelical Christians for his views on the sanctity of life," the article noted, as it assured readers that the con-
gressmen pushing for Koop "believe he is by far more qualified than others whose names have been mentioned."[19] Yet Koop soon became the center of controversy, as the moral and political battles of the 1980s played out in his confirmation hearing.

Over the course of eight months, Congress, political and health agencies, and media outlets alike debated Koop's qualifications for the ap-
pointment. Critics focused on his outspoken stance against abortion, which they argued was out of step with the legal decision rendered by the Supreme Court in *Roe v. Wade* and well to the right of the majority of Americans at the time. Progressive groups such as Planned Parenthood, the National Organization for Women, and the National Abortion Rights Action League denounced his nomination. Even the American Medical Association (AMA) withheld its support. The AMA had already opposed Reagan's appointment of Pennsylvania's Republican senator Richard Schweiker as secretary of Health and Human Services. Early on, Schweiker marked his shift to the right of his predecessor Patricia Roberts Harris when he opposed the promotion of sex education programs, in-
cluding those that taught teens about contraceptives, despite an epi-
demic of pregnancy among teenagers. Now the AMA refused to back Koop as well.[20]

Furthermore, while Koop's successful career as a pediatric surgeon demonstrated his skill with handling individual patients, many questioned whether he could serve as a spokesperson for *public* health. Dr. William McBeath, executive director of the American Public Health Asso-
ciation, lauded Koop as a "distinguished pediatric surgeon" but worried he was "otherwise almost uniquely unqualified" to be surgeon general.[21] In Congress, Democratic representative Henry Waxman of California spoke most frankly against Koop's appointment. "Dr. Koop frightens me," he admitted: "He does not have a public health record, he's dogmatically de-
nounced those who disagree with him and his intemperate views make me wonder about his, and the Administration's, judgement [*sic*]."[22]

The *New York Times* agreed. Titled "Dr. Unqualified," the *Times* editorial lauded Koop's work as a pediatric surgeon but underscored his lack of public health experience. Past surgeon generals, almost without exception, the article continued, have possessed experience specifically within the field of public health. That Koop had shown no evidence of such experience, along with the fact that he technically was older than the legally permitted age to assume the position, suggested that the Reagan administration's interest in Koop had to be found elsewhere: "That 'elsewhere' may be his anti-abortion crusade." The *Times* concluded with its hope that Congress would reject the appointment, for not to do so "would be an affront both to the public health profession and the public."[23]

Following months of contentious hearings, in November 1981 Koop was finally confirmed as surgeon general, the pulpit from which he would famously campaign against smoking in the early 1980s, and from which he would soon preach the gospel of sex education to combat AIDS. And as it turned out, it was Koop's conservative followers who would eventually turn their backs on him, while liberals would praise his stance against big tobacco and his pragmatic approach to AIDS prevention.

Koop's Campaigns: Smoking and Baby Doe

By most accounts, Koop turned out to be quite skilled in his new post. The first "celebrity surgeon general," he reinstated the practice of wearing the position's ceremonial military uniform (Figure 2.2). Together with his forceful and at times controversial public health campaigns—not to mention what *Time* dubbed his "Old Testament beard" and "preacher's voice"—this look made Koop a highly visible figure in the Reagan era.[24]

Koop waged two of his most significant battles as surgeon general in the first years of his tenure, when he fought against smoking and in support of the rights of disabled children. In 1982, he released the *Surgeon General's Report on Smoking and Health*, his first official act following confirmation. The report focused on the connection between smoking and cancer, but it also highlighted broader public health concerns. Almost a third of the American populace smoked, leading to 400,000 deaths annually and about $13 billion spent each year on health care expenses. "If I were a smoker of a pipe, cigars, or cigarettes, and were reasonably intelligent and had read this report," Koop thundered at the press conference held upon the report's release, "I would long since have quit."[25]

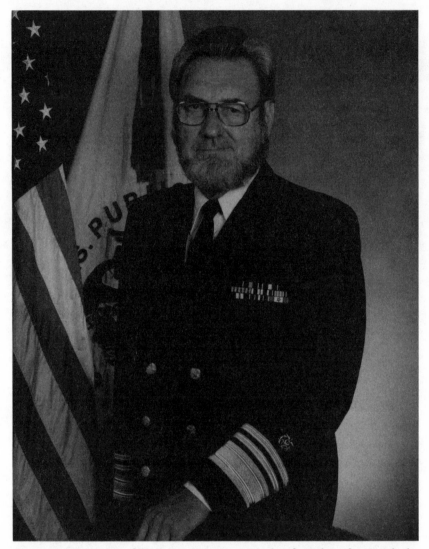

FIGURE 2.2 Portrait of C. Everett Koop wearing his formal uniform with the Public Health Service. (Courtesy of the National Library of Medicine.)

The report launched Koop into the public spotlight yet again. He testified before Congress on behalf of a new requirement that replaced the generic surgeon general's warning on cigarettes with a series of rotating warnings on the specific dangers of smoking. These included heart disease, cancer, emphysema, and risks to the unborn children of pregnant women. In 1984, Koop kick-started the Campaign for a Smoke-Free America by the Year 2000. Two years later, he ensured that warning labels would also appear on smokeless tobacco products and drew attention to the dangerous effects of secondhand smoke.

Koop's wide-ranging campaign appeared to be successful. During his tenure in office, the percentage of smokers dropped from 33% to 26%. While the tobacco industry spit fumes, Koop continued to hit home the connections between smoking and health risks such as cancer and heart disease. The mainstream press also warmed to Koop, who garnered widespread support for his campaign. With all this national attention, Koop recalled, "I began to see the valuable ways in which the Surgeon General's position could be used to advance the health of the nation with moral suasion," a tactic that would prove even more promising in his later campaign for AIDS education.[26]

But if Koop's anti-smoking campaign was a popular and media success, the case of Baby Doe pulled him back into the thick of culture wars politics. Baby Doe was born in a hospital in Bloomington, Indiana on April 9, 1982 and diagnosed with Down syndrome as well as esophageal atresia, a condition in which the esophagus was separated from the stomach, making it impossible for the infant to absorb food. The obstetrician notified the mother that her newborn would have only a 50% chance of surviving the surgery to correct the esophageal atresia and would still require medical attention for the rest of his life. The doctor recommended allowing the baby to die of natural causes. Going against this advice, a pediatrician at the hospital and the mother's family physician recommended immediate surgery. Presented with conflicting medical opinions, the parents decided to allow the child to die naturally. This decision ignited a fury of legal action, as the hospital's attorney called for a judicial hearing to decide Baby Doe's fate.

Superior Court Judge John Baker first heard the case. In his opinion, since the parents had been presented with two legitimate medical options, it was their right to decide between them. The Monroe County Child Protection Committee as well as the Indiana Supreme Court supported the decision. Three attorneys for the hospital then attempted a different approach to enforce the treatment of Baby Doe. They sought to declare the infant a neglected child under the Indiana Child in Need of Services statute. But the acting judge held once again that there had been no violation, and the power to decide the infant's future remained with the parents. Finally, an attorney acting to save Baby Doe filed an appeal with the United States Supreme Court, for which Justice John Paul Stevens was to hear the request. But time had run out: Baby Doe died on April 15, before the justice could make a decision.[27]

The controversy over Baby Doe's case took on new life in national media and in political debate. The central fault lines pitted the rights of parents and physicians against the rights of the disabled child. This heated debate (exacerbated by the case of "Baby Jane Doe" the following year) would quickly involve the surgeon general in a campaign to pass the "Baby Doe Law," which amended the 1984 Child Abuse Law to include withholding food, water, or medical treatment from disabled children, especially those with intellectual disabilities. By his own account, Koop's frustration with the death of Baby Doe and his efforts to protect the rights of children with disabilities derived both from his calling as a pediatric surgeon and from his Christian faith; he considered his support for newborns a logical extension of his pro-life position.[28]

The case of Baby Doe presented difficult terms for public debate. Koop recognized the complex dimensions of this situation, even as he fought to protect the rights of disabled children on moral and medical grounds alike. If Koop discovered the power of moral suasion while at work in his anti-smoking campaign, he drew upon his own righteous discontent in the fight for the rights of disabled children as much as for the unborn. In the controversy surrounding Baby Doe, and in his anti-smoking campaign, Koop revealed his deep concern for human life, a compassion rooted as much in his Christian faith as it was in his medical training. The two, in fact, often went hand in hand for the surgeon general. The emergence of the AIDS epidemic would test his medical, political, and moral resolve once more.

AIDS in the Age of Reagan

While Koop remained occupied with his anti-smoking campaign and the controversy surrounding the case of Baby Doe, a new infection was sweeping through urban gay communities in Los Angeles, San Francisco, and New York. Medical researchers with the Centers for Disease Control and the National Institutes of Health began to suspect a new disease on the horizon. By August of 1982, they had named it AIDS.

The AIDS crisis struck at an auspicious moment in the advancement of medical research. Immunology and virology—the two medical fields that would become most involved in HIV/AIDS research—had only recently reached a state advanced enough to understand HIV, the retrovirus that nearly all researchers by 1984 agreed caused the condition known as AIDS.[29] Though optimistic about such quick gains in understanding the disease, even by the mid-1980s researchers did not expect a vaccine or cure anytime soon. AZT, the most promising antiretroviral drug, was still going through trials. It was difficult to obtain and often disappointing for those able to get it. Politically, the epidemic surfaced at an unpropitious time for minority populations and those without health care. As the disease spread through urban communities throughout the 1980s, Reagan's policies for economic and social reform scaled back funding for health care and medical research. The receding role of the state in such matters combined with national homophobia and racism to stymie the government's political and public health response. Years passed before a clear national spokesperson emerged in the figure of Surgeon General Koop—and even then never officially.

In the first years of the epidemic, the American people received mixed and often inaccurate information about AIDS. Coverage in the mainstream press was initially scarce, as editors and journalists shied away from reporting on a disease that appeared to target gay or bisexual men, drug users, sex workers, and Haitians. As the epidemic continued to spread, however, more and more it appeared to threaten the American mainstream. That made for good news. Media outlets sensed not only the threat, but also the potential for higher ratings. They increased coverage of AIDS, but in doing so often fell back on sensationalist rhetoric and poorly interpreted medical information.[30] Coverage shifted from emphasizing gay men with AIDS and condemnations from the Christian Right to the emergence of AIDS among heterosexuals. News coverage found a new category of "AIDS victim" among hemophiliacs, mostly children, who contracted HIV through blood transfusions. A number of stories depicted them as "innocent victims" or even what Diane Winston has called "AIDS martyrs."[31] These were people unfairly burdened by a disease associated with sexual sin but whose personal sufferings could teach everyone lessons about AIDS.

Ryan White, who contracted HIV from a blood transfusion, would become the most famous martyr, though he often spoke against the moral rhetoric of innocence versus guilt implicit in this naming. After being diagnosed in 1984 at the age of 13, White gained national attention when he attempted to return to his public school in Kokomo, Indiana. Medical experts at the time confirmed that he posed very little risk to others, but a number of parents and teachers nonetheless pressured the school to ban White from attending. White eventually won this protracted battle (and would in 1990 become the namesake of the largest federally funded program for people with HIV/AIDS in the United States), though his family would have to move to another town to escape harassment.[32] His case demonstrated both the fears many Americans had about AIDS as well as their lack of information. In the absence of a clear and focused national response, many Americans grew ever more frustrated and afraid, and they directed their anger towards people with HIV and AIDS.

In the early years of the epidemic, gays and lesbians formed numerous grassroots organizations to fill the vacuum left open by Reagan's silence. They included more conventional service organizations as well as activist groups, such as Gay Men's Health Crisis (GMHC) and ACT UP (the AIDS Coalition to Unleash Power) in New York City. At first, service and activist organizations often overlapped: the very existence of such organizations relied upon and enacted community-based AIDS activism. Together, service organizations and activist groups pressured local and national governments to provide care for those who had contracted HIV and to sponsor prevention programs for those at risk. In the absence of a fully committed response from the government, these groups often took it upon themselves to provide such information and care. Toward this end, they developed sophisticated educational approaches that contained often explicit, sex-positive information about safe sex and HIV prevention that was targeted at the populations most at risk.[33]

During this period—the first five years of the AIDS epidemic—Koop monitored CDC reports and the response of the Public Health Service from the sidelines. Despite his position as surgeon general, for which Congress mandated him "to inform the American people about the prevention of disease and the promotion of health," Koop lamented that he was "completely cut off from AIDS."[34] His immediate superior, Assistant Secretary for Health Edward Brandt, informed Koop that he would not be assigned to cover AIDS, and indeed Koop would not speak publicly about the epidemic until Reagan's second term. This is not to say that the Public Health Service, or other branches of the federal government, was not taking steps to confront the AIDS crisis. In 1983, Brandt created an Executive Task Force on AIDS to respond to the growing epidemic, though Koop was not a member. The history of the White House's response to AIDS is more complex. Journalist Randy Shilts most famously documented the Reagan Administration's slow and inept response to the crisis in his 1987 account *And the Band Played On.* He underscored how political games slowed the pace of research and cost more lives in the delay of medical advancement. More recent historical work on the Reagan

Administration's response has augmented Shilts' original description and revealed the religious battles raging behind closed doors.[35]

AIDS in the White House

The Reagan era ushered in not only a new national leader, but also a new White House staff that included a number of anti-gay conservatives, chief among them Pat Buchanan, Gary Bauer, and William Bennett. This shift consequently curtailed the already limited access that gay and lesbian leaders had to aides within the previous administration. As historian William Turner puts it, "[R]ather than having highly sympathetic White House and executive-agency staffers serving under a largely indifferent president who supported the basic logic of civil rights, suddenly activists faced hostile staffers serving under a largely indifferent president who opposed the basic logic of civil rights."[36] The records of meetings about AIDS called by White House staffers demonstrate this shift.

The first occurred on June 21, 1983, and included two gay activists, Virginia Apuzzo and Jeff Levi, both from the National Gay Task Force (NGTF). They were joined by Judi Buckalew, special assistant to the president for public liaison, and staff members from Health and Human Services. According to Apuzzo, this was the first meeting between the gay and lesbian community and the new administration, and their goal was to get acquainted with one another and to share concerns about the epidemic. But the new administration quickly soured on these gay leaders, turning their attention instead toward another political constituency: religious conservatives. A second meeting called in August included no representatives from the gay and lesbian community. Those in attendance included Faith Ryan Whittlesey of the Office of Public Liaison and two of her staff members; Judi Buckalew, who attended the previous meeting; and Morton Blackwell, who served as special assistant to the president as the public liaison for religion. They met with two religious conservatives who had called the meeting to discuss the administration's response to AIDS as a public health issue. Howard Phillips, the national director of the Conservative Caucus, favored a strategy that would place information about AIDS within the context of public condemnation of homosexuality, describing it as a moral wrong. The final person in attendance, Dr. Ron Goodwin of the Moral Majority, did not go quite so far. But he joined his colleague in calling on the Office of Public Liaison to encourage the administration to close gay bathhouses, to require blood donors to provide detailed sexual histories, and to become "more visible and vocal" in its fight against AIDS.[37]

This meeting highlights the extent to which information about AIDS would be politicized within the Reagan White House and among national leaders more generally. The various agencies of the government responding to the AIDS crisis established different approaches that often pitted public health experts against Reagan's political advisors. Efforts to provide education about AIDS proved the main target of such battles and revealed the new administration's conservative religious concerns about homosexuality. As historian Jennifer Brier explains, while public health leaders attempted to gain control of the epidemic, they had to wrestle with "many of Reagan's domestic advisors and aides [who] wanted to bend what they called 'AIDS education' to fit the model of social and religious conservatism that posited gay men as sick and dangerous."[38]

One of the central battles emerged around two competing general approaches to dealing with the epidemic. AIDS activists joined many liberal and moderate religious organizations, as well as public health experts, in insisting upon a strong state-based approach that would acknowledge the need to preserve people's basic civil rights. Religious and political conservatives, on the other hand, considered any accommodations to protect civil liberties in the face of AIDS to be political pandering to liberals, especially gay activists. Illustrating this belief, nine Republican congressional representatives, including William Dannemeyer, Robert Dornan, and Newt Gingrich, wrote a letter to the president attacking what they viewed as a liberal response to the crisis and calling for "common sense guidelines that address the problem and ignore the politics." Specifically, they called for the closing of bathhouses and mandating that all AIDS cases be reported to the CDC.[39]

In a separate letter to the assistant secretary of Health and Human Services, Gingrich underscored the need to refrain from tempering medical advice with worries about "political" problems. In this approach, Brier has argued, the term "political" came to represent an opposition to what conservatives took as the best, or even the commonsense, public health or medical approaches, ones that consistently foregrounded health at the expense of civil liberties. "In this case, Gingrich argued that closing bathhouses or mandating reporting of AIDS was a more reasonable policy than trying to provide sex education at bathhouses or keeping the names of people who tested positive for HIV anonymous," writes Brier: "Here, the commonsense arguments betrayed a particular stance on AIDS, one that sought to make the public healthy by restricting the civil rights of those believed to be sick." The Reagan administration followed Gingrich's advice.[40]

In its strategy to address AIDS, the administration made social conservatives William Bennett, the secretary of education, and Gary Bauer, the undersecretary of education, the White House's key spokespeople. They worked together to formulate a strategy that emphasized "morality, local control, and a strong executive branch." Despite the initial connection between AIDS and the gay community, as well as earlier responses within this community to discuss HIV and to educate people about safe sex that had proved effective, Bennett and Bauer sought to marginalize any approaches that supported behavior that they deemed immoral. In an internal memo, Bauer wrote that the Department of Education needed to focus on the idea that "heterosexual sex within marriage is what most Americans, our laws and our traditions consider the proper focus of human sexuality."[41] It was within this framework that Bennett and Bauer hoped to place AIDS education.

Koop's Call to AIDS Education

As it turned out, Bauer and Bennett would not be the administration's only spokespeople on AIDS. By the summer of 1985, Koop had grown recalcitrant about the need for the surgeon general to speak out. Up to that point, he had been turning down a growing number of requests to address the crisis. That summer an anonymous, conservative campaign even sent telegrams to the HHS secretary's office calling for Koop to be "unmuzzled" in regard to AIDS. The campaign leaders apparently hoped the conservative Reagan appointee would speak against protections for gay civil rights and in favor of stricter public health measures—they expected Koop, if unmuzzled, to side with Bennett and Bauer.

By this time, Brandt had left his post as the assistant secretary for health, and a new acting secretary, James O. Mason, heeded Koop's call for a central spokesperson. He installed the surgeon general as a member of the AIDS Task Force, effectively empowering Koop to speak out. By the end of that year, Koop began to hear rumors that President Reagan planned to call on him to write a report on AIDS for the American people. The announcement came from Reagan during an unusual visit to the Department of Health and Human Services. At the meeting, held on February 5, 1986—now almost five years after the first reported cases of what became known as AIDS—Reagan declared the epidemic a top priority and asked the surgeon general to prepare a report. Koop started his work the next day, and for the following two years, as he tells it, AIDS would take over his life.[42]

Koop recounts in his memoir how he knew from the beginning that if he were to write what he considered an unbiased report on AIDS, he would have to limit the number of political forces that could provide input or that could potentially hold it up. Much of this resistance, he suspected, would come from the White House. "A large proportion of the president's constituency was anti-homosexual, anti-drug abuse, anti-promiscuity, and anti-sex education," Koop recalled: "these people would not respond well to some of the things that have to be said in a health report on AIDS." To avoid political delays, Koop sought permission from recently appointed Secretary for Health Otis Bowen to bypass the normal clearance process for his report.[43]

Following months of research, on October 22, 1986 Koop released *The Surgeon General's Report on Acquired Immune Deficiency Syndrome*. It presented the best medical information available to date about HIV and AIDS and sought to alleviate the fears of the American people. The thirty-six-page report called Americans to fight the epidemic as a unified group rather than condemning certain populations disproportionately affected by the disease who some felt "deserved" the illness (though they go unnamed, this would surely include homosexuals and drug users). By saying this, Koop attempted to move the rhetoric of the AIDS epidemic beyond its association with homosexuality and drug use, away from the idea that it was the just desserts for immoral behavior. As he noted, "We're fighting a disease, not people."[44] The report also opposed compulsory testing for HIV and quarantines for those testing positive, ideas favored by some conservative leaders in Congress and the White House. But Koop's report went even further than anyone had anticipated from the evangelical surgeon.

The *Surgeon General's Report on AIDS* represented a strong shift away from the conservative impulses of Bennett, Bauer, and other members of the political and Religious Right. It called for a comprehensive education campaign that would teach about sexual activity and the use of condoms. One passage in particular drew attention from the media and ignited yet another firestorm of controversy for the surgeon general. According to the report,

> Education concerning AIDS must start at the lowest grade possible
> as part of any health and hygiene program. The appearance of AIDS
> could bring together diverse groups of parents and educators with

opposing views on inclusion of sex education in the curricula. There is now no doubt that we need sex education in schools and that it include information on heterosexual and homosexual relationships. The threat of AIDS should be sufficient to permit a sex education curriculum with a heavy emphasis on prevention of AIDS and other sexually transmitted diseases.[45]

The mainstream media applauded Koop's report but homed in on his discussion of sex education.[46] A review in the *Los Angeles Times* illustrated the media's focus in its choice of headline: "Koop Urges AIDS Sex Course in Grade School."[47] Almost immediately, Koop's discussion of sex education stirred debate.

A number of gay rights leaders and AIDS activists were relieved to see that Koop did not fall in line with conservative Christian denunciations of sexual immorality, even if they still found the report too moderate. Gil Gerald of the National Coalition of Black Lesbians and Gays wrote to Koop, "To be quite honest the report and your statements exceeded our expectations." While noting the report could have said more about how AIDS impacted racial minorities, Gerald commended Koop's support for sex education and his stance against mandatory mass testing and quarantine for people with AIDS.[48] Paul Kawata, executive director of the National AIDS Network and board member of the National Minority AIDS Council, explained: "Given who Koop is and what he represents in the New Right agenda, he was up front about education and outreach." And speaking on behalf of the National Gay and Lesbian Task Force, Urvashi Vaid lauded Koop's stance on sex education, though she hoped that such curricula would be "value-free," which was not to be the case.[49]

Koop would meet more resistance in the gay press following a forum on HIV/AIDS held at Harvard University's Kennedy School of Government, where he shared the stage with the *Boston Globe*'s Loretta McLaughlin. An article on the event in *Gay Community News*, Boston's weekly gay magazine, captured Koop's emphasis on sexual monogamy and the lessons of morality. It also reported McLaughlin's criticism of the federal government for its sluggish and inept response to the AIDS crisis. She faulted Koop's report in particular for failing to call for more money. "If we are sincere about teaching children about AIDS, why wasn't there a great call for funds?" she asked. Koop more or less folded, admitting that his influence was limited to "moral suasion and borrowed money."[50] Conservative reaction was even more hostile.

Writing in the *Washington Post*, Christian Brahmstedt complained of Koop's "blatant disregard and neglect of moral teaching" in his call for sex education. Brahmstedt thought Koop missed an opportunity to present an agenda more along the lines of what Catholic Secretary of Education William Bennett had been promoting: one that placed AIDS in a moral context and condemned immoral, risky behavior. Conservative commentator William F. Buckley, Jr., likewise slammed the surgeon general's stance on sex education, while Rowland Evans and Robert Novak penned a factually misleading and sensationalistic attack on his call for AIDS education in secondary schools. Phyllis Schlafly, founder of the Eagle Forum, proved one of Koop's most ardent critics. The AIDS report, she fumed, "looks and reads like it was edited by the Gay Task Force." Schlafly even accused the surgeon general of advocating for third-graders to learn the rules of "safe sodomy." Koop was baffled. "Why anyone paid attention to this lady," he bemoaned, "is one of the mysteries of the eighties." Airing his frustration to reporters, Koop continued, "I'm not Surgeon General to make Phyllis Schlafly happy. I'm Surgeon General to save lives."[51]

Koop anticipated attacks from the political right, but he was disconcerted by the failure of many of his friends in the Christian Right to understand his position. Reflecting on the responses to his report, he noted:

> Castigation by the *political* right, although disappointing and unpleasant, did not unduly upset me; after all, castigation seemed to be their business. But I did feel a profound sense of betrayal by those on the *religious* right who took me to task. My position on AIDS was dictated by scientific integrity and Christian compassion. I felt my Christian opponents had abandoned not only their old friend, but also their own commitment to integrity and compassion.[52]

Koop's position on condoms and sex education strained ties with longtime allies, including his friend Carl Anderson, a White House aide, and many evangelical conservatives who viewed his position as a betrayal of their shared moral values. The surgeon general complained that his fellow Christians often failed to see moral messages in his AIDS campaign. After an interview on the Christian Broadcasting Network's *The 700 Club*, Koop penned a letter to Pat Robertson, the founder of the network and host of its flagship program. He complained that the interview "did not provide a forum for discussion of the Christian concepts underlying my report" and that the segment suffered from poor reporting, including the misrepresentation of facts. Much of this could have been avoided, he quipped, had *The 700 Club* staff bothered to read his 1986 report.[53]

Some conservative Christians attacked Koop more directly. In *AIDS: A Special Report*, published by Summit Ministries in 1986, David Noebel, Wayne Lutton, and Paul Cameron included an appendix, "AIDS Warning: The Surgeon General's Report May Be Hazardous to Your Health." In a section titled "Koop Chickens Out," they accused the surgeon general of ignoring the key threat posed by sexual immorality, particularly homosexuality. Koop's "pro-homosexual bias" came through in his refusal to castigate gay men, they charged, and his report was also "littered with unscientific, allegedly 'authoritative' statements" about the disease, most of which let gays off the hook. They concluded their anti-Koop screed with a list of steps to be taken. First off, they suggested, "our public health authorities must be made to realize that their first responsibility is to protect the public's health, not the perceived 'civil rights' of homosexuals or drug abusers." For these writers, gays and lesbians (and drug users) fell outside the bounds of moral citizenship. While this statement might sound extreme today, it was not at the time. Noebel, Lutton, and Cameron cited the recently released Supreme Court decision in *Bowers v. Hardwick* (1986) as proof that "sodomy is not protected by the Constitution." This ruling would not be overturned until 2003's *Lawrence v. Texas*. They also recommended that "no printed matter involving homosexual activity or paraphernalia or child sexual activity should have access to the U.S. mails under penalty of law," recalling Anthony Comstock's Victorian campaign against obscenity.[54] Little did they know at the time that Koop, who had already refused the former suggestion through his AIDS report, would a couple years later violate the latter through his AIDS mailer.

Koop's AIDS report also deepened opposition within the White House. Conservative aides pressured Koop to remove references to condoms from all future publications of the report and took steps to promote their own approach to AIDS education. Koop expected as much. In an interview with *Time*, he recalled, "the White House doesn't like the C word. But if you don't talk about condoms, people are going to die. So I talk."[55] He was right about condoms but still underestimated the depth of opposition from within the White House.

The president, for one, seemed not to have learned much from Koop's report. Speaking about the epidemic in February of 1987, Reagan leveled with Americans: "let's be honest with ourselves. When it comes to preventing

AIDS, don't medicine and morality teach the same lessons?"[56] Other White House insiders attacked Koop directly. Secretary of Education William Bennett characterized one of Koop's AIDS lectures in a note to Bauer as "straight homosexual propaganda, lifted out of their tirades."[57] In 1987, Bennett released his own report through the Department of Education called "AIDS and the Education of Our Children: A Guide for Parents and Teachers." It warned that education about condoms could promote further sex among teenagers and called instead on parents and teachers to "[t]each restraint as a virtue" and to "[p]resent sex education within a moral context."[58] His position echoed calls for sex education by social hygienists in the early twentieth century. Unlike the stricter Victorian anti-sex ideology, this approach comprehended the need for some sort of education about sex, yet feared that too much education, and too little moral framework, would corrupt not only young minds, but also society at large.[59]

Gary Bauer also composed an alternative AIDS strategy. In December 1986, he drafted an education policy for school children contending that AIDS education "should not be neutral between heterosexual and homosexual sex." "Homosexuals should not be persecuted," he submitted, "but heterosexual sex within marriage is what most Americans, our laws and our traditions consider the proper focus of human sexuality." According to Bauer and his co-author John Klenk, all federally sponsored AIDS education materials should "encourage responsible sexual behavior — based on fidelity, commitment, and maturity, placing sexuality within the context of marriage." Ignoring Koop's recommendations, Reagan approved this new language in a document subsequently delivered to every federal agency.[60] To borrow a term from Jennifer Brier, its rhetoric proved infectious. Within months, Senator Jesse Helms, a perennial opponent of AIDS funding, passed legislation that echoed Reagan's policy by regulating the content of AIDS publications funded by the federal government. Helms' amendment prohibited the CDC from using government funds to "promote, encourage, and condone homosexual sexual activities or the intravenous use of illegal drugs."[61]

But Koop's message on AIDS did not end with his report. The Public Health Office (PHO) soon began efforts to produce a trimmed-down version of the AIDS report that would be cheaper to produce and more accessible to most Americans. After delayed support from the White House, Congress empowered the PHO to produce and distribute a brochure on AIDS "without necessary clearance of the content by any official," thereby ensuring White House politics would stay out of it.[62] The final pamphlet, called *Understanding AIDS* (Figure 2.3), was ready to go by May 1988. Koop's office printed 107 million copies, enough to be mailed to nearly every household in the United States, making this the largest mailing sponsored by the federal government at the time.[63]

In six pages, *Understanding AIDS* described how AIDS was contracted and—perhaps more importantly—how it was *not* spread, thereby easing fears among many Americans worried that HIV could be spread through casual contact, kissing, donating blood, or mosquito bites. It also outlined

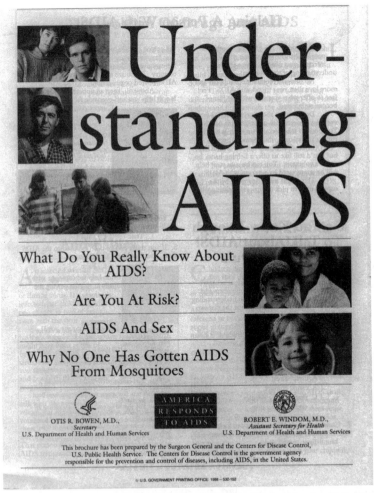

FIGURE 2.3 Cover page of *Understanding AIDS*, published by the U.S. Department of Health and Human Services and distributed to American families in 1988. (Courtesy of the National Library of Medicine.)

the types of behavior that put one at risk, which included needle sharing, anal sex "with or without a condom," oral and vaginal intercourse without protection, and sex with multiple partners. The brochure even included a section called "What Is All This Talk about Condoms." It prescribed condoms as the best protection against HIV, aside from abstinence, and provided advice about how best to use them.[64]

With such wide reception, the brochure was sure to draw criticism. Gary Bauer complained that the pamphlet promoted condoms and sexual promiscuity among the nation's youth. He also insisted that its discussion of how AIDS could and could not be transmitted was medically inaccurate. But mostly, Bauer was dismayed that the brochure discussed sexual matters, including anal and oral intercourse, which he thought were sure to offend most Americans.[65] Beyond critics on the Far Right, the pamphlet got generally positive reviews.[66] Moreover, it marked Koop's greatest and final major endeavor as an AIDS educator during his tenure as surgeon general, from which he would retire in October 1989.

AIDS, Morality, and the Surgeon General

If Bauer's attacks on Koop's AIDS brochure may have exuded the rhetorical excess expected of culture wars critique, his recognition of the magnitude of the mailing—and the novelty of discussing sexual behaviors like oral and anal intercourse, along with the proper use of condoms—was well-founded. The surgeon general's brochure, along with media coverage of the AIDS epidemic, brought discussions about sex into every household in America, even those that had remained relatively shielded from or indifferent to the sexual revolution of the previous two decades. Political cartoonist Gary Brookins captured this sentiment for readers of the conservative-leaning *Richmond Times-Dispatch*. His cartoon (Figure 2.1) featured an older white couple—represented as rural, if not the epitome of down-home country. The husband, wearing suspenders and smoking a pipe, strolls up to his wife, who has passed out on the ground in front of the mailbox. Beside her lies a flier. The husband remarks, "I take it the Surgeon General's 'AIDS' pamphlet came today." Such representations were by no means limited to newspapers in the Bible Belt. The *Los Angeles Times* ran Ralph Dunagin's political cartoon (Figure 2.4) depicting a white mother clad in a dress and pearl necklace that recalls images of the all-American suburban housewife of the 1950s. The mother is heading out the door but turns back. She instructs her two sons not to open the mail while she's gone, for fear that Koop's pamphlet might arrive. As these illustrations suggest, this little brochure was not only the largest public health mailing the government had ventured to date, but also the most extensive public effort to educate "real" Americans about sexuality.[67]

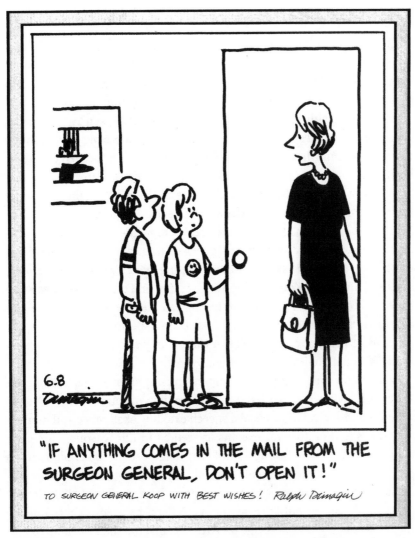

FIGURE 2.4 Ralph Dunagin's political cartoon, titled "If anything comes in the mail from the Surgeon General, don't open it!" ran in the *Los Angeles Times* in 1988, shortly after the release of the pamphlet *Understanding AIDS*. (Ralph Dunagin: ©1988. Distributed by TCA/MCT Reprints. Courtesy of the National Library of Medicine.)

As a self-described conservative evangelical, Koop was an unlikely poster figure for comprehensive sex education. Historians have described Koop's education campaign as rising above the moral, or even moralistic, approach taken by religious and social conservatives within the Reagan administration. "Koop's beliefs made him the perfect candidate to write a special report on AIDS that would emphasize morality, defined as a commitment to heterosexual marriage as the key institution of the American family and nation, rather than condoms and sex education," writes Jennifer Brier in her brilliant history of the AIDS epidemic: "Much to the disappointment of many conservatives, Koop failed to live up to their expectations."[68] Jonathan Engel effuses that Koop "steadfastly refused to overlay the epidemic with a moral taint," by performing his primary role "as a public health officer as opposed to a moralistic sentry." Narrating government debates about AIDS policy, Robert Self slots Koop among those espousing what he calls the "liberal view," which focused on public health and a concern for rights, rather than the "conservative view," characterized by "sexual discipline and public order."[69] While there is some basis for this interpretation, Koop's work belies this bifurcation. Reading his religious activism alongside his AIDS campaign—indeed, reading his AIDS work as a kind of religious activism translated into the terms of morality—revises this skewed understanding, which not only historians, but also journalists, Koop's conservative critics, and even sometimes Koop himself have shared. It demonstrates instead the extent to which the surgeon general's work on AIDS both arose from a specific moral perspective founded in post-1960s conservative Christianity and codified this sexual morality in national AIDS education.

Even Koop complained that the press misrepresented his position on sex education when it focused on his promotion of condom use. "Often I would spend several minutes of a speech extolling abstinence and monogamy (for social and moral reasons as well as health reasons)" Koop explained: "And then at the end I would say that those foolish enough not to practice abstinence or mutually faithful monogamy should, for their protection and their partner's protection, use a latex condom." "Usually the press would repeat only the last phrase," Koop recalled: "That annoyed me."[70] Reading Koop's message on AIDS against the rhetoric of the political and religious right, one can understand how the impression arises that his stance was sound and relatively objective medical advice, unmarked by moralism. But our interpretive options are not so limited. The Far Right did produce moral and even moralistic rhetoric about AIDS, but so did

Koop. In fact, so did AIDS activists and public health workers. It would be inaccurate to hold that emphasizing condoms and sex education is in itself not, or at least could not be, a moral endeavor. That is, it would be an interpretive and historical mistake to associate morality only with conservative religious positions, thereby opposing it to an assumed secular liberal position unmarked by normative assumptions and ethical projects of its own. Morality, religion, and secular liberalism are far more complicated, especially in regard to sexuality.[71]

In order to ascertain the moral tenor of Koop's AIDS message, it helps to read his work not only against activists on the Right such as Bennett and Bauer, but also alongside his public lectures on AIDS, including his efforts to reach out to churches and synagogues through these lectures. We should also read his sex education project against efforts already under way among gay and AIDS activists to promote alternative, "sex-positive approaches."[72]

Koop's Moral Appeal

During his time as surgeon general, Koop maintained that his faith informed his approach to public health. Yet he consistently distanced his specific positions on AIDS from his religious views, arguing that his position was not a moralistic one. There is little reason to believe Koop was not sincere about this point, even if he was mistaken in his self-assessment. Though he did not allow his religious beliefs to dominate his formation of an AIDS policy as his colleagues in the White House did, Koop nonetheless remained preoccupied with the question of sexual morality and with the role of churches and synagogues in the formulation of AIDS education. In fact, Koop's first printed interview on AIDS appeared not in a government publication or mainstream newspaper, or even in a publication that targeted the gay community, which was most at risk of infection and in need of information. Rather, it appeared in the leading evangelical magazine *Christianity Today* in November 1985.[73]

In the interview, Koop addressed basic questions about AIDS—what public fears were warranted, how contagious was it, and what would his role be in addressing the epidemic. He also responded to questions about whether AIDS was a homosexual disease (he said that it was not), whether he would address the moral aspects of HIV transmission, and what challenges Christians faced ministering to people with AIDS, given that they viewed the behavior associated with its transmission as sinful. In response to the latter two questions, Koop affirmed that his statement on AIDS was a public health position, but that "it is interpreted by people who don't like prohibition of a permissive sexual lifestyle as a moral statement." He maintained that, as a public health officer, "I'm not entitled to a moral opinion in a situation like his. But the public health opinion that I give happens to coincide with a moral position of a very large segment of the country." Koop compared the church's challenge to ministering to "AIDS victims" to the challenges faced in ministering to unmarried pregnant women. Though difficult, the church would have to develop the appropriate care and compassion to fulfill its mission.[74] Koop walked a thin line in this interview between moralist and public health officer. But the attempt to keep these two positions separate ultimately proved impracticable.

Early on, Koop witnessed the pernicious role that anti-gay crusaders like Paul Cameron played by calling for extreme measures in the face of the AIDS epidemic, including quarantine and mandatory testing for homosexuals. "I could see where these people were coming from," Koop recalled in his 1991 memoir, "but I could not agree with them." He continued:

> I strongly disapproved of the forms of behavior responsible for most AIDS transmission: promiscuity, homosexual behavior, sex outside of marriage, and drug use. My Christian faith forms the basis for my moral standards, and I knew that the practice of homosexuality was anathema to most Christians, who believe that it, along with much that we humans do, is sinful.[75]

Though Koop found sexual promiscuity and homosexual behavior morally troubling, he professed two central obligations that he possessed as a Christian and as physician: to save lives and to alleviate suffering. He also felt compelled to speak to the Christian community in particular. "Knowing what Christians believe," Koop explained, "I felt I was in a unique position to understand their point of view." He hoped that he could reason with members of the pro-life movement with whom he had worked in the past, "people who knew me and had supported my confirmation." Ultimately, Koop aspired to draw his religious supporters into his AIDS campaign:

> I saw a unique opportunity for these groups to join together to produce a morally based sex education program that would conform to their moral standards and also serve to protect a generation of

youngsters from AIDS. I hoped that we could work together after the release of the report to unite morality and science.[76]

Perhaps more than any surgeon general before him, Koop made a concerted effort to draw religious communities into the fold of public health programming.

Koop's first efforts could be seen through the groups he met with in formulating his 1986 report on AIDS. Unlike White House conservatives, he sought a broad array of opinions when he was conducting his research. At the press conference during which the report was released, as well as during his subsequent lectures, Koop made a point of mentioning the diverse organizations with which he consulted. They included the expected slew of medical and health organizations, but also gay rights groups such as the National Coalition of Black Lesbians and Gays and religious organizations like the United States Catholic Conference, the National Council of Churches, the Synagogue Council of America, and representatives from the Southern Baptist Convention.[77] Most of the groups applauded Koop's final report. Rabbi Henry Michelman of the Synagogue Council of America, for instance, thanked Koop for consulting with his organization and ensured him that they would do their best to work with the surgeon general in the future.[78]

Koop's meeting with representatives from the Southern Baptist Convention also proved beneficial. The surgeon general found them to be "delightful, but very naïve about AIDS. I think they were shocked by what we had to tell them, about how the virus was sexually transmitted." Koop realized they might be uncomfortable with his call for sex education, so he challenged them to write their own sex education program for the members of their denomination.[79] Larry Braidfoot, writing on behalf of the Christian Life Commission of the Southern Baptist Convention, applauded Koop's commitment to authoring a "candid, factual report." He assured Koop that his organization would continue to inform their constituency about AIDS and "strive to contextualize the problem within our Christian tradition's emphasis on monogamy, sexual fidelity, drug-free living, and resistance to promiscuous life-styles."[80] Far from the vicious rhetoric flung by Bennett, Bauer, and others on the Far Right, Braidfoot's cooperation illustrated a more measured, but no less moral, evangelical response, one that better represented the official statements of most evangelical denominations regarding AIDS in the mid-1980s, including the National Association of Evangelicals.[81]

Koop's meeting with members of the Christian Life Commission suggested an opening for the surgeon general to make headway among evangelical Christians who were receptive to hearing him out, even if they did
not agree with his positions. Chuck McIlhenny, pastor of First Orthodox
Presbyterian Church in San Francisco, for instance, wrote to Koop to support his fight against the AIDS crisis and "to encourage your stand against
promiscuity." But McIlhenny pressed Koop on his "conspicuous silence as
a Christian" in regard to the condom debate. While he agreed in part with
the surgeon general's stance on condoms, he implored Koop to consider
what he leaves out of his message about AIDS:

> It seems to me that your main message against AIDS is the mes-
> sage of Christ and his saving power not just as a personal belief but
> as the public answer to AIDS. I recognize your official public health
> position in the government and that your concerns are not limited
> to the Christian community but I find it difficult to understand how
> you can be so silent when you know what other people need to hear:
> repentance from sin and change in their moral life through Christ.

McIlhenny pushed Koop to take his private Christian views into the public
sphere. The surgeon general had already espoused "the whole gospel of
safe sex through condom education," but now it was time to share the
gospel of Jesus Christ. "Which gospel will you identify with in public
office?" he asked.[82]

Koop responded by thanking McIlhenny and sharing a copy his 1986
report, directing the pastor toward the list of further reading about the
epidemic. He concluded his letter by citing their different vocations: "We
Christians have a responsibility to show biblical love and compassion to
the victims of this terrible disease, and to teach those within our sphere of
influence concerning its causes, its prevention and its consequence."[83]
Such encounters opened Koop's eyes to the need for education about the
AIDS crisis among America's religious communities. It was also an opportunity to shore up his political and religious quarrels with former supporters. Following the release of the 1986 *Surgeon General's Report on
AIDS*, Koop would embark on a lecture circuit among religious groups to
share his message, one that increasingly blurred the lines between the
gospel of condoms and the gospel of Jesus, as the surgeon general's
sphere of influence came to encompass that of the itinerant public health
preacher.

Koop's Parable for Wise and Foolhardy Virgins

Koop's first stop was Liberty University, where he was invited to speak by his friend Jerry Falwell, founder of the Moral Majority, on January 18, 1987. Despite Falwell's fulminations against homosexuals, and his infamous declaration that AIDS was a punishment from God, Koop recalled his friend as "one of the most understanding and far sighted members of the religious community in reference to AIDS."[84] Koop presented his lecture to an audience of students at Liberty, and it was also broadcast live on southern television networks.

In the lecture, Koop described the details of homosexual sex that he thought necessary to understand the history and transmission of AIDS, a point he made explicit for an audience he assumed to be naïve about such details. He then stressed two messages. First, monogamy. "My advocacy of monogamy may sound like a morality lesson," the surgeon general explained, "but it also happens to be good science. In containing the epidemic of AIDS, science and morality advance hand-in-hand toward the same goal." Koop's second message was for people who did not yet have a partner, and his advice to them was caution. He called "fool-hardy" all those people "who will not be abstinent or will not achieve a faithful monogamous relationship and, therefore, will expose themselves and others to the AIDS virus." His reluctant advice to such foolhardy people was the following: "Don't have sex with someone who could carry the virus of AIDS [. . .] a person who, for example, practices high-risk behavior. That includes homosexuals, intravenous drug users, prostitutes and other persons who have many different sex partners." Finally, Koop continued, if you do have sex with such a person, "a decision that could have serious health consequences—then, if you're a man, at least use a condom from start to finish. If you're a woman, make sure your partner uses a condom."[85]

Here Koop favored abstinence and monogamy, not simply as scientific measures to prevent the spread of AIDS, but as moral lessons—anything else was "fool-hardy." Koop advanced this opinion among secular organizations as well. Speaking to the Annual Meeting of the National School Boards, he stated, "I believe children should be taught to be abstinent until they grow up, assume the role of a responsible adult, and find a mutually monogamous relationship. That doesn't seem to be too far-fetched. In fact, it was considered the norm for this country and a return to such a norm would insure the end of sexually transmitted AIDS."[86] In this instance, Koop referenced America's ostensibly moral past, before the sexual revolution of the 1960s and 1970s eroded what used to be the norm—good kids who remained abstinent until happily married. Koop's vision of this moral past was shortsighted. If Alfred Kinsey's infamous reports on human sexuality were not convincing enough, historians have amply demonstrated that this notion of an idyllic, moral America is more fantasy than reality. By nearly all demographic measures, "including divorce rates, age at marriage, and number of children per family," writes Robert Self, "the 1950s and 1960s stand out as historical exceptions to longer trends."[87] Koop's vision of this moral past may have proven more aspirational than factual, but its rhetorical power persisted.

The surgeon general further illustrated his fidelity to conservative morality in an address to the National Religious Broadcasters, an association representing over 650 evangelical Christian radio and television broadcasters.[88] He stressed the importance of "good values," which included developing children's sense of personal responsibility and strengthening the concept of the family.[89] Koop also countered accusations that he advocated a form of sex education lacking moral prescription: "I've been attacking sex education curricula that just teach technique and don't mention responsibility and morality." "And I took that position," he continued, "before some of my critics knew there was such a thing as sex."[90] The surgeon general did not retreat from his position on safe sex, including condom use, but he qualified his support: "You will hear a lot about 'safe sex' and how this or that technique is a way of containing the AIDS epidemic. But the safest approach to sexuality for adults is to choose either abstinence or faithful monogamy."[91]

Drawing his speech to a close, Koop pleaded for more compassion for people with AIDS, but he made a telling distinction in the process. "A large number of truly innocent people are being infected by the AIDS virus and they are going to die," he explained. "Who are they? They are . . . the wives of bisexual men . . . they are the spouses of I.V. drug users . . . they're the wives and husbands of promiscuous spouses," he declaimed. But perhaps worst of all, "I'm afraid we must also count the babies born to I.V. drug users or otherwise infected mothers," Koop concluded: "They are the most innocent victims of all." Much has been written on the construction of innocent versus guilty victims of AIDS: gay men, drug users, and female sex workers have not fared well in this economy of blame and innocence, which Koop reproduced here. But he did not stop short of showing compassion for gay men as well, as he refused to sidestep the question of homosexuality. "[Y]ou can't avoid it, if you're going to discuss AIDS," he warned his religious audience. His advice for them was to "please remember that one of your fundamental teachings has been to 'separate the sin from the sinner.' You may hate the sin . . . but you are to love the sinner."[92]

Koop reaffirmed his commitment to sexual values when speaking before the Christian Life Commission of the Southern Baptist Convention in Charlotte, North Carolina, in March 1987. "The reason people have become so interested in my views on education," he remarked, "is that the issue goes to the heart of each person's own system of moral and ethical values . . . or lack thereof."[93] For evangelicals such as Koop, moral and ethical values were fixed in advance and detailed in the Bible, and one either had them or didn't. This assumption allowed him to construct both an argument for moral truth regarding sexuality as well as a distinction between those communities (or persons) that possessed these moral and ethical values and those that did not. He began his lecture, for instance, by reminding his audience of their previous efforts in teaming up for moral causes, including the Baby Doe case and the fight against pornography. "I would have to say that nothing is a more powerful weapon against this disgusting material," Koop argued, "than the honest truth about human sexuality." For the surgeon general, true sex was moral—loving, benign, and non-commercial. This understanding of sex could only lead to contempt for pornography. He linked this point to his education campaign: "I believe that a child who is given the facts about his or her own sexuality— in a matter-of-fact yet caring manner—is a child who will feel more secure as an evolving adult and will have only contempt for pornography." The same logic held for AIDS, a problem more pressing as the geography of contagion shifted. "It is no longer primarily a disease attacking the homosexual communities of San Francisco, Los Angeles, and New York City," Koop explained: "It is now appearing in all 50 states and among heterosexuals. And that means the rest of us."[94] By invoking "the rest of us," Koop marked his Southern Baptist audience apart from northern and western urban dwelling homosexuals, an assumption that marked as well the implausibility that his Christian audience could be among *them*.

The Morality of Public Health

I underscore these speeches for three reasons. First, they illustrate the extent to which Koop reached out to religious organizations, including politically and theologically conservative groups known for their opposition to homosexuality. Koop himself noted how unusual it was for a surgeon general to take seriously the involvement of religious groups, but he did not shy away from challenging religious conservatives to discuss homosexuality, sex education, and AIDS. Perhaps more revealing, however, was that Koop focused his educational efforts on religious (and mostly white evangelical) groups rather than gay and lesbian communities, racial minorities, or drug users. Apart from his initial meetings with representatives from the National Coalition of Black Lesbians and Gays, Koop's archive suggests little contact with gay and lesbian community representatives, despite the disproportionate toll AIDS took on this population, and despite the well-established network of AIDS service organizations that had developed, often within the gay and lesbian community itself, by the mid-1980s.[95] The surgeon general's efforts to save America from AIDS led him not to those populations most at risk, but to those most likely to renew the moral fabric of the nation. Koop made this point most clearly when he spoke not to Christians, but to Jews.

Addressing the 59th General Assembly of the Union of the American Hebrew Congregations, the surgeon general argued that AIDS was not like other diseases.[96] This one would not be overcome by scientific research and clinical practice alone, he stated: "The final victory over the disease of AIDS will much more likely spring from the impelling force of compassionately committed, ethically motivated, and courageously reverent men and women with little or no medical background at all." Koop situated the AIDS epidemic in a specific moral context. "People get AIDS" he explained, "because they do things they ought not do." If his audience did not know who "they" were, he clarified:

> As I'm sure you know by now, the majority of the victims of AIDS—
> about 66% of them—have been homosexuals or bisexual males.
> For several terribly tragic years a great number of them engaged in
> certain harmful sexual practices with many anonymous partners.
> The worst of these practices, from a medical point of view, is anal
> intercourse, also known as sodomy.[97]

"For health and medical reasons," he noted, "they ought not to have done that." Yet it had become clear that most Americans, Koop assured his audience, "are rendering the same verdict for clearly social and moral reasons: 'Those men did something they ought not to have done. And so they got AIDS.'"[98]

Koop did not target sodomy alone. He also emphasized the need to recognize drug users at risk for infection alongside the growing prominence of AIDS among blacks and Hispanics. He then conflated drug use, race, and improper behavior: "In other words, 90 percent of the people who have the disease of AIDS contracted it because they did things that most people believe ought not be done: they either recklessly engaged in sodomy or they swapped dirty needles while 'shooting' dangerous drugs."[99] Koop's speech provides an unusual entrance to the religious and cultural politics of the 1980s, a period that witnessed a further relaxing of denominational divisions as new "others" came to the fore. Speaking as a Christian (he calls himself a "gentile" at one point) to an audience of Reform Jews, Koop positioned Jews and Christians in a common struggle—a moral battle—against the sinful behaviors of homosexuals, drug addicts, and (one is left to infer) blacks and Hispanics.[100] The rhetoric of the speech re-enacts the racial and religious realignments that occurred following the Second World War, through which Jews were incorporated as both religious and ethnic minorities into the fabric of a nation founded on "Judeo-Christian" principles.[101] "But," Koop concluded, "the question I must ask is this: 'Would we nevertheless work for and plead for their lives? If we had the opportunity, would we have a dialogue with the Lord to save them all, as Abraham did for the inhabitants of Sodom?'"[102] Salvation from AIDS lay in the hands of religious communities.

My second point is that Koop's language requires a more complicated reading of his position on sex education, including his own contention that his approach was that of a public health officer, not a moralist. The line between the two, already permeable in his AIDS report, blurred in his speeches—as promiscuous students and adults became "fool-hardy," as personal responsibility and family values became the cornerstone of sex education, and as morality and medicine bent toward one another to justify this approach. If Koop differed from other conservative Christians, it was less on the question of *when* to have sex or *how* to do it, than that of *who* would continue, pragmatically speaking, to have sex with whom. Since some men were not likely to stop having sex with other men, Koop maintained, he had to address them. Unlike Bennett and Bauer, the surgeon general stopped short of denouncing "homosexuality" through the language of public health, restricting his moralizing against homosexuality to his lectures to more conservative, often-religious audiences. As a Christian, he maintained the sinfulness of homosexuality, but as the nation's public health leader, he saw the need to resist stigmatizing gays and lesbians. Koop departed from his conservative contemporaries in at least three other ways as well: in his call for a state-sponsored public education program, in his support for comprehensive sex education in public schools, and in his insistence on the need to mention condoms as a last-ditch preventative measure. But these positions far from established Koop as an unbiased public health leader, not to mention the liberal activist—or gay agenda supporter—his critics accused him of being.

Rather, through his pamphlet and lectures, Koop joined Bauer and Bennett in preaching the gospel of abstinence and monogamy, which became not only the markers of safe sexuality, but also definitive of sex deemed moral and healthy—a claim backed by the imprint of the state and presented through the logic of public health. Through Koop's mass mailing, the state called upon the American people to be compassionate toward the sick. In educating Americans, *Understanding AIDS* also imagined and reproduced the American mainstream as straight, caring, concerned, and moral: in a word, normal. Most Americans could see themselves reflected in the pamphlet's photos, leading happy lives free from disease. So long as they had monogamous sex, or no sex at all, the pamphlet told them, they would be safe. If they ignored such warnings and still had sex, they were instructed to use a condom during every sexual encounter "from start to finish."[103] While well meaning, these instructions no doubt left some readers to wonder—when is it that sex starts and did lesbians need to heed such advice? Koop used similar language in his speeches following the release of his first report, though he often directed his instructions to men, stating, "if you're a man, at least use a condom from start to finish." We see here one of the difficulties that arises when translating from particular speech, intended for a religious audience presumed to be heterosexual, to the general speech intended for the broader American population. While the language of the pamphlet struggles to be inclusive, it betrays the normative understanding of sex that Koop and other members of the PHO held.

Moreover, heterosexuality did not need not be specified, as Bauer and Bennett wanted, because it was already presumed in the flier's visual presentation. This point would have been abundantly clear to gay men looking for representations of themselves in the pamphlet: they were notably absent, despite composing the largest number of AIDS cases to date and remaining one of the populations most at risk of infection. Paula Treichler quips that "gay men looked for themselves in vain among the target groups pictured in the mailer's photos and had to settle for the construction worker whose hard hat might—in a stretch—be seen as an effort at gay iconography."[104] The mailing was never for them, as gays (and lesbians) were scripted outside of moral citizenship. If the moral message of *Understanding AIDS* remained implicit, Koop's lectures clarified his position—and by extension, the position of the government's public health program.

Finally, the rhetoric of responsibility and morality was not limited to positions that advocated abstinence and monogamy, as Koop assumed, nor to the religious communities to which he reached out. In the first years of the epidemic, gay and lesbian AIDS activists debated issues of personal responsibility and the ethics of sex, including promiscuous sex. They developed what have since been called sex-positive approaches to curb the spread of AIDS—approaches that have succeeded in lowering rates of infection in gay communities.[105] In San Francisco, for instance, the Sisters of Perpetual Indulgence, a performance-based queer protest group drawing upon religious camp and gender drag, produced a safe-sex brochure called *Play Fair!* A year later, AIDS activists Michael Callen and Richard Berkowitz authored another early safe sex pamphlet, "How to Have Sex in an Epidemic," which they handed out in New York City in 1983. Both of these pamphlets resisted the sexual moralism glimpsed in calls to limit sex partners or to stop having sex. But they also went a step further in articulating new moral approaches to sex. Take, for instance, Callen and Berkowitz's section on "Ethics and Responsibility." "Since we are a community," they wrote, "taking responsibility for our *own* health during sex ultimately requires that we protect our *partners'* health as well as our own."[106] Callen and Berkowitz called neither for monogamy nor for gay men to stop having sex, but for mutual care and widespread safer sex practices. Their discussion of safe sex included the use of condoms, but they also reflected on other types of sexual practices that gay men could engage in without exchanging bodily fluids.[107]

Douglas Crimp took these calls a step further. In "How to Have Promiscuity in an Epidemic," he criticized the sexual moralism and panic of those who called men to limit sexual practices, including leaders of the Christian Right and some gay and AIDS activists. Crimp espoused the political value of promiscuity itself. The stakes for queer activists like Crimp were clear: sexual moralism and medical panic should not curb the political and social gains made by gay activists since the 1960s. AIDS was not a wake-up call, as some gay leaders have since framed it, for gay men and lesbians to come of age, give up their promiscuity, and become responsible members of society.[108] Rather, as Crimp put it, "AIDS showed anyone willing to pay attention how genuinely ethical the invention of gay life had been," which included an ethics of responsibility that followed from queer sex itself.[109] Like Koop, and like Bauer and Bennett, these AIDS activists recognized the moral ramifications of sex and provided a moral prescription for sexual engagements they deemed healthful and responsible. Read against this call for a responsible safe sex program, Koop's strategy—which focused on abstinence, monogamy, personal responsibility, and the family—appears not simply "morally based," but also far more like the conservative Christian positions characteristic of the 1970s and 1980s than it has been given credit for.

In the end, Koop was not merely offering a "middle road" between the Christian Right and the AIDS activist, often gay, Left. And he was not just applying medical principles to a public health issue. He was also engaged in a project of moral reform: his target was the "sexual revolution" and his prescription a return to a golden age of sexual innocence. This was a project he shared with many evangelicals—indeed, with many Americans—despite his resistance to adopting fully and explicitly the Christian Right's moral rhetoric, including fulminations against homosexuality. My point here is not simply to criticize Koop's moral approach to sex education or the idea that any moral approach is undesirable, but rather to color in the overlooked moral presuppositions of the government's major public health spokesperson on AIDS. Far from neutral, Koop's approach placed AIDS education within a specific moral framework, one that would come to dominate public discussions not only of AIDS, but of sexuality more generally. It is a framework that has also fueled the rise of abstinence-only morality campaigns that have gained influence in the last three decades.[110]

Reflecting on Koop's tenure as surgeon general, an author for *Time Magazine* described the physical appearance of the pediatric surgeon-turned-national AIDS educator as making him look like "Moses come down from Mount Sinai to deliver commandments eleven through twenty." Koop's likeness to the biblical prophet went beyond mere visual appearance, as the article continued: "Smoking? It's an addiction that will kill you. Sex? Only in marriage. AIDS? The best preventative device is a monogamous relationship; the second best, a condom."[111] One of Koop's greatest accomplishments was not to spare medicine and public health of moral politics, but instead to translate public health into no less than a religious and moral commandment itself.

Chapter Three

Ecclesiastical Authority

AIDS, SEXUALITY, AND THE AMERICAN CATHOLIC CHURCH

"Sometimes I believe the greatest damage done to persons with AIDS is done by the dishonesty of those health-care professionals who refuse to confront the moral dimensions of sexual aberrations or drug abuse."
—CARDINAL JOHN J. O'CONNOR, "Who Will Treat the Victims of AIDS?"

"Sexual techniques and sexual morals are closely related."
—MARCEL MAUSS, "Techniques of the Body"

IN THE WINTER of 1985, *New York Magazine* asked feminist writer Gloria Steinem to name the worst things about New York City. She offered two. Cardinal O'Connor made her list "because his experience as a military chaplain is turning New York into an armed camp, men against women, anti-abortionists against pro-choice." The other worst thing she mentioned was AIDS—"because it is a human tragedy that is made even worse by human bias."[1]

Steinem's comment proved prescient. Installed as the Archbishop of New York the previous year, O'Connor irritated many of New York's liberal politicos from the start. Few were surprised that a Roman Catholic bishop denounced abortion.[2] But O'Connor went further. Along with a growing number of Catholics, he elevated abortion to one of the central moral issues—if not the most pressing topic—of the day. This conviction arose together with a new sense of confidence among the Catholic leadership in the second half of the twentieth century, a confidence that led the bishops to exercise greater authority in American public life. As the new archbishop soon discovered, his ecclesiastical authority could be used to support the local and national pro-life movement, part of a broader trend that sociologist of religion José Casanova has called "public Catholicism."

In *Public Religions in the Modern World*, Casanova distinguishes between the "social Catholicism" of the early twentieth century and the advent of "public Catholicism" by the 1980s. Social Catholicism emerged from the efforts of a small number of liberal bishops as part of the broader, and mostly Protestant, social gospel movement. These leaders focused on the concerns of Catholic working men and their families, including the many Irish and Italian faithful immigrating to America's bustling cities. Beyond the local, often "ethnic" parish, however, Catholic laity took little part in the movement. And most American bishops proved unenthusiastic in their support. It was not until after the Second World War that Catholics shifted from a predominantly ethnic mindset toward a national one. As sociologist Will Herberg has famously argued, American Catholics joined mainline Protestants and Jews to form the trifecta of "Protestant-Catholic-Jew," part of the Christian-Jewish heritage constitutive of the now dominant "American Way of Life." The election of the first Catholic President of the United States in 1960 affirmed Catholic acceptance at the national level and, along with the modernizing efforts of the Second Vatican Council, paved the way for the bishops to address American public life.[3]

Among the most important manifestations of this public Catholicism, argues Casanova, were the American bishops' progressive-leaning pastoral letters on nuclear warfare and economic justice. But it was their role at the forefront of the pro-life movement—especially following the 1973 Supreme Court case *Roe v. Wade*—that most defined the American Church's public role by the time O'Connor began his new post.[4] In the emerging culture wars, the bishops' alignment with cultural conservatives on the issue of abortion also energized many pro-life lay Catholics. But this hardline position on abortion muffled other long-standing moral concerns, such as world peace and economic justice. By the 1980s, the American bishops had found their voice in national politics, but it strained under the deepening split between liberal and conservative members within the Church and in American society more generally—especially, as Steinem observed, when it came to growing divisions between pro-life and pro-choice proponents.

What Steinem couldn't have known in 1985 was that O'Connor's penchant for controversy regarding abortion would soon merge with the other "worst" thing about New York: the AIDS crisis. The epidemic, and its historical ties to the gay community, prompted the American Church to extend its newfound public voice to issues of public health and sexual morality. O'Connor infuriated AIDS activists and members of the gay and lesbian community in the latter half of the decade when he spoke against the use of condoms as a preventative measure in the fight against HIV infection. But resentment had already been building. Earlier, the cardinal had publicly criticized political candidates who supported abortion rights and opposed citywide anti-discrimination measures aimed at securing civil rights for gays and lesbians. For many progressives, O'Connor represented all that was wrong with the Catholic Church, or at least the church hierarchy—its increasingly intransigent stance against abortion, birth control, and condoms; its opposition to homosexuality; and its insistence on promoting universal moral proclamations in American public life. As O'Connor preached Catholic morality from his pulpit at St. Patrick's Cathedral, gays, lesbians, and AIDS activists joined pro-choice feminists like Steinem in their frequent attacks on the political prelate and the church.

The tensions building in New York City rehearsed a local politics of Right versus Left, but they were not particular to Gotham. They reflected a series of overlapping struggles central to the history of the American nation itself: political battles that pitched religious conservatives against secular liberals, ongoing tensions between church and state, and long-standing brawls between Protestants and Catholics, in which the former have periodically deemed the latter unfit for American democracy. This chapter turns to O'Connor and the Archdiocese of New York to demonstrate how the American Catholic Church became involved in political debates concerning AIDS programming and education in the 1980s. O'Connor proved a central figure in this history for two reasons. First, he began his post in New York in 1984—at a high point for AIDS hysteria—thus placing him at the center of the epidemic and at the helm of arguably the most important archdiocese in the United States. Second, O'Connor represented a developing movement within the American Church hierarchy that took hardline conservative stances on issues of sexuality and the family and readily asserted the church's influence in local and national politics. Under his leadership, the American bishops addressed the epidemic as a concern for all Americans, not just Catholics. By defining the epidemic in terms of sexuality, the American bishops re-inscribed AIDS as a social epidemic, but more importantly as a national moral crisis.

Outside the church hierarchy, numerous Catholic sisters, priests, hospital care workers, theologians, and lay Catholics also responded to the epidemic by providing spiritual and medical care. While many operated with the positions of the church hierarchy in mind, a great number found ways to work within and against official church teachings, secretly or openly, as they came to terms with the AIDS epidemic on the ground.[5] Still, we cannot lose sight of the force that the hierarchy exerted. The American bishops spoke with great rhetorical and material authority, especially in regard to education and health policies. Their response to the AIDS crisis in the 1980s demonstrates the reach as well as the limitations of this ecclesiastical authority, both within the American Catholic Church and in local and national politics.

Awash in a Sea of Controversy: Public Catholicism in New York City

By his own account, O'Connor's appointment to one of the most powerful positions in the Catholic Church was quite unexpected. Ordained in 1945, he served as a Navy chaplain during the Korean and Vietnam wars. In 1972, he became the first Catholic appointed senior chaplain at the United States Naval Academy in Annapolis, Maryland, and rose to the position of Navy Chief of Chaplains based in Washington, D.C., three years later.[6] In 1979, Pope John Paul II advanced O'Connor to auxiliary bishop of the Church's Military Ordinariate, now called the Archdiocese of the Military Services. This position placed O'Connor under his mentor and friend Cardinal Terence Cooke and made him responsible for all Catholic members of the armed forces. The Vatican promoted O'Connor once again in 1983, when he became the Bishop of Scranton, Pennsylvania. He had held this post only eight months when the Holy See tapped him to succeed Cooke as the Archbishop of New York City—or as Pope John Paul II called it, "the Capital of the World."[7]

When Archbishop Pio Laghi, the apostolic delegate to the United States, first delivered the news, O'Connor noted, "I thought it was a joke."[8] Moving to New York involved a number of new responsibilities, and the prelate worried about his own lack of experience.[9] With about 360,000 Catholics in the metropolitan area, the Scranton diocese paled in comparison to New York, the fourth largest diocese in the nation with about 1,839,000 faithful.[10] O'Connor would oversee three hundred Catholic elementary and secondary schools, eleven colleges and universities, and an

estimable health care system that included eighteen hospitals, two nurs-
ing schools, fifteen homes for children, and eleven homes for elderly and
disabled patients.[11] In the month leading up to his installment in March
1984, O'Connor foreshadowed what his tenure in New York might be like.
"I think every bishop has a responsibility to evaluate every political issue
from a moral perspective. [. . .] If there are moral implications, he must
address them," O'Connor explained: "Sometimes, however, you express a
moral position best by silence."[12] As it turned out, the new archbishop
would be remembered for many things, but his moral silence would not
be one of them.

Soon after moving to New York, O'Connor took on key battles against
local gay activists by opposing anti-discrimination laws intended to protect sexual orientation. These political battles between the archbishop and
New York's gay and lesbian community inevitably shaped the religious
politics of AIDS, as we will soon see. Perhaps more than any other issue,
though, abortion brought Catholic Church leaders and laity alike into the
arena of American politics. O'Connor's religious and political stance
against abortion defined the tenor of public Catholicism in the 1980s and
set the stage for later fights with gay and lesbian and AIDS activists.

During a news conference on June 24, leading up to the November
1984 presidential election, O'Connor stated, "I don't see how a Catholic
in good conscience can vote for a candidate who explicitly supports abortion."[13] Repeated in the press, this line hit a nerve among a number of
New Yorkers, including Governor Mario Cuomo, who interpreted
O'Connor's comment as a plea for fellow Catholics in New York to vote
against Democrats who supported a woman's constitutional right to have
an abortion.[14] Bishop James Malone, president of the United States Catholic Conference (USCC), issued a statement on "Religion and Politics"
that appeared to confirm not only the governor's suspicions of political
partisanship, but also fears that the church was singling out abortion as
a key issue ahead of the 1984 election. Malone affirmed that while the
USCC published opinions on public policy issues based on Catholic
moral teaching, "it does not take positions for or against political candidates." He encouraged Catholics to take part in public debate and to bring
their faith into those discussions, noting that, on a number of issues,
much room existed for "sincere disagreement." But room for disagreement did not extend to the matter of abortion. "[W]ith regard to the immorality of the direct taking of innocent human life (e.g., by abortion or by
direct attacks on non-combatants in war)," the bishop declared, "our views

are not simply policy statements of a particular Catholic organization, the U.S. Catholic Conference." Echoing O'Connor, he continued: "We reject the idea that candidates satisfy the requirements of rational analysis in saying their personal views should not influence their policy decisions; the implied dichotomy—between personal morality and public policy—is simply not logically tenable in any adequate view of both."[15]

The political mood worsened that September, when O'Connor responded to remarks by Democratic vice presidential candidate Geraldine Ferraro, who served New York's 9th District in the House of Representatives. She raised eyebrows upon referring to the Catholic position on abortion as "not monolithic," pointing to the variety of opinions that existed on this topic, even among Catholics. O'Connor brought up the topic at a convention sponsored by the Pennsylvania Pro-Life Commission. He explained, "Geraldine Ferraro has said some things about abortion relevant to Catholic teachings which are not true." According to the archbishop, Ferraro "may be intensely sincere on everything she's doing. I can't judge that. As an officially appointed teacher of the Catholic Church, all I can judge is that what has been said is wrong—it's wrong." Ferraro made it seem as though Catholics had grounds to disagree over Catholic teaching with regards to abortion. O'Connor corrected her. "There is no variance," he clarified: "there is no flexibility."[16]

Governor Cuomo could not have disagreed more with the archbishop. His rebuttal came later that month in a speech delivered at the University of Notre Dame that the *New York Times* lauded as "one of the most anticipated exercises in theology ever presented by a member of the laity."[17] "The Catholic Church has come of age in America," Cuomo announced to the audience of one of the country's most revered Catholic institutions: "The ghetto walls are gone, our religion no longer a badge of irredeemable foreignness." Cuomo rehearsed the history of anti-Catholic discrimination in America. Once found threatening to American democracy, Catholic Americans now blended into the fold, accepted as equals in the American melting pot of white, European ethnicities and Judeo-Christian religions. "This new-found status," he asserted, "is both an opportunity and a temptation."[18] The temptation was that the bishops would overreach in their exertion of moral influence. Issues like abortion raised important questions about "public morality" not just for Catholics, but for all Americans. While Cuomo confirmed his private opposition to abortion, as governor he recognized that not all Americans held this position. And further, he respected their right to hold this contrary view. "[T]hose who endorse legalized abortions [. . .] aren't a ruthless, callous alliance of anti-Christians determined to overthrow our moral standards," he explained:

> In many cases the proponents of legal abortion are the very people who have worked with Catholics to realize the goals of social justice set out in papal encyclicals: the American Lutheran Church, the Central Conference of American Rabbis, the Presbyterian Church in the United States, B'nai B'rith Women, the Women of the Episcopal Church.[19]

The question was then: how would the Catholic Church respond to this context of pluralism?

In the past, Cuomo explained, the church's moral principles were not uncompromising. The church accepted "that in our pluralistic society we are not required to insist that all our religious values be the law of the land." Yet abortion was treated otherwise, Cuomo charged—in a way that did not fit into the historical precedent the church had set.[20] Previously, the Catholic Church had followed a central rule of thumb: the translation of morality into politics was not a "matter of doctrine," but rather "a matter of prudential political judgment."[21] It privileged pragmatism over dogma. Cuomo offered the example of the bishops' position regarding slavery before the Civil War. While individual bishops denounced slavery, the church fell short of formal opposition. This silence was not a moral failure, the governor insisted; it was a pragmatic decision not to prevent marginalizing Catholics who already occupied a compromised political position amid rabid anti-Catholic sentiment. "Church teaching on slavery and abortion is clear," he proceeded: "But in the application of those teachings—the exact way we translate them into action, the specific laws we propose, the exact legal sanctions we seek—there was and is no one, clear, absolute route that the Church says, as a matter of doctrine, we must follow." Cuomo insisted that he was not calling for "religious quietism." He instead implored the church to take up Cardinal Joseph Bernardin's "seamless garment" argument, in which the great number of issues affecting human life, including poverty, disease, and warfare, would not take a backseat to the single issue of abortion.[22]

While Cuomo's speech resonated with many lay Catholics—and non-Catholics—he did not convince the archbishop of New York. "I will never believe for one minute that there is free choice on the issue of human life," O'Connor responded during a televised newscast.[23] He did not consider his position out of line with Catholic thought in any way, historically or otherwise. In his public lectures, the cardinal denied singling out abortion and upheld the importance of all matters of life. He even applauded Bernardin's "consistent ethic of life," though he worried that the argument had been misinterpreted to imply that all life issues ought to be weighed equally.[24] For O'Connor, this simply wasn't the case. "There is danger in the seamless garment," he claimed during an interview that followed the 1983 release of the American bishops' statement on nuclear war: "The danger is in losing the focus. We are all concerned about nuclear war, but it is a potential slaughter. Abortion is the slaughter that is taking place all around us."[25] O'Connor may have supported all life issues in theory, but he maintained his priorities in politics.

The debate between Cuomo and O'Connor reflected key moral and political disagreements brewing in the city and suggested growing division even within the Catholic hierarchy. By referencing Bernardin's consistent ethic, Cuomo played up one of the central fault lines emerging in the Catholic hierarchy between moderate bishops and their politically conservative opponents. By the 1980s, a new push for theological orthodoxy was under way, largely as a reaction to the reforms made during the Second Vatican Council.[26] A growing number of American bishops, including O'Connor, Cardinal Bernard Law of Boston, and Cardinal John Krol of Philadelphia, underlined abortion and sexual immorality as the major issues facing the church. Moderate bishops like Bernardin, on the other hand, insisted that the church keep sight of a broader range of problems, including global poverty and the need for nuclear deterrence, rather than prioritize abortion or sexual morality over other issues.

This political bifurcation within the Catholic Church coincided with two other historical shifts. First, the American political system witnessed a significant rearrangement when Reagan's election in 1980 ushered religious conservatives into the Republican Party, in large measure by appealing to evangelical and Catholic opposition to abortion. Second, shoring up this alignment of pro-life politics with the Republican Party pushed some church leaders into political debate, such as when they began to speak against pro-life Democrats. It accompanied and even fueled a broader transformation in how the American bishops engaged with public policy—one that marked the emergence of "public Catholicism" in the 1970s and 1980s.[27]

While the Catholic leadership gained confidence speaking in the American public sphere in the second half of the twentieth century, their speech has been marked by "two radically different forms of moral discourse." José Casanova demonstrates this split by comparing two kinds of religious participation in the public sphere. The bishops' pastoral letters on nuclear warfare and economic justice—*The Challenge of Peace: God's Promise and Our Response* (1983) and *Economic Justice for All: Catholic Social Teaching and the U.S. Economy* (1986)—evinced one style of participation, while their role in the fight against abortion displayed another.[28] Casanova discerns three inconsistencies that arise between these two forms of speech. He calls them *semantic, performative,* and *procedural* differences.[29]

First, semantic inconsistency. The bishops would not entertain the possibility of moral ambiguity on the question of abortion, a point reflected in the USCC position mentioned above. Casanova contrasts this refusal with discussions of the Catholic tradition of just war, in which killing could be justified under some conditions. Why was it, he asks, that the church was willing to accept a just war but not something like a "just abortion?"[30] Casanova next points to performative inconsistencies. The bishops intended their pastoral letters on the economy and nuclear warfare to provide policy recommendations and to foster public deliberation. But with regard to abortion, "the church seeks to translate immediately its normative recommendations into law."[31] In addition, while the bishops played a key role in organizing the right to life movement and mobilizing Catholics to fight against abortion, they did not demonstrate similar efforts to mobilize the Catholic laity in response to other social concerns, such as the peace movement, nuclear deterrence, or economic justice. Finally, there were procedural inconsistencies. The bishops formulated their moral arguments in the pastoral letters differently than those in their statements on abortion. The letters constructed moral discourse inductively, paying attention to "the signs of the times." In drafting their letters, the bishops referred both to Catholic tradition and to authorities outside the church, thereby displaying their willingness to open moral discourse to public discussion. But with abortion, Casanova asserts, the church made no appeal to social context, such as the changing role of women in society or advances in medical research and technology. Neither did the bishops demonstrate an openness to consult women or to consider the issue from their perspective.[32]

Historically, Catholic leaders have proved more evenly "progressive" on economic and foreign policy issues than the American population at large, including lay Catholics, but more resoundingly "conservative" in regard to issues of sexual morality and the family.[33] Situated within this context, then, is the further tension between conservative bishops, such as O'Connor, and more moderate leaders like Bernardin. Often the distinction between their positions has had less to do with strict theological teachings about sexual morality or abortion—about which most agreed—than with the emphasis they placed upon these issues within their dioceses, the degree to which they engaged political issues, and the different modes of rhetoric they employed in making their arguments.

O'Connor's impulse to jump headfirst into controversial political issues could be seen in his statement that Catholics of good conscience ought not vote for pro-choice candidates and in his subsequent scuffles with Ferraro and Cuomo. Certainly, the archbishop's anti-abortion campaign partly explains why one *New York Times* reporter labeled him "the most visible and outspoken Roman Catholic Bishop in the nation."[34] To translate this into Casanova's terms, O'Connor proved one of the most active bishops in the new "public Catholicism."

The Cardinal, the Church, and the Battle over Gay Rights

If O'Connor's views on abortion frustrated many of the city's pro-choice activists and Democrats, his outspoken opposition to gay rights cast the archbishop as downright bigoted in the eyes of many more New Yorkers, especially members of the city's gay and lesbian population. As with abortion, the trouble was not so much with the archbishop's specific views about homosexuality, which followed Catholic teachings that most New Yorkers would respect, if begrudgingly, on the grounds of religious freedom. But unlike his predecessor Cardinal Cooke, who worked behind the scenes to fight abortion and gay rights, the newcomer from Scranton placed himself, and by extension the Archdiocese of New York, at the forefront of battles against the city's gay rights measures. The church's take on homosexuality was not the only factor that influenced how O'Connor and other Catholics approached the emerging AIDS epidemic, but it demonstrates how the bishops, the gay community, and the press wedded these issues together. Broader issues of sexual morality shaped not only the church's response to AIDS education, but also the significant (and sometimes anti-Catholic) backlash from AIDS activists and the mainstream press.

Civil rights protections had become a key issue for gays and lesbians since the 1970s, when the fight for gay rights accelerated in the political sphere.[35] On April 25, 1980, a few years before O'Connor arrived in New

York, Democratic Mayor Edward Koch issued Executive Order 50, which prevented organizations from entering into contracts with the city unless they agreed not to discriminate on the basis of sexual orientation in their hiring practices. The order risked impacting some of the city's religious organizations, such as the Salvation Army and Catholic Charities, which had long held contracts with the city to provide health care and social services for New Yorkers who the city could not reach. Hundreds of millions of dollars in public money were at stake. The Archdiocese of New York alone held contracts with the city to provide social services, including childcare, that amounted to more than $60 million.[36]

The archdiocese made little issue of the new order under Cardinal Cooke. But O'Connor refused to comply with the new requirements. When the archdiocese's contracts came up for renewal, he challenged the order in New York's State Supreme Court. O'Connor claimed that the archdiocese had not discriminated against anyone on the basis of sexual *orientation*, which, he explained, the church did not consider sinful in itself. Rather, he refused to condone or hire *practicing* homosexuals. Koch's order overstepped the city's reach by interfering with church teaching, O'Connor contended, and provided "a classic illustration of the way in which the City can upset the Church-State balance by attempting to exercise excessive jurisdiction."[37] The archdiocese eventually won the case. State Supreme Court Judge Alvin F. Klein ruled on September 5, 1984 that Koch's order exceeded his powers as mayor because it required legal protection beyond anything already guaranteed by city or state legislation. The city challenged the ruling, but the Court of Appeals finally overturned Koch's order on June 28, 1985.[38] Activists would have to go through the City Council to pass anti-discrimination legislation.

O'Connor's fight against Executive Order 50 certainly didn't win the new archbishop any friends in the gay and lesbian community, but it was his vocal opposition to the anti-discrimination bill proposed in the City Council that irreparably damaged his standing with regard to gay and lesbian issues—and which drew renewed accusations that the Catholic Church was stepping over the line in political matters. Gay rights activists had been pushing such a bill for over a decade, but longtime Council Majority Leader Tom Cuite, a staunch opponent of gay rights, repeatedly prevented the bill from coming up for a vote in the General Welfare Committee. By 1986, Cuite had resigned, and the new Majority Leader Peter Vallone vowed to permit the bill to go to the floor.[39] When Koch introduced a new version of the gay rights bill to the City Council on January

23, 1986, supporters sensed a real chance for victory. The new bill prohibited discrimination based on sexual orientation in housing, employment, and public accommodation, adding sexual orientation to the existing protected categories of race, gender, creed, marital status, age, and national origin in the city's human rights laws.

Like its predecessors, the bill drew criticism from many of the city's religious organizations, including the Salvation Army, the ultra-Orthodox Jewish movement Agudath Israel, and the Archdiocese of New York. Gay rights leaders and other supporters of the bill anticipated religious opposition. Andrew Humm, spokesman for the Coalition for Lesbian and Gay Rights, declaimed from the steps of St. Patrick's Cathedral that Cardinal O'Connor was "step[ping] up efforts" to defeat the bill and waging "an all-out war."[40] Even before Koch introduced the bill, O'Connor had called upon Catholic officials "to join him in opposing any proposal which would seem to endorse lifestyles contrary to Church teaching, force employers to hire a quota of homosexuals, or require schools to include lessons on homosexuality in their curriculum."[41] Though the cardinal would not issue a formal statement for several weeks, the archdiocese warned New York's Catholics about the impending bill and all that it might entail.

Yet the bill enjoyed widespread support from key politicians, including Governor Cuomo, and other religious leaders. The Episcopal Bishop of New York, Rev. Paul Moore, Jr., joined Rabbi Balfour Brickner of the Stephen Wise Free Synagogue in supporting the anti-discrimination measure. "[T]here's been so much religious pressure on this issue," Moore stated during an interview, "not only from the Cardinal but from conservative Jewish leaders, that Rabbi Brickner and I thought it important to say we speak for many Christians and Jews who are for the bill."[42] Moore had also spoken against O'Connor's earlier opposition to Executive Order 50. Throughout the decade, he provided a liberal religious voice that countered the cardinal's stances on issues like homosexuality and abortion.

The *New York Times* also lauded the initiative. Responding to criticism of the bill, the newspaper of record ran an editorial asking whether the city's homosexuals "really need this added protection?"[43] "The regrettable answer," the *Times* responded, "is yes"—because too many members of the gay and lesbian community feared exposing their sexual identification, which could lead to lost housing or jobs. Critics of the bill, the editorial continued, mistook the "defense of homosexual rights" as "a declaration of support for homosexual ways of life." But, the *Times* noted, the bill explicitly denied support for any specific community or group and even included an exemption for religious groups under a long-standing agreement that allowed religious institutions to retain their own criteria in hiring practices.[44]

The Cardinal, the Times, *and the Anti-Religious Threat*

The *New York Times* editorial struck a nerve with O'Connor, who responded in the archdiocese's weekly magazine *Catholic New York*. His column "What Kind of Mischief Is This?" reflected the tensions building in the city between the archdiocese and the mainstream media, which he characterized as anti-religious, if not anti-Catholic. It also displayed the rhetorical strategies the prelate employed to build opposition to the bill. The problem, O'Connor stated, was "the way the editorial disposes of those who may possibly disagree with its judgment."[45] He protested that the *Times* "implie[d] with little subtlety that disagreement with the proposed bill is the result of 'bigotry' that 'is often hard to prove.'" "It is an ugly thing to call someone a bigot, isn't it?" O'Connor asked: "Ugly, but extremely effective." Moreover, figuring out who these "bigots" were proved confusing. The answer came in the editorial's final paragraph, he continued, "where we read that '. . . the proposed law yields much to religious scruples about homosexuality, notably those of some Catholic and Orthodox Jewish leaders.'" O'Connor took offence to this claim: "Is it paranoid to make the connection between 'bigotry' and 'some Catholic and Orthodox Jewish leaders?'" He suggested it was not.

O'Connor underscored the term "scruple," defined as "a *doubt* arising from difficulty in deciding what is right, proper, etc." This definition would make the editorial's statement false, he asserted, since the Orthodox Jewish leaders with whom he had spoken, like leaders in the Catholic Church, had no doubt whatsoever concerning the moral status of homosexuality. Another meaning of "scruple," he continued, could suggest that religious leaders worried unnecessarily about some trivial concern. This meaning left the cardinal asking whether the editorial meant that "anxiety over the proposed bill is foolish because the bill is unimportant, or concerns trivial matters? Is anxiety groundless, or even neurotic?" O'Connor concluded with another meaning that would imply that religious leaders "care 'scrupulously' about morality and society"—meaning with great care and attention.[46] O'Connor's article is significant for two reasons. His misreading of the editorial suggests his anxieties about the representation of

the Catholic Church in the *Times*. It also demonstrates the rhetorical arguments the cardinal made to express his opposition to the gay rights bill.

The *New York Times* editorial did not refer to those who opposed the
bill as bigots, as O'Connor contended. Rather, it targeted discrimination
against homosexuals in daily affairs that were not related (or which the
Times thought ought not be related) to their sexual status, such as housing, employment, and public accommodations. The paragraph reads:

> The bill would add "sexual orientation" to the categories of race,
> creed, gender, marital status, age and national origin already cov-
> ered by the city's human rights laws. It would make sexual habits
> legally irrelevant to many private as well as official transactions, af-
> fording at least some protection against a bigotry that is often hard
> to prove.[47]

The editorial employed the term "bigotry" here to describe acts of discrimination against homosexuals; it did not explicitly address the people who were
discriminating or the religious leaders referenced several paragraphs later.

O'Connor also appeared concerned about the editorial's statement that
the bill made exceptions for religious groups. "It would also be nice to
know what the editorial means by 'yielding much' to 'religious scruple,'"
O'Connor wrote: "Surely it can *not* mean merely what it says, namely, that
the bill 'incorporates the human right[s] law's long-standing religious exemptions.' How in the world can a bill 'yield' what is already law?"
O'Connor's confusion here is curious, but instructive. The previous week,
Catholic New York had printed nearly the exact line with which O'Connor
takes issue in its story about the bill. As it explained: "Sponsors of the bill
tried to address the objections of the Cardinal and others by citing language that would prohibit quota systems for homosexuals, exempt religious organizations and their agencies from the law and not permit sexual
activity with minors—which is already illegal."[48] True, some of the "yielding" might have been legally redundant, but the bill included such language precisely to appease O'Connor and others who feared it would
impose gay rights on the church.

The *New York Times* editorial finally backed the bill because of its moderate stance as a civil rights bill, rather than a political ploy:

> This is not a bill "validating" homosexuality, as some opponents
> fear and some homosexuals would prefer. It is a civil rights bill,

affirming protections that belong to all citizens and reinforcing the right of some not to have the revelation of their homosexuality devalue citizenship. New York has much to gain and nothing to fear from this bill's passage.[49]

Even the Catholic Church had spoken out against the very forms of discrimination the bill sought to eliminate. Given the actual text of the editorial, O'Connor's column perhaps did appear paranoid, as he suggested, but it also accomplished important work of its own. It provided readers of *Catholic New York* a subtle example of how the mainstream media discriminated against religion. It suggested, in other words, that the *Times* betrayed the presumed secular, liberal agenda against traditionalist religious leaders—leaders who it not only condemned, but also mocked by calling them "bigots." Whether or not this was true proved, in the end, beside the point.

Shortly after this column appeared, O'Connor joined Brooklyn's Bishop Francis Mugavero in a statement opposing the gay rights bill, citing "compelling moral and social reasons" for their intervention.[50] O'Connor and Mugavero affirmed their opposition to the harassment of homosexuals and "all arbitrary and invidious discrimination directed against" them. They further urged "proper respect for the rights of all persons." Still, they feared the bill exceeded these protections:

> We believe it is clear that what the bill primarily and ultimately seeks to achieve is the legal approval of homosexual conduct and activity, something that the Catholic Church, and indeed other religious faiths, consider to be morally wrong. Our concern in this regard is heightened by the realization that it is a common perception of the public that whatever is declared legal, by that very fact, becomes morally right.[51]

The bishops claimed the bill was unnecessary, since the rights of homosexuals "can be protected by legitimate application of existing laws"—a claim gays and lesbians living in New York who had been fighting for such protections eagerly disputed. The bishops also charged that the bill violated the rights of non-gay members of society. "In purporting merely to protect the rights of homosexuals," O'Connor and Mugavero explained, "the bill has the effect of violating the rights of nonhomosexuals." They reasoned that although the bill "appears" to impact only gays and lesbians, "in fact, it does have potential for grave harm to all society" and especially "for our children."[52] *Catholic New York* picked up on the claim that the bill would violate the rights of "nonhomosexuals," that is, "the rights of all for whom homosexual behavior is improper by making such behavior a protected, and therefore sanctioned, way of life." The editors issued a call to action: "Catholics and all others who consider such activity to be morally wrong," they declared, shared "an obligation to speak out against legislation such as this."[53]

The editors of *Catholic New York* took another swipe at the legislation a month later. They described the need "to review some of the key elements involved" in the gay rights bill in order "to separate fact from fiction."[54] The first fact they noted was that the bill's effects would go well beyond the suggestions of its proponents. Not merely protecting civil liberties, it would "grant recognition and approval to homosexual conduct and activity." The column also claimed that supporters of the bill misconstrued evidence in arguing for why the bill was necessary. The editors cited a report released by the Human Rights Commission of New York City, which reported some 474 complaints of violence and discrimination against homosexuals in the previous year. Most of those complaints concerned violence or *threats of violence*, which, the editorial contended, were two very different things—a distinction too quickly overlooked by the bill's supporters. Further, the editors pointed out that existing laws already addressed violence against anyone, thereby rendering this bill unnecessary.[55] One problem with the editors' point here was that the report they cited attempted to show that discrimination against homosexuals existed, which it clearly did. It was not arguing for laws prohibiting violence against homosexuals, which did already exist. The editorial conflated the two.

But if the reasoning of the editors' or the bishops' arguments was not always consistent, it nonetheless resonated with the newspaper's readers, demonstrating the reach of the rhetorical messages carried in *Catholic New York*. Kevin O'Reilly of the Bronx penned a letter to the editor that echoed the language employed in the paper's discussion of the gay rights bill. "The principal objection to the homosexual rights bill," he stated, "is that the bill, in effect, proclaims that is it a matter of moral and societal indifference in our community whether a person practices, advocates or promotes sexual deviancy." The problem with offering this class of people legal and social protection, he claimed, was that then "anyone who makes distinctions on that basis is the moral equivalent of a racist or religious bigot."[56] The bill, in other words, made good moral citizens out to be bigots. Once again, tradition was under attack.

The archdiocese redoubled its opposition as the City Council's vote drew closer. On March 11, Franciscan Brother Patrick Lochrane, who served on the board of directors of the Health and Hospitals Corp and as director of St. Barnabas Hospital in the Bronx, released a statement from the archdiocese. "We believe that the primary purpose of this bill is to achieve legal approval for homosexual and bisexual conduct and activity," he proclaimed, "something that is totally abhorrent to people of almost every religious persuasion."[57] The day before the vote, O'Connor spoke against the bill during the morning service homily at St. Patrick's. "Divine law cannot be changed by Federal law, state law, country law or city law," the cardinal insisted: "even by passage of legislation by the City Council."[58] O'Connor rebutted claims that the church's fight against the bill was an effort to impose Catholic morality on all New Yorkers. "The response to that is easy," he retorted: "Let not any legislature impose anyone else's morality on society or on the Catholic Church."[59]

O'Connor also distributed a statement against the bill to every parish in Manhattan, the Bronx, and Staten Island. He directed church officials to read it aloud or hand out copies during Mass. The statement reiterated the cardinal's arguments and exhorted Catholics to contact their City Council representatives to urge them to vote down the bill. But some members of the city's Catholic community resisted O'Connor's message. While the archdiocese pushed forward in condemning the legislation, a crowd of priests, nuns, lay people, and other activists from the Catholic Coalition for Gay Civil Rights and the Sisters in Gay Ministry gathered outside of St. Patrick's Cathedral. Among them was Father Robert Sinski, chaplain at Long Island College Hospital, who demanded that "other legitimate Catholic opinions be heard." Sister Jeannine Gramick from the National Coalition of American Nuns protested that O'Connor "has failed in his responsibility as a teacher" regarding the right to respect deserved by gays and lesbians.[60]

Despite opposition from O'Connor, the City Council approved the gay rights bill, which Mayor Koch signed into law on April 2, 1986. Amendments to the final bill clarified that homosexuality would not be taught in schools and that exemptions would remain in place for religious organizations—both were concessions to conservative opponents. *Catholic New York* nonetheless decried the bill's passage as "a defeat for common sense," and the archdiocese had begun seeking legal council to fight the bill even before the vote.[61] By the mid-1980s, O'Connor's vocal opposition to Executive Order 50 and the gay rights bill didn't merely mark him as a conservative Catholic leader. Many New Yorkers feared O'Connor's potential influence over millions of Catholic votes in the city, his clout with local politicians, his position as supervisor of eighteen Catholic hospitals, and his willingness to take such outspoken stands on key issues. This made the cardinal "one of the worst things about New York" not only for Gloria Steinem, but for the city's gay and lesbian community and their supporters as well. And it foreshadowed the political controversies the cardinal and his archdiocese would soon ignite with regard to AIDS.

AIDS and the Politics of Sex
in the Archdiocese of New York

In November of 1985, *Catholic New York* ran an article reflecting upon the Catholic Church's response to the AIDS crisis in New York City. It lauded the efforts of New York's Cardinal Terence Cooke to help break down the "shameful wall of official reticence" concerning AIDS in the early 1980s. At the time, a number of local and state politicians kept silent, refusing to acknowledge a disease associated with gay men and drug users. In 1983, Cooke opened one of the earliest conferences on AIDS in the city or anywhere for that matter. The conference was organized by Kevin Cahill, a senior member of the New York City Board of Health and director of the tropical disease center at Lenox Hill Hospital in Manhattan.[62] Cooke's invocation granted public legitimacy and respectability to the conference, which brought together medical and public health experts along with members of the health care community. His presence foreshadowed the major role the Archdiocese of New York would play in the epidemic in the ensuing decade, particularly under the leadership of Cooke's successor, Cardinal O'Connor.

"We don't damn anyone," O'Connor announced during the third annual Mass for Health Care Workers sponsored by St. Patrick's Cathedral on October 13, 1985. "When we learn someone is ill with the disease, our doors open," he insisted. The cardinal acknowledged the social stigmas attached to AIDS that had led some medical care workers to turn patients away.[63] Indeed, the numerous Catholic hospitals, hospices, and medical care centers within the Archdiocese of New York did open their doors to people with HIV and AIDS, and the archdiocese itself had already contributed $50,000 to St. Vincent's Hospital in Greenwich Village for research and care. Even more, the archdiocese had recently opened a shelter in Manhattan for people with AIDS and planned to work with Mother Teresa to open new hospices for children, the homeless, and prisoners living with the disease.[64]

One of the archdiocese's most significant contributions included a treatment facility at St. Clare's hospital in the Clinton neighborhood of Manhattan. The first specialized AIDS unit in New York, the Spellman Center, opened late in 1985 with twenty beds—it eventually expanded into the city's largest treatment center for people with AIDS and one of the largest in the United States.[65] Along with St. Clare's, New York's Catholic hospitals found themselves at the forefront of AIDS care, making O'Connor one of the city's most influential figures in fighting the epidemic. Even the White House took notice.

In the summer of 1987 President Reagan appointed O'Connor to his Presidential Commission on HIV. Proposed by Reagan's conservative aide Gary Bauer, the commission proved contentious from the start. Bauer envisioned the committee as a vehicle for conservatives in the White House to regain control over public policy regarding the AIDS crisis, especially in the context of his disagreements with the surgeon general. The president allowed Bauer to take the lead in choosing committee members, and he did so with an eye toward underlining the White House's policies of promoting "local control" and "responsible sexual behavior based on fidelity, commitment, and maturity, placing sexuality within the context of marriage."[66] From the start, Bauer prioritized candidates' conservative bona fides over their expertise in AIDS. To the chagrin of many AIDS activists, no one with HIV or AIDS was among the thirteen appointed to the commission, which also included only one openly gay person, geneticist Frank Lily—and he was appointed despite Bauer's opposition. Dr. Eugene Mayberry of the Mayo Clinic was selected to lead the commission, though he quickly departed (along with Dr. Woodrow Meyers) because he felt the commission was too ideologically compromised to accomplish its goals.

O'Connor's appointment was one of the many that sparked protest among AIDS and gay and lesbian activists. Over three hundred protestors gathered in New York to oppose his nomination. Gay rights activist Andrew Humm called the cardinal's appointment "an indication that the commission is not to be taken seriously."[67] O'Connor initially defended his appointment to the panel, citing the time he had spent visiting with patients with AIDS under the care of hospitals in the archdiocese. But as political troubles within the commission began to arise, he briefly considered abandoning his post. He worried that his responsibilities in New York, including his work with AIDS patients, would take up too much of his time, but he also feared the panel might be "simply heading in the wrong direction." In the end, O'Connor decided to remain on board.[68]

After Mayberry's departure, retired naval officer Admiral James Watkins took charge of the commission, which delivered its report in the summer of 1988.[69] To the surprise of many critics, the relatively moderate—if not progressive-leaning—report focused on the social conditions of poverty that led to drug use and to the spread of HIV into impoverished and minority communities. It called for substantial increases in government spending along with the need for a national and state-led approach to fight the epidemic. Underscoring the structural reasons for poverty and drug use, the statement avoided much of the victim-blaming that marred other representations of AIDS. But this focus also sidelined discussion of the most aversely affected group—gay men. The report downplayed issues of sexuality and sex education, thereby avoiding the political controversies then occurring in New York City—controversies in which O'Connor played a leading role.

New York City's Condom Debate

The autumn of 1986 witnessed a "storm over contraceptives," as the *New York Times* dubbed it. Members of the city's Board of Education learned that nine high school health clinics offered contraceptives to students.[70] The clinics arose less because of fears concerning AIDS than because of the escalating rate of teenage pregnancy, and they were strongly supported by Schools Chancellor Nathan Quiñones and Mayor Koch. The Board of Education was pushing to mandate a sex education program for the city's thirty-two school districts and unanimously approved one a short time later. But vocal opposition to the existing clinics and to the proposed education programs quickly arose, much of it from members of the Archdiocese of New York.

An editorial in *Catholic New York* called the plan "A Bad Mistake," as the archdiocese joined other religious groups opposing the board's decision, which it decribed as "valueless."[71] Auxiliary Bishop Edward Egan, the archdiocese's vicar for education, led vociferous opposition to the city's sex education curriculum, and indeed the city suspended the distribution of condoms in the wake of such public outcry. Egan argued at a meeting of the Priests' Council of the archdiocese that the Board's campaign "inculcate[s] a specific morality" with a "do exactly as you please way of thinking," a position which he equated with "a religion" (and later that spring re-termed "a new irreligion"). "If our religion is not allowed to be taught," he cried, "neither should this."[72] Egan joined John Woosley, the archdiocese's director of the Office of Christian and Family Development, in prompting priests to urge school boards in their individual districts to challenge the Board of Education's decision and to demand sex education programs that would promote abstinence until marriage.[73]

Under Egan's leadership, the archdiocese magnified its opposition over the course of that winter and spring. During a City Council meeting, Egan complained that the city's sex education program would teach children that promiscuity was fine—that is, so long as children prevented pregnancy with birth control or solved it through abortion, he quipped. "The new rule is [that] promiscuity is acceptable no matter what your age," he charged, "as long as you use drugs and devices to avoid pregnancy and as long as you are willing to kill what is in the mother."[74] The council was meeting to decided between two proposals, one to resume the distribution of contraceptives and another to end it altogether.

In addition to attacking school-based education campaigns, the archdiocese slammed the city's new television advertisement campaign to prevent the spread of HIV/AIDS through the promotion of condoms. The commercials shied away from presenting gay men, but depicted (ostensibly straight) adult women considering whether or not to have sex and the benefits of using condoms. An editorial in *Catholic New York* called this "condom campaign" the city's "latest misguided attempt" to fight AIDS. "For the most part," it continued, the epidemic has spread "because of excessive sexual activity," which the promotion of condoms would further encourage. The editorial implored the government instead to "reinforc[e] a call to traditional values and lives of chastity" and for a "return to sexual normalcy—to monogamy, to chastity, to abstinence."[75]

O'Connor also decried battles with the city over safe sex programming and condom ads, which he called "'safe sex' propaganda" and "a dangerous but popular cliché." "Nothing would do but that the television stations hawk condoms to kingdom come," O'Connor complained: "that they be scattered around 'shooting galleries' like campaign leaflets, and all be stashed into cereal boxes for little kids to discover as prizes. I can't accept that." He regretted that his friend and sometimes ally Mayor Koch

was also on the "condom bandwagon."[76] Despite Koch's position, the archdiocese's opposition to condoms clearly held sway at City Hall.

After meeting with Bishop Egan, Mayor Koch backtracked. He announced later that summer that the city would sponsor a new advertising
campaign targeting teenagers that would focus on promoting abstinence.[77]
The campaign reflected a more conservative approach to fighting AIDS by
emphasizing personal responsibility, a shift conveyed in its title, "Don't
Ask for AIDS, Don't Get It." Koch explained that the new focus on abstinence arose because "there are people for religious reasons who believe it
is morally wrong to use condoms or to engage in sexual intercourse if you
are not married." "It is not a kook position," he continued, "and now we
have to address it."[78]

By November 1987, New Yorkers could already sense the influence of
the archdiocese, not only in the politics of abortion and homosexuality, but
now too in the life and death matters of AIDS care and prevention. While
the archdiocese and the city's gay and AIDS activist communities fought
against the growing crisis, they upheld quite different moral and political
positions regarding sexuality, and especially homosexuality. These local
battles would soon be eclipsed by the national conversation on AIDS that
the American bishops initiated the following month, when they released a
controversial statement on the epidemic. That statement prompted two
years of debate within and beyond the church hierarchy concerning a variety of issues, not least among them Catholic stances on contraception
and homosexuality and the political role that the church ought to play in
the context of America's pluralistic democracy. They raised the vital question of how the church should enter into modern political debates to best
achieve its mission.

AIDS, Homosexuality, and the Catholic Church

O'Connor and other Catholic bishops situated AIDS within the church's
teachings on sexuality and contraception. Throughout the 1970s and
1980s, the church hierarchy developed nuanced theological positions
regarding how to care for homosexual persons and to support the pastoral needs of their family members.[79] Cardinal Joseph Ratzinger, Prefect
of the Congregation for the Doctrine of the Faith, penned the church's
most important statement on homosexuality in October 1986, only
months following the political ruckus set off in New York by the gay
rights bill.[80]

In "Letter to the Bishops of the Catholic Church on the Pastoral Care of Homosexual Persons," he called attention to how "the issue of homosexuality and the moral evaluation of homosexual acts have increasingly become a matter of public debate, even in Catholic circles."[81] The Vatican had briefly addressed homosexuality in its 1975 "Declaration on Certain Questions Concerning Sexual Ethics," in *Persona Humana*. That statement distinguished homosexual acts from a homosexual "tendency" or "orientation," which in some individuals could be considered innate. While individuals who expressed this tendency should be treated with understanding, the statement explained, homosexual acts could not be morally justified.[82] The 1986 letter registered this distinction, but worried that many Catholics remained confused about homosexuality, some even taking the previous statement to imply that homosexuality itself was neutral or good.[83]

Ratzinger's letter insisted that hate speech or violence used against homosexuals was "deplorable" and must be condemned by the church, before it clarified the earlier position.[84] While homosexual acts (as opposed to homosexual inclination) were sinful in themselves, neither the act nor the tendency was benign. Even the tendency gestured toward "intrinsic moral evil." "Although the particular inclination of the homosexual person is not a sin," the letter reasoned, "the inclination itself must be seen as an objective disorder."[85] Ratzinger called for special concern in this matter, fearing that some might be led to think that living out a homosexual tendency is morally acceptable. The letter clarified, "It is not."[86] Ratzinger then proceeded to homosexual rights, which he feared were gaining momentum.

The letter decried efforts both from within and from outside the church to characterize homosexuality as a "harmless, if not an entirely good thing." It described the "deceitful propaganda" of the "pro-homosexual movement" along with "an effort in some countries to manipulate the Church by gaining often well-intentioned support of her pastors with a view to changing civil-statutes and law."[87] Ratzinger warned his fellow bishops to be cautious of such threats, including any attempts to challenge the church's teaching with regard to sexuality.[88] He also requested that the bishops employ "special care" in designating pastoral ministers who were fully faithful to the church's teaching. Lastly, the letter called on church authorities to stop supporting organizations that "seek to undermine the teaching of the Church, which are ambiguous about it, or which neglect it entirely." "Even the semblance of such support," the cardinal warned, "can be gravely misinterpreted."[89] No longer, in other words, could the church harbor any disagreement on the topic of homosexuality. This statement had direct repercussions for many gay and lesbian Catholics. Following its call, Catholic churches, including those in the Archdiocese of New York, closed their doors to pro-gay Catholic groups such as Dignity, preventing such dissenters from holding special services on church grounds.

The letter also addressed the issue of homosexuality in relation to broader social and political concerns. Though the Vatican condemned violence against gays and lesbians, the letter argued that such condemnations should not lead to acceptance:

> The proper reaction to crimes committed against homosexual persons should not be to claim that the homosexual condition is not disordered. When such a claim is made and when homosexual activity is consequently condoned, or when civil legislation is introduced to protect behavior to which no one has any conceivable right, neither the Church nor society at large should be surprised when other distorted notions and practices gain ground, and irrational and violent reactions increase.[90]

According to this reasoning, the claim that homosexuality should be considered normal—or the passage of legislation that might have this effect, such as New York's gay rights bill—could itself lead to increased violence and discrimination against gays and lesbians. Many critics of the church were troubled by how this statement tethered violence against homosexuals to the fight for gay rights. Increased violence would arise not because society needed time to accept such changes and to become comfortable with gay rights—a fair expectation, many would agree—but because the acceptance of one type of disorder (homosexuality) would lead to the acceptance of others, namely violence. Condoning one kind of disorder, the letter suggested, would produce another.

Ratzinger drew further criticism from gay and lesbian activists for suggesting that homosexuals were hurting themselves. They pointed to the indirect but telling reference to the AIDS epidemic in his letter. "Even when the practice of homosexuality may seriously threaten the lives and well-being of a large number of people," Ratzinger declared, "its advocates remain undeterred and refuse to consider the magnitude of the risks involved." Here the cardinal suggested that the AIDS epidemic ravaging the gay community arose not from a virus communicated through sex, but from homosexual acts themselves. In other words, he suggested a moral causation lurking behind the AIDS epidemic, one similar to that identified by some evangelicals.[91]

While the "Letter to the Bishops of the Catholic Church on the Pastoral Care of Homosexual Persons" addressed the AIDS crisis only implicitly, it suggested a link between violence and risk on the one hand, and homosexual behavior on the other. Over the next few years, the American bishops would make a stronger connection between homosexuals and AIDS as they tackled the question of the church's role in responding to the epidemic—a task that involved the bishops in discussions about sexuality and AIDS education that proved more controversial than even they had expected.

The American Bishops Confront AIDS

Writing in the Jesuit weekly *America* in June of 1986, Michael G. Meyer, who had worked with various religious groups in Washington, D.C., to address AIDS, chastised the American Church for its lethargic response to the epidemic. The church, he accused, "has made little attempt to address the problems of the vast number who are facing death and are afraid to die." While over 1300 cases of AIDS had been reported in San Francisco alone, for instance, the Archdiocese of San Francisco hosted only a fifteen-bed hospice—a clear symbol of the church's "reticence." Meyer called for a national response to the crisis. "If service is to be efficient and effective," he argued, "dialogue must begin on a national level within the Church."[92] More specifically, he called upon the American bishops to form a committee on AIDS as part of the United States Catholic Conference (USCC), which would produce a statement to jump-start conversation about AIDS at the highest level. The church heeded his call.

In December 1987, the administrative board of the USCC released "The Many Faces of AIDS," the first national Catholic statement on AIDS. Two years later, the bishops revisited their position on AIDS in a second statement, released by the National Conference of Catholic Bishops (NCCB).[93] Both affirmed the church's long-standing imperative to care for the sick, including those with HIV/AIDS and without regard for how it was contracted. The statements illustrated fluency in the latest medical and scientific information available to their authors. The bishops placed the AIDS crisis within the broader Catholic tradition of concern for human dignity, offered clear steps to curb the spread of HIV, and provided instruction for members of the church on how to care for people with HIV/AIDS.[94] Furthermore, the statements declared that AIDS was not a divine punishment for human sins, namely homosexual sex and illicit drug use, and roundly condemned legal and social discrimination (including discrimination within medical practice and insurance coverage) against marginalized populations affected by the disease.

The major distinction between the two statements arose in their positions regarding condom use as a preventative measure. The earlier statement drew considerable press attention for conceding the need for education about the use of condoms, though it stipulated such discussions should take place only under specific circumstances and always within the broader moral context of Catholic teachings on sexuality. For some readers, Catholic and non-Catholic alike, this position heralded a promising new turn in Catholic teaching on contraception. But others argued that it produced a central misunderstanding in Catholic teaching that demanded quick redress. A number of conservative American bishops, O'Connor among them, sided with the latter position and called for an amendment to "Many Faces." Two years later, "Called to Compassion and Responsibility" stood as a correction to the earlier position. It affirmed that Catholic teachings about contraception had not changed and left no room for tolerance regarding the issue of condom use.

Taken together, the two statements demonstrate an important disagreement concerning church teaching on condoms. Even more, they provide a window into new battles sparked by the AIDS crisis that raged within the church hierarchy and among Catholics more broadly over both sexual morality and the role the church ought to play in the emerging culture wars. Toward this end, these statements demonstrate the bishops' continued boldness in speaking about political issues of concern for American society as a whole, rather than for Catholics alone—the performance of "public Catholicism" that Casanova described. But their public voice was not monolithic.

Two central tensions emerged in the Catholic statements on AIDS. The first arose in the use of *medico-scientific* versus *moral-religious* epistemologies to discuss AIDS care and prevention. The second pitted the language of *pluralism* espoused by the first statement against the language of *universalism* more strongly pronounced in the second. Both tensions were tied to debates over sexuality. In fact, these statements reveal how the American bishops continued to draw attention to the role of homosexuality in the AIDS crisis, despite their own references to the spread of HIV among populations not necessarily defined by homosexuality, particularly drug users. The statements shifted seemlessly in discussions of prevention from addressing AIDS to describing homosexuals and immoral sexual acts, as they often collapsed the former into the latter. Lastly, the tensions present both within and between these major statements were not peripheral to their messages—they were essential to the work that they performed (and continue to perform) in constituting the American Church's formal positions on AIDS, sex education, and homosexuality.[95]

Drafting the "Many Faces of AIDS"

In 1987, the United States Catholic Conference, the administrative arm of the American Catholic Church, formed an ad hoc committee to research and write "Many Faces." Over the summer and fall of that year, committee members Bishop William Hughes, Cardinal Joseph Bernardin, Bishop Raymond Lessard, and Bishop Anthony Bosco drafted several versions of the statement, which they also submitted to a two-day consultation on July 15–16 in Washington, D.C. The conference included Catholic theologians as well as experts from the Centers for Disease Control, members of the Catholic Health Association, and representatives from existing diocesan AIDS and hospice programs.[96] Following this meeting, the committee submitted another draft of the statement for discussion at the administrative board meeting scheduled in late September. Shortly after, board members approved an updated version of the statement through a voice vote at which no vocal dissent was recorded.[97]

Released in early December of 1987, "Many Faces" addressed itself to "sisters and brothers in the Lord and all people of good will." It established the importance of its call: "The Church confronts in this disease a significant pastoral issue," one complicated only more so because the "etiology" of AIDS, its prevention, and care for those affected by it "present society with serious moral decisions." The epidemic raised questions about the responsibilities of church members and society-at-large in caring for people with AIDS and HIV and what steps ought to be taken to prevent new infections. "How we make these choices with their moral implications," the statement continued, "will affect both the present generation and, most likely, future ones as well."[98] The statement included three major sections, which covered facts about AIDS, methods of prevention, and reflections on how to care for people affected by the disease. It concluded with an appendix containing a series of questions and responses meant to guide fellow bishops and members of the church.

Taken as whole, "Many Faces" offered an informed contribution to the growing medical and social discourse on AIDS. The bishops offered six major reflections. They affirmed that AIDS was a human disease, not a divine punishment, and must be understood through medical and scientific studies. They declared that the church and society ought to "stand in solidarity" with those affected and provide "compassion and understanding, along with pastoral care and medical and other social services."[99] They also emphasized that the church must clarify Catholic moral teachings on human sexuality, a point about which I will elaborate shortly. Next, the bishops condemned violence and discrimination against people with AIDS. Fifth, "Many Faces" called members of the church to work with the public to prevent the spread of the disease by promoting educational programming, which "should include an authentic understanding of human intimacy and sexuality as well as an understanding of the pluralism of values and attitudes in our society." Finally, the statement argued that people with HIV must themselves live in such a way that avoids spreading the virus to others.[100] In offering these reflections, the bishops sought to contribute the church's particular expertise in dealing with the moral questions raised by the epidemic, a dimension that would in turn have repercussions for medical and political discourses. Though the bishops called for care and compassion for people with AIDS, condemned discrimination, and elaborated upon the need for education, the statement's most controversial claims dealt with sexual morality.

The longest section of "Many Faces" was devoted to methods to prevent AIDS and thus, by extension, devoted the morality of sexual conduct. It demonstrated the central tensions within the statement itself. The bishops' insistence upon fidelity to medical and scientific facts concerning AIDS reached its limit when set against the church's tradition of moral reasoning. That is, in the end, it proved impossible to separate medical facts from religious or political claims about AIDS. The statement also demonstrated the difficulty the bishops faced in addressing both Catholics and the broader American public. The authors of "Many Faces" struggled to situate the universal moral positions promoted by the church within the pluralistic context of American society. Their attempts to work within this setting resulted not merely in textual tensions within this statement, but also prompted disagreement among many conservative-leaning American bishops upon its publication.

The Sexuality of "Many Faces"

Though conceived as a text about AIDS, "Many Faces" is at least as much a statement about sex—and what its authors saw as the declining moral status of American sex in particular. By 1987, the AIDS crisis had ravaged gay male communities throughout the United States. Towards the end of the decade, the public face of AIDS began to shift from mostly white, gay men to gay, bisexual, and straight African American and Latino men and women. The bishops recognized this shift as well. In "Many Faces," they attempted to remove AIDS from its popular representation as a "gay disease" in order to illustrate its broader reach. But the statement nonetheless recast AIDS as a disease of sexual immorality and drug use.[101]

Early in the statement, the authors sketch four of the "many faces of AIDS" with which they had come into contact in their ministry work. They start with Mary and Phil, a young professional couple who had recently married. Asked to donate blood for a friend, Mary soon discovered that she had contracted HIV from a previous partner. John, the second face of AIDS, was a young man raised in the inner city by a single mother. He contracted HIV after turning to drugs. Peter, the next example, was a rising business professional in his late twenties who was homosexual. He contracted the virus sexually, after which his employers fired him. Finally, the bishops describe Lilly, a 15-month-old child who contracted the disease from her mother, a drug addict who had abandoned her. These faces presented common typologies of people who could develop AIDS—the good couple with an unfortunate past, the gay man, the drug user, and the innocent child who contracted HIV through her mother.

While the statement did not specify the race of these four "faces of AIDS," it emphasized how they each contracted the disease and suggested their moral fault or innocence. The statement implied that some forms of contraction were sinful, even as it pressed the reader not to confer judgment. "What does the Gospel tell us about these representative faces of AIDS?" it asked. That God shows compassion and is not vengeful, the statement answered: that such diseases are not restricted only to a few social groups, and that Jesus "proclaimed to those most in need the good news of forgiveness."[102] Here the representative faces of AIDS were marked as sinful, as their disease continued to carry not merely social but now moral stigma as well, a stigma already in need of forgiveness. The statement then addressed AIDS prevention, eventually narrowing its focus to sexual conduct.

Once again, "Many Faces" prefaced its remarks with a nod toward the diversity of opinion in modern America. "We speak to an entire nation," the bishops wrote, "whose pluralism we recognize and respect." The authors recognized that many people would not heed their calls to stop using drugs and to practice sexuality in a way consistent with Catholic teachings. Yet they included these people in their message as well, describing how the church cared even for those who placed themselves or others in danger of contracting HIV. This included "drug users and their partners, children born and unborn, and persons involved in sexual conduct which is physically dangerous or morally wrong." The bishops' major concern was with people's "moral and physical well-being, not their condemnation, however much we might disagree with their actions."[103]

"Many Faces" nonetheless contended that "the best source of prevention" could only arise from the promotion of "an authentic and fully integrated understanding of human personhood and sexuality" and by eliminating of the causes of drug use.[104] Education and encouragement designed to correct immoral behavior proved central to this endeavor. But it is also important to note the bishops' general focus on the dignity of human life. To prevent AIDS, they argued, "we must deal with those human and societal factors which reduce or limit the quality of human life." One key factor was poverty, which caused people to "turn to drugs or reach out for short-term physical intimacy in a mindless effort to escape the harsh conditions in which they live."[105] To deal with this epidemic, in other words, the bishops called for attention to the societal mechanisms that might lead people to engage in risky behavior.

The statement next turned to the question of sex and the need for a better understanding of the nature of human sexuality. "Every person, made in God's image and likeness," the bishops explained,

> has both the potential and the desire to experience interpersonal intimacy that reflects the intimacy of God's triune love. This reflection in human love of the divine love gives special meaning and purpose to human sexuality. Human sexuality is essentially related to permanent commitment in love and openness to new life. It is most fully realized when it is expressed in a manner that is as loving, faithful and committed as is divine love itself.[106]

Here, the bishops established two key suppositions in the Catholic understanding of authentic human sexuality: first, that sex should unite one man and one woman through faithful commitment and love and, second, that it should be open to the possibility of procreation. The bishops promoted this position not merely for Catholics, but for "all people." "Human sexuality, as *we* understand this gift from God," they continued, though now framing this position as their particular stance, "is to be genitally expressed in a monogamous heterosexual relationship of lasting fidelity in marriage." The bishops clarified this point: "unless, as a society, we live in accord with an authentic human sexuality, on which our Catholic moral teaching is based, we will not address a major source of the spread of AIDS." Alternative solutions, they warned, would provide only a stopgap and would augment "the trivialization of human sexuality that is already so prevalent in our society." For this reason, the bishops explained, they opposed what was "popularly called 'safe sex.'"[107]

"Many Faces" offered two reasons for not supporting efforts to teach "safe sex." First, safe sex trivialized human sexuality, "making it 'safe' to be promiscuous." And second, they argued, the notion that sex could be "safe" in such instances was itself misleading. Citing a study from the National Academy of Sciences, the authors suggested that "safer" would be a more accurate description than "safe."[108] The bishops reaffirmed their commitment to education about sexuality and AIDS, including the church's support for legislation that would provide information about the epidemic to the American public. Even more, they recognized the need for such efforts to go beyond "mere biological education." Americans, and children especially, needed to be educated about sexuality. But, they claimed, "we also have a responsibility as religious leaders to bring analysis to bear upon moral dimensions of public policy."

The authors of "Many Faces" insisted that information about AIDS must be presented within a broader moral context. And that moral context must include consideration of "the consequences of individual choices for the whole of society." They elaborated, for instance, that any proposed legislation or education guidelines must respect parents' rights to be the first to educate their children about matters of sexuality. But the bishops also recognized the controversial nature of sex education as well as the questions it raised regarding the potential for religious morality to upset the constitutional separation of church and state. The need to respect this separation, they submitted, would make efforts to legislate Catholic views of sexuality problematic. Still, they maintained, "we are willing to join other people of good will in dialogue about how such a fuller understanding of human sexuality might be communicated in our public schools and elsewhere."[109] The bishops further conveyed their optimism that "there are certain basic values present in our society which transcend religious or sectarian boundaries" and from which common ground could be found.

The bishops sought a compromise with reigning medical opinion, which supported efforts to teach about safe or safer sex education, including the use of condoms. "Because we live in a pluralistic society," they explained, "we acknowledge that some will not agree with our understanding of human sexuality." Public education campaigns had to address a broad spectrum of society, many members of which, the bishops allowed, would not abstain from sex outside of marriage or with same-sex partners and who would not stop using illegal intravenous drugs. Given this pluralistic setting—and the pressing need for instruction—the bishops made specific allowances for education that could include discussions of condom use. The key passage from "Many Faces" asserted:

> In such situations educational efforts, if grounded in the broader moral vision outlined above, could include accurate information about prophylactic devices or other practices proposed by some medical experts as potential means of preventing AIDS. We are not promoting the use of prophylactics, but merely providing information that is part of the factual picture. Such a factual presentation should indicate that abstinence outside of marriage and fidelity within marriage as well as the avoidance of intravenous drug abuse are the only morally correct ways to prevent the spread of AIDS. So-called 'safe sex' practices are at best only partially effective. They do not take into account either the real values that are at stake or the fundamental good of the human person.[110]

This position is restated in a set of potential questions included in an appendix. The question concerned whether health professionals working within Catholic hospitals could provide information about safe sex. Once again, the bishops advocated Catholic teachings about sexuality and responded that Catholic health care workers "should be unequivocal about the moral teaching of the Church in their programs and personal counseling." Such agencies should not promote the "'safe-sex' approach." But, they continued, it would be "permissible [. . .] to speak about the practices recommended by public health officials for limiting the spread of AIDS in the context of a clear advocacy of Catholic moral teaching." The first step for health professionals would be to invite those at risk or already infected "to live a chaste life." If it is clear that the patient will not do so, the bishops added, "then the traditional Catholic wisdom with regard to one's responsibility to avoid inflicting greater harm may be appropriately applied."[111] The bishops justified this position by appealing to the tradition of the toleration of the lesser evil, as explained by Thomas Aquinas in the *Summa Theologica*, a long-standing source for Catholic thought.[112]

"Many Faces" garnered very favorable press coverage, though many reporters singled out the statements on contraception. One headline in the *New York Times* announced "U.S. Bishops Back Condom Education as a Move on AIDS." Such headlines proclaimed what seemed to be a major shift in Catholic teaching, burying the fact that the statement allowed for such education only under very specific circumstances.[113] They also sparked the ire of many American bishops, especially those belonging to the conservative wing of the American Church. The bishops pointed back to "Many Faces" as the real culprit, however. Because it lacked clarity about Catholic moral teaching, some bishops would complain, the USCC statement had resulted in "widespread [and] considerable confusion" and "misinterpretation" among members of the press and many Catholics themselves.[114]

The Bishops Debate "Many Faces"

Cardinal O'Connor was one of the first bishops to criticize "Many Faces," which, he wrote, has led to "serious confusion." He affirmed the call to care for people with AIDS and support for prevention and treatment programs. "It is apparent, however," he explained, "that some portions of the text have been construed as supporting toleration for certain educational approaches which I cannot accept as applicable within my area of church jurisdiction and responsibility, the Archdiocese of New York." O'Connor took aim at the statement's bend to pluralism. As he understood from discussions with Archbishop John May, the president of the NCCB, the administrative board's statement was meant to confirm that any education about condoms must be presented within the context of Catholic teaching, which held, according to O'Connor, that "the use of prophylactics is immoral *in a pluralistic society or any other society.*"[115] During a press conference following his morning Mass on December 13, O'Connor outright opposed the statement's position that condoms could be mentioned as part of the complete factual picture regarding AIDS in accord with the church's teaching concerning tolerance for the lesser of two evils. The cardinal described the report as a "grave mistake" and insisted that "[n]othing will change" in his archdiocese in regard to AIDS care: "There will be no teaching about condoms" at Catholic schools, hospitals, or elsewhere in New York.[116]

O'Connor was not alone in his criticisms of the statement or in his idea of what exactly Catholic tradition would and would not allow regarding information on condoms as a preventative measure. A group of seventeen bishops, among them O'Connor's ally and fellow conservative Cardinal Bernard Law of Massachusetts, issued a statement decrying the media confusion that followed the release of "Many Faces." "We wish to make it clear," they wrote, "that the only proper expression of genital sexuality is one that is open to procreation within marriage." They drew a fine distinction: "We cannot approve or seem to approve distribution of information regarding contraceptive devices and methods which might lead some to think that they could in good conscience ignore or contradict this teaching."[117] The Archdiocese of Military Services also faulted the media, citing an article in *Time* from December 21, 1987, which stated, "The bishops will now reluctantly accept the publicizing of information on the devices [condoms] in public education campaigns and school classes."[118] The bishops countered that "the church does not accept even reluctantly the promotion of condoms as a preventative against AIDS" and that "the only morally acceptable and medically safe way to prevent the spread of AIDS is chaste, sexual abstinence."[119] The bishops of Metropolitan Washington came to a similar conclusion. "It is never morally permissible to employ intrinsically evil means to achieve a good purpose," they argued: "No Catholic pastor or counselor is ever free to advocate the use of contraceptive devices."[120]

Cardinal John Krol of Philadelphia joined his recently named successor Archbishop Anthony Bevilacqua in a statement expressing similar criticism, but they also referenced a statement released by the NCCB only a month before concerning school-based clinics. As they pointed out, that statement was approved by the full body of American bishops (unlike "Many Faces") and clearly opposed any programs that promoted condoms as part of safe or safer sex education. Krol and Bevilacqua pushed the matter further, attacking not merely the USCC statement's muted tolerance of such education, but also what they viewed as its genuflection to American pluralism. They asserted, "pluralism should not be used as a pretext for giving a diluted message or a double message about moral responsibility."[121] According to Krol and Bevilacqua, the bishops best served society—even a pluralistic one—by promoting the universal teachings of the church without compromise.

Archbishop J. Francis Stafford of Denver offered one of the bishops' most detailed arguments against the USCC's AIDS statement, which he considered flawed from both a "theological and canonical point of view." Stafford underscored two points. He insisted that the statement exceeded the powers and purpose granted the USCC, which was formed as a civil body but had now issued a doctrinal statement, thus stepping on the toes of the NCCB. Stafford's larger point dealt with the theological problems contained in "Many Faces." He faulted the statement for misapplying the principle of toleration of the lesser of two evils. He argued that the authors failed to understand that the passage from Aquinas they cited focused on the possibility that human government, rather than the church, could tolerate lesser forms of evil. "The principle as articulated by Aquinas permits toleration of social evil by civil authority," Stafford concluded, "but not toleration, and still less real or tacit cooperation in its transmission, by the bishops and the Church community." The statement also failed to verify the key claim that would be necessary even if the lesser evil were tolerated: "that AIDS constitutes a danger so clearly threatening to the common good that it justifies 'toleration of error,' i.e., laws and social policies which promote prophylactic use."[122]

As dissent mounted from Stafford and other bishops, the authors of "Many Faces" and the president of the USCC defended their choice of language. They were joined by a number of other bishops who voiced their full support for the statement, including its discussion of AIDS education. Supporters of the statement also suggested new reasons why the church could not remain silent on the use of contraceptives. Bishop William Hughes, who headed the ad-hoc committee that drafted "Many Faces," underscored the "special importance" of AIDS prevention. He offered two reasons for this. Echoing the original statement, he appealed to the "pluralistic society" within which the church operates and the fact that many people would not follow its teachings. Even more, he continued, AIDS demanded special weight: unlike other sexually transmitted diseases, this one was fatal. For these reasons, he concluded, the bishops "believed they could not object to education programs that presented all important facts that could help in decreasing the spread of this fatal disease."[123] Hughes thus offered a practical response to the situation at hand, which represented not a relaxing of Catholic moral positions or a reconsideration of their truthfulness, but rather acknowledgment of the fact that the church's position on the prevention of sexually transmitted diseases was one among others in a diverse country. Though he admitted the moral superiority of the church's teaching, upholding this position alone, for the sake of clarity, was not worth risking the lives of the many people who failed to heed its message.

Daniel Pilarczyk, USCC vice president and archbishop of Cincinnati, agreed with his colleague. "Are we going to talk about condoms and 'safe sex' practices when we teach about AIDS? Yes, we are, because they are part of the whole picture. There is no point in pretending such things do not exist," he argued. "Are we going to give detailed information about how to use condoms and advocate their use as a means of preventing the spread of AIDS?" he asked: "No, we are not. We are going to talk about them, but talking about something does not constitute advocacy." As it turned out, the question of whether or not just talking about condoms constituted advocacy was a matter of disagreement. As we saw with Ratzinger's letter on homosexuality, for instance, the "mere semblance of support" could be called into question. Pilarczyk did not bend to this fear. "In my judgment none of this is particularly controversial," he concluded: "It is simply good sense."[124]

Archbishop John May of St. Louis, who served as president of the NCCB (and thus the USCC as well), also defended the statement on AIDS. He recognized that some media reports had misrepresented "Many Faces" and reemphasized what the original statement made clear: that Catholic teaching on contraception had not changed. "But," he continued, "many health officials have recommended the use of condoms to reduce the risk of transmitting or acquiring the AIDS virus, and we acknowledge that this fact will be part of comprehensive factual presentations on the disease." May added another argument to the mix—that failing to address condoms in sex education "would leave people to learn of them from factually misleading campaigns designed to sell certain products or to advocate safe sex without reference to a moral perspective." In other words, it would behoove the church to offer this information first, in order to take the opportunity to place it within the church's own moral and religious context.[125]

Cardinal Joseph Bernardin agreed. The way he phrased this point, though, betrayed the moderate or even conservative position regarding contraception offered in "Many Faces." Writing in his archdiocese's newspaper *The Chicago Catholic*, Bernardin worried that "some are reading into the document certain things which are not there." In drafting "Many Faces," neither he nor the other bishops suggested changes in church teaching.

The selections from the text that had caused controversy, he further explained, addressed "*public* educational programs . . . *not* what is taught in Catholic schools on this matter, as some have implied." Moreover, the bishops' position regarding public education programs called specifically for education that privileged chastity and monogamous marriage as the "only appropriate responses." It called for such programs to provide "*accurate*" medical information, which, Bernardin insisted, "clearly states that there is no such thing as 'safe sex.'"[126] Not all people would follow such teachings, he reasoned, so programs that provided such education could include a discussion of contraception—but only after offering these other reflections on sexual morality.

Finally, reflecting May's point, Cardinal Bernardin emphasized that many students would already be exposed to safe sex through "flawed education programs." He suggested that to combat such misinformation teachers should discuss condoms and safe sex "*in order to point out their medical inaccuracy and moral failure.*" The point of such discussion would not be to promote condoms but rather "to teach why prophylactic approaches are wrong and, therefore, not to be followed."[127] Bernardin's defense of "Many Faces" demonstrated not merely how the statement upheld the church's moral stance, but also how teaching about condoms, far from compromising Catholic tradition, would help undermine the purportedly faulty logic of "safe" or even "safer" sex. From his view, "Many Faces" looked even more conservative regarding AIDS prevention than its progressive detractors claimed.

Taken together, the reactions from the American bishops revealed different layers of disagreement. Some accused the mainstream press of misreading the original statement but nonetheless upheld its reflections as promoting traditional Catholic teaching on sexuality. Other bishops found the statement itself unclear or ambiguous and faulted its argumentation as either unclear or theologically inaccurate. But the American bishops also found themselves the object of scrutiny in the wider context of the Catholic Church. For the first few months following the release of "Many Faces," the Vatican was officially silent on the statement and on AIDS prevention generally. But church authorities in Rome soon began to contest the statement's controversial claims.

Monsignor Carlo Caffarra, head of the John Paul II Institute for Studies of Matrimony and Family and adviser on moral theology to the Pope, rejected the logic of "Many Faces" under the strict terms of Catholic moral reasoning. "Even the smallest moral wrong is so much greater than any physical wrong," he explained. "I know this is hard for some to accept when the dangers are great," he qualified, "but the church is here to combat moral wrongs." Public health reasoning was beside the point, he maintained: "it is a fundamental precept that ethical judgments are not based on whether a form of behavior is good or bad for a man's health." The Vatican's chief spokesman, Joaquin Navarro-Valls, concurred. "From the church's point of view," he explained, "saving a life is not the foremost value on a moral issue."[128] Though it would sound wrong to many ears, in other words, moral reasoning itself was no sentimental or practical matter of saving lives. The church's work was not medical treatment but moral teaching—in this economy of reason, moral compromise could not be accepted.

The following spring Cardinal Ratzinger, speaking on behalf of the Congregation for the Doctrine of the Faith, formally entered the discussion. On May 29, 1988, he issued a letter outlining the Vatican's concerns. It was forwarded to Archbishop May, president of the NCCB, and later distributed to all of the bishops in the United States.[129] Ratzinger reminded the bishops of the import of documents released by national conferences, statements that can easily generate worldwide reaction and repercussions. Given such influence, he recommended that national bishops consult the Holy See in advance of releasing such statements. Ratzinger next addressed what he considered the moral problem central to "Many Faces," which was the question of whether it allowed for teaching about condom use. The cardinal cited an article on AIDS prevention published in *L'Osservatore Romano* that March:

> To seek a solution to the problem of infection by promoting the use of prophylactics would be to embark on a way not only insufficiently reliable from the technical point of view, but also and above all unacceptable from the moral aspect. Such a proposal for 'safe' or at least 'safer' sex—as they say—ignores the real cause of the problem, namely, the permissiveness which, in the area of sex as in that related to other abuses, corrodes the moral fiber of the people.[130]

This statement suggested that sexual permissiveness—rather than viral infection—remained "the real cause of the problem" of HIV infection. The answer to such moral laxity thus could not be found in the promotion of condoms or indeed any form of safer sex. Cardinal Ratzinger also denied the relevance of the appeal to the toleration of lesser evil, since "one would not be dealing with simply a form of passive toleration but rather with a kind of behavior which would result in at least the facilitation of evil."[131] He thereby sided with the conservative critics of "Many Faces," and, with this letter, the Vatican made its presence felt among the American bishops. The American Church responded accordingly.

The American bishops decided to revisit the issue of AIDS, this time during a full-session meeting held at St. John's University in Collegeville, Minnesota on June 24–27, 1988. Cardinal Bernardin addressed his colleagues at a private meeting held on the final day of the conference. He steered the focus away from why "Many Faces" was misunderstood and toward "the fact of the controversy and the great need—pastorally and ecclesially—to resolve it as quickly as possible."[132] He called on his colleagues to avoid splitting into sides over the issue and instead to work to "resolve the problem itself, whether real or perceived, whatever the cause, regardless of numbers" in order to restore unity to the American Catholic Church.

Though some bishops had called for a retraction of the first statement, Bernardin disagreed. He worried such a move would be "imprudent," if not "disastrous," as it would suggest that "the entire document is flawed and that the entire Administrative Board was in serious error."[133] Bernardin proposed instead that the bishops draft a new document, a move supported by all the members of the original task force that authored "Many Faces." In preparing the new statement, he also recommended that the new committee be in contact with Cardinal Ratzinger and the Holy See. The bishops approved Bernardin's proposal and began drafting the American Church's second statement on AIDS.

Recalling "Compassion and Responsibility"

During their national meeting in November 1989, the full conference of American bishops overwhelmingly approved "Called to Compassion and Responsibility: A Response to the HIV/AIDS Crisis."[134] The statement affirmed many of the points articulated in "Many Faces," including the need to respond to the epidemic by citing the best available medical and scientific information, the need for care and compassion for people with HIV or AIDS, and the need for educational programs to help combat widespread misunderstanding and ignorance. But the 1989 statement also marked an important departure—that difference could be seen in its articulation of moral authority.

"Called to Compassion" rejected language about American pluralism. Instead, the bishops legitimated their position by appealing to the special resources offered by the church. Entering into "public dialogue regarding HIV infection," the statement offered, "we are conscious of the social responsibility of the Church" as an "expert in humanity." Referencing *Gaudium et Spes*, a decree of the Second Vatican Council about the role of the church in the modern world, the bishops stated: "The Church enters into this conversation in the conviction that 'faith throws a new light on everything, manifests God's design for man's total vocation and thus directs the mind to solutions which are fully human.'" The bishops thus prefaced their reflections by clear reference to church doctrine and to the knowledge revealed not through science but through God. "Indeed, only God," they argued, "provides a fully adequate answer to these questions. This He does through what He has revealed in Christ His Son."[135] More than "Many Faces," the new statement underscored particular religious and moral arguments about the AIDS crisis and about sexuality—and that the church was the body best equipped to formulate them.

The bishops thus addressed the moral questions posed by AIDS— questions all the more important, they suggested, because AIDS was "not only a biomedical phenomenon but a social reality rooted in human behavior."[136] Focusing on the social dimensions of AIDS allowed the bishops to remove the disease from the medical context in which most public health experts and many mainstream gay and AIDS activists understood it. The bishops instead characerized AIDS as "a product of human actions in social contexts" that are "shaped by larger cultural and social structures."[137] This move allowed them to elevate the importance of moral approaches to ending the AIDS crisis.

In making this argument, the bishops echoed a number of Left-leaning AIDS theorists and activists and a handful of social critics of medicine.[138] That is, they sounded more like Cindy Patton, Dennis Altman, and other AIDS activists in calling attention to the political construction of medical knowledge and public policy, rather than Randy Shilts or Jonathan Engel, who championed medical and scientific actors whose march of progress was hindered only by political disruptions. The Leftist theoretical position framed the epidemic not as arising from moral laxity regarding sex and drugs (as the bishops maintained), but at least in part from a long history of social and political oppression and marginalization.

To argue for social factors, then, moved the bishops away from mainstream medical and activist opinion, which urged the public to think of

AIDS as a public health problem and medical concern—a viral infection. This mainstream argument emerged as a response to the broader social perception that AIDS resulted from homosexuality, and it sought to disconnect the disease from this social stigma. But as we can see with the example of the bishops, voicing a medical or a social understanding of AIDS did not immediately mark a particular political stand. Constructivism was not to progressivism, in other words, as biology was to a moderate or conservative position. Both depended on context for their political significance. To be clear, my argument does not assume an objective scientific or medical position flanked by either progressive or conservative political constructions of AIDS. Medical knowledge must be understood in its social and political context. But the Catholic case study counters arguments that posit a progressive constructivist view against an objective (usually understood as moderate or conservative) medical view. The Catholic position adds another constructivist understanding: the moral genesis of AIDS.

The bishops cited several social factors that contributed to the AIDS crisis, including the cultural acceptance of "[c]asual sexual encounters and temporary relationships," which amounted to no less than "the toleration of exploitation"; increasing acceptance of homosexuality; conditions of economic poverty that spurred drug use; and commercial incentives that led to the promotion and marketing of sex entertainment, including the promotion of condoms and pornographic material.[139] For the bishops, these social factors led to illegal drug use and to sexual behaviors that not only transferred the virus—as public health experts and most AIDS activists also maintained—but also constituted the epidemic itself, which was every bit as much moral as biological. Hence, the bishops insisted that a central problem in fighting AIDS was precisely "the refusal to discuss publicly the direct link between sexual activity and intravenous drug use on the one hand and HIV/AIDS on the other." Their argument was not merely one moral position among others, but represented truth. "Silence about the connection between these forms of behavior and HIV/AIDS," they urged, "is not only intellectually dishonest, but it is unfair to those at risk."[140]

The bishops singled out the fact that "public campaigns often promote solutions which are contrary to morality and against human dignity."[141] One such solution included needle exchange, which sought to decrease rates of HIV infection among IV drug users by offering clean needles. While a number of public health leaders supported this effort, many political and religious conservatives, including President Reagan and the Catholic bishops, opposed it. Clean needle programs targeted poor minority populations, reflecting the movement of AIDS from the gay ghetto to the inner city. The bishops nodded to this transition, declaring the "critical importance" of recognizing that AIDS had shifted towards becoming a disease of poverty that would "be disastrous for African Americans and Hispanics."[142] But AIDS was still "a disease of homosexual men," and "Called to Compassion" emphasized the importance of sexual morality, including the promotion of chastity and of fidelity within heterosexual marriage. Despite the shifting demographics of the AIDS crisis, the greater portion of the statement was given to discussing Catholic positions on the prevention of sexual, and especially homosexual, transmission.[143]

"Called to Compassion" reiterated Catholic teaching on sexual morality. But it was more emphatic than "Many Faces" in upholding the claim that proper sexuality involved the union of one man with one woman that included the possibility of procreation. The statement thus recalled the church's opposition to homosexual sex. This privileging of heterosexuality was not any sort of departure, to be sure. My point is that the bishops (and other Catholic writers) often made rhetorical choices about the extent to which they would foreground the church's positions regarding sexuality. "Called to Compassion" offered a much stronger rebuttal for what the bishops designated as sexual sins than did their previous statement. Indeed, it focused on sexuality more than any other topic regarding AIDS and spent far more pages developing its theology of sexuality than did "Many Faces."

The NCCB statement included a subsection devoted to "AIDS and Homosexuality" under the heading "A Call to Responsibility." The bishops maintained the church's distinction between homosexual inclination versus actions and urged homosexuals to form stable, chaste relationships. The statement equated homosexual sex itself with unsafe sex, thereby collapsing the moral argument against homosexual sex with the medical data on safe versus risky forms of sex. The bishops noted as a "matter of grave concern" that, although many homosexuals altered their sexual behaviors to practice safer sex, "fewer may be choosing to live chaste lives. This further underlines the critical importance of the Church's teaching on homosexuality." The passage directs the reader to a footnote, which cites a 1989 study from the University of California, San Francisco, reporting that many gay men were "relapsing" into unsafe sex practices.[144] In its reasoning here, "Called to Compassion" collapsed two distinct statements of fact to underscore the importance of the church's teaching on homosexuality: first, that fewer homosexuals were choosing to lead chaste lives, and second, as the footnote signaled, that more gay men were relapsing into unsafe sex practices. The bishops were far clearer in their discussion of the proper form that sexuality should take.

Describing the importance of human integrity, the bishops explained the biblical precedent for complementarianism:

> In God's plan as it existed in the beginning (Gn. 1:1, 17) we find the true meaning of our bodies: We see that in the mystery of creation man and woman are made to be a gift to each other and for each other. By their very existence as male and female, by the complementarity of their sexuality and by the responsible exercise of their freedom, man and woman mirror the divine image implanted in them by God.[145]

Beyond privileging this focus on heterosexual coupling (and, consequently, gendered norms for men and women), the bishops offered an elaborate discussion of "the challenge of chastity" and problems with prevention efforts that focused on safe sex. This discussion also further evidenced the statement's shift away from addressing the needs of a pluralistic society and towards its reliance on the church as authority.

According to the bishops, "human integrity requires the practice of chastity" as a way to foster "self-control" over one's sexuality and to better equip oneself to love another person in a way that goes beyond "the mere desire for physical pleasure."[146] The value of chastity, the bishops continued, was not limited to the faithful. "While chastity has special meaning for Christians, it is not a value only for them," they explained: "All men and women are meant to live authentically integral human lives."[147] The bishops defined the church's relationship to pluralism quite differently here than they did in "Many Faces." They allowed no space, figuratively or in the text, for the fact that some people would not be chaste (the point is never raised), but instead appealed to how *all* men and women *ought* to live. By not acknowledging difference, they did not have to extend their discussion beyond the question of proper behavior. The difference between "Many Faces" and "Called to Compassion" became more striking in the new statement's position regarding prevention.

Under the subsection "AIDS and the Use of Prophylactics," the bishops argued that the "safe sex" approach "compromises human sexuality and can lead to promiscuous behavior." It offered nothing more than a "quick-fix" for the problem of AIDS. This was true not merely because the use of condoms was "technically unreliable," the bishops charged, but also (and more importantly) because "advocating this approach means in effect promoting behavior which is morally unacceptable."[148] "Campaigns advocating 'safe/safer' sex," they continued, "rest on false assumptions about sexuality and intercourse. Plainly they do nothing to correct the mistaken notion that non-marital sexual intercourse has the same value and validity as sexual intercourse within marriage."[149] In this passage, the bishops revised the USCC's specific allowance for the discussion of condoms. They made no reference to the sexual behaviors in which some people, especially those who were not members of the church, would continue to participate. In effect, they confronted the pluralistic setting of the United States not through acknowledgment or compromise, but by clarifying and hardening the church's unequivocal position against the use of prophylactics.[150]

Whether this position was good church teaching remained a matter for debate. Some moral theologians argued that the position articulated in "Many Faces" was perfectly consistent with Catholic teaching, if not even "moderate," and that the hardline stance taken in "Called for Compassion" represented more a conservative turn than fidelity to church tradition. David Hollenbach, S.J., associate professor of moral theology at Weston School of Theology, defended "Many Faces" in America, calling it "entirely consistent with Catholic moral teaching and tradition," including its discussion of the toleration of the lesser of two evils. In fact, he argued, the statement did not go far enough—the bishops should have "positively counseled" the use of condoms. Bela Somfai, S.J., offered one of the more creative rationales for the use of condoms in AIDS education in an earlier article. He contended that condoms used by men having sex with men to prevent HIV infection could not possibly prevent conception, since procreation was already impossible in same-sex sex. Using condoms in this instance was not, strictly speaking, a contraceptive act; hence, its moral evaluation could not be mirrored on the church's opposition to birth control.

The American bishops' decision not to acknowledge the pluralistic setting of the modern United States in "Called to Compassion" had at least three rhetorical effects: it distanced the NCCB statement from the previous one; it affirmed the church's focus on what the bishops perceived as consistency over compromise; and it offered a specific exercise in authority. The quotation cited previously, for instance, mentioned "false assumptions" about sexuality, but the bishops never articulated nor disproved such assumptions. In this case, by withholding an argument—which is made even more significant given that the statement itself is a prolonged argument—the bishops emphasized the extent to which alternatives to their position were indeed obviously in error, beyond even need of consideration. They generated textual authority precisely through the refusal of acknowledgment—or, to put it differently, through their performative erasure of the reality of American pluralism and the existence of alternative sexual practices.

"Called to Compassion" represented more than a shift in the American Church's approach to AIDS and its willingness, conveyed by its predecessor, to "join in dialogue with people of good will." The new statement dropped any discussion of pluralism and removed its analysis from the immediate context of AIDS. It offered instead an uncompromising moral position at odds with the current medical and scientific advice concerning prevention. The bishops offered moral truth, which they based on their authority as the church and reasoned through appeal to theological principles that seemed increasingly irrelevant for many Americans (and indeed for a good number of Catholics among them). For countless AIDS activists and many members of the church itself, the American bishops also sacrificed for the sake of a consistent moral vision the church's reputation as a reasonable contributor to the public discussion concerning AIDS. In the pragmatic spirit of American politics, moral consistency for its own sake appeared arcane.

***

A week after the U.S. bishops approved "Called for Compassion," the Vatican hosted its first conference on AIDS, which brought together over a thousand representatives from almost ninety countries. The lineup included a slew of church authorities, scientists, theologians, and health care experts, among them American biomedical researcher Robert Gallo, the famed, if controversial, co-discoverer of HIV. Despite the Holy See's previous displeasure with the American bishops over their 1987 statement, two years later the Vatican and the American Church seemed to be on the same page, as the three-day conference was opened by none other than the esteemed Archbishop of New York.

O'Connor did not mince words over the church's stance on AIDS prevention. "The truth is not in condoms or clean needles," he averred: "These are lies, lies perpetrated often for political reasons on the part of public officials." O'Connor also bemoaned the reluctance of health care workers to dissuade their patients from behaviors that caused AIDS, including drug use and "homosexual acts."[151] In the two short years since the publication of "Many Faces," the American Church had once again established itself in the good graces of the Vatican. It did so by replacing compromise with absolutism, pluralism with universal truth, and science with morality. "Good morality," the cardinal testified at the Vatican, "is good medicine."[152]

Chapter Four

Protest Religion!

ACT UP, RELIGIOUS FREEDOM, AND THE ETHICS OF SEX

"I believe that nothing is more important for us than that we recognize that we are bound and sworn to that which horrifies us most, that which provokes our most intense disgust."
—GEORGES BATAILLE, "Attraction and Repulsion II"

"There is nothing that is sacred in itself, only things sacred in relation."
—JONATHAN Z. SMITH, "The Bare Facts of Ritual"

"Our words are the currency of our existence, the funds we spend to fight the disease, the blood that is spilled in the demonstrations, the tears shed and the semen ejaculated by and for our lovers."
—RAFAEL CAMPO, "AIDS and the Poetry of Healing"

"THREE YEARS AGO," wrote Cardinal O'Connor in a 1992 column in *Catholic New York*, "members identified as belonging to a coalition which rejects Church teaching on homosexual behavior and abortion desecrated the Blessed Sacrament in St. Patrick's Cathedral."[1] O'Connor was referring to the Stop the Church demonstration organized by two activist collectives: the AIDS Coalition to Unleash Power (ACT UP) and the Women's Health Action and Mobilization (WHAM!). On December 10, 1989, they staged a mass protest at O'Connor's cathedral that drew over four thousand demonstrators. They targeted the church hierarchy's public opposition to homosexuality, abortion, and safe-sex education. Media accounts of the protest underscored one particular action that occurred within the cathedral: a young man crumbled the sacred host. "Much of this desecration and more," O'Connor added, "was televised at a later date in a production called 'Stop the Church.'"[2]

Filmed guerrilla-style by ACT UP member Robert Hilferty, the documentary *Stop the Church* followed members of ACT UP and WHAM! as they organized the demonstration, starting with a meeting held to plan the protest. It captured footage of the protest outside of St. Patrick's Cathedral as well as disruptions within.[3] The documentary did not show the desecration of the host specifically, as O'Connor had thought. But it did record protesters falling into the aisles as part of a mass "die-in," while others shouted at the cardinal as he began his homily, calling him a murderer. The documentary received national press in 1991 when the Public Broadcasting Station announced it would air the film as part of its *P.O.V.* (Point of View) series. PBS later pulled the film after facing protests from local stations and members of the Catholic Church, including most prominently Archbishop of Los Angeles Roger Mahoney.[4] The documentary, subtitled in the opening credits "A Robert Hilferty Inquisition," incited accusations of Catholic-bashing and reanimated much of the controversy that had surrounded the original protest.

The 1989 protest captured in the documentary was the first major action of the Stop the Church movement—and the one that garnered the most media attention—though smaller and less disruptive demonstrations continued in the years following.[5] Only a week before O'Connor penned his 1992 column, a woman attending services at St. Patrick's once again crumbled the host. O'Connor noted that he could not be sure her act was related to the larger protests. But now he feared acts of sacrilege might happen again, as protesters once more threatened to demonstrate at St. Patrick's. The point of his article, O'Connor clarified, was not to condemn such protests, as he would never "deny for a moment the right of *peaceful* protest."[6] Rather, he intended to speak of the divine nature of the consecrated host, which was no less than "the Son of God, the One who was born for us as an infant on the first Christmas Day, the One who was beaten and crucified and suffered and died for us on the cross."[7] Focusing on the Eucharist allowed O'Connor to divert attention away from the political reasons for such protests and to define religion as something outside of politics. He depicted demonstrators attacking not only the religious freedom of Catholics, but even Christ himself. "What has *He* done to be treated with contempt?" the cardinal asked.

O'Connor understood the Holy Communion as sacred, set apart from any of the profane or political reasons that could prompt a demonstration. In Catholic thought, this sacrament reenacts the Last Supper, as the wine and bread are transubstantiated into the blood and body of Christ. It demonstrates what historian of religion Robert Orsi calls an "abundant event," a manifestation of divine presence in this world.[8] For O'Connor, such an event could hardly have anything to do with *politics*. "Is the Holy Eucharist to be used to divide, to express hatred, to politicize?" he asked. Set apart from politics, the Eucharist fell beyond the limits of what the cardinal considered a reasonable object of protest. "In my judgment," he declared, "such desecration bespeaks either madness, or hatred equivalent to madness, or something so inexpressible as to border on demonic." In other words, there was simply no rational argument for these protests. O'Connor's characterization of the activists—gays and feminists "bordering on demonic"—found further confirmation beyond the church.

New York Post columnist Ray Kerrison expressed the outrage of many of New York's religious. "In all my life," he wrote, "I have never witnessed a spectacle quite like that which shook St. Patrick's Cathedral yesterday when radical homosexuals turned a celebration of the Holy Eucharist into a screaming babble of sacrilege by standing in the pews, shouting and waving their fists, tossing shredded paper and condoms into the air and forcing squads of cops lining the aisles to arrest them." Kerrison characterized the protest as a battle between indulgent secularists and the righteous church. "In an age jaded with self-indulgence, secularism, indifference and civic cowardice," he continued, few public figures were willing to "lift their voices" in order "to defend virtue and protect the sacred."[9] In this struggle, he confirmed, Cardinal O'Connor stood alone.

Stop the Church quickly became one of ACT UP's most notorious demonstrations.[10] For critics, activists were not merely targeting the Catholic leadership's positions on AIDS and abortion; they were attacking the Catholic Church itself. Such accounts represented the protest as a battle between secular activists and sacred tradition—homosexuals and feminists against innocent parishioners and the church. Building on a history of battles between Christians and the gay rights movement, religion and homosexuality have often appeared antithetical to one another. The protest at St. Patrick's Cathedral registered for many as one of the most explosive manifestations of this division.[11] In this case, critics leveled another charge against the protesters. The staunchly anti-religious activists exceeded the bounds of peaceful protest, crossing into the territory of disrespect, if not anti-Catholicism. More than disturbing religious freedom, they attacked religion itself, exemplified by the desecration of the host.

This chapter places the protest at St. Patrick's within the broader histories of AIDS activism and American religious politics.[12] Stop the Church was not merely a protest against religion, the Catholic Church, or even Cardinal O'Connor. It was a demonstration against a particular ethic of sexuality, that is, the moral approach advanced by leaders of the Catholic Church that focused on monogamous and procreative heterosexuality. But it was also a demonstration for an alternative ethics of sexuality, one that promoted safe sex, the right to sexual self-determination, and the political value of sexual pleasure. This approach was rooted in the sexual liberation movements of the 1960s and the development of gay sexual cultures in the 1970s. The Stop the Church protest, and subsequent representations of the demonstration in secular and religious media, stirred debates over morality, religious freedom, and the politics of AIDS and of sexuality. These debates increasingly posited the religious freedom of American Catholics against the sexual freedom of gay AIDS activists. Construed in this way, the demonstration became a case study of the American culture wars and the battle to define American citizenship and public morality.

ACT UP and the Ethics of Safe Sex

The Stop the Church demonstration occurred at the height of ACT UP, the direct-action AIDS activist organization founded in New York City in March 1987. Earlier gay community responses to the AIDS crisis laid the groundwork for this organization. In 1982, when newspapers began carrying stories of a rare cancer and rising rates of infection with pneumonia among homosexual men, writer Larry Kramer called a meeting to discuss what measures the gay community could take. In a climate marked by urgency and fear, this meeting sparked the formation of Gay Men's Health Crisis (GMHC), the first and soon the largest AIDS service organization in the United States. GMHC became a leader in AIDS fundraising and the promotion of safe-sex materials in the 1980s and 1990s and demonstrated the power of grassroots responses by New York's gay community to combat the new epidemic.[13]

In the years following the formation of GMHC, the collective sense of urgency and fear shifted more toward urgency and anger. Gay and lesbian and AIDS activists accused the government of neglecting the epidemic for political reasons, as year after year passed without President Reagan speaking to the nation about this crisis primarily affecting gay men and intravenous drug users. Even the United States Surgeon General, the nation's leading spokesperson for public health issues, was silent on AIDS until 1986. The effect of this government neglect was striking, as the number of people diagnosed with AIDS increased by the day. The number of deaths would skyrocket from 451 in 1981 to 50,628 in 1995, before the introduction of highly active antiretroviral therapy.[14] By the mid-1980s it was already clear that the AIDS crisis demanded a greater political response.

In 1986, a group of activists and artists formed the Silence = Death campaign to raise awareness of AIDS as a political issue. ACT UP would later adopt this slogan (Figure 4.1), which has become emblematic of the organization and of political activism regarding AIDS in general. That same year witnessed the formation of the Lavender Hill Mob, one of the first gay direct-action groups, which provided an important link between gay activism and AIDS activism. The group was formed when activists broke off from the Gay and Lesbian Alliance Against Defamation (GLAAD), after becoming disenchanted with its genuflection to political respectability. In one of their first actions, the Mob protested the Supreme Court's decision in *Bowers v. Hardwick*, which upheld the constitutionality of state laws banning sodomy, effectively criminalizing gay and lesbian relationships. In his concurring opinion, Chief Justice Warren Burger appealed to the long tradition of "Judeo-Christian" moral condemnation of gay and lesbian sexual practice.[15]

With this sense of urgency and anger soaring, members of the gay community soon began to criticize GMHC for becoming overly professionalized. As it gained respectability and influence, the AIDS service organization shied away from overt political action. One of the co-founders of GMHC, Kramer soon became its leading critic. In January 1987, he penned an open letter to Richard Dunne, executive director of GMHC, chastising the organization's persistent failure to address "the political realities of this epidemic: THERE IS NOTHING IN THIS WHOLE AIDS MESS THAT IS NOT POLITICAL!"[16] Coupled with his abrasive and over-the-top rhetorical style, Kramer's insistence on making AIDS a political issue irritated members of GMHC who had seen him as a potential liability from the group's beginning. In fact, GMHC had expelled Kramer from its board shortly after its founding. By the mid- to late 1980s, however, his rhetoric struck many within the gay community as exactly right. AIDS was as much a political crisis as a medical one, and any effective organizing had to contend with both aspects.[17]

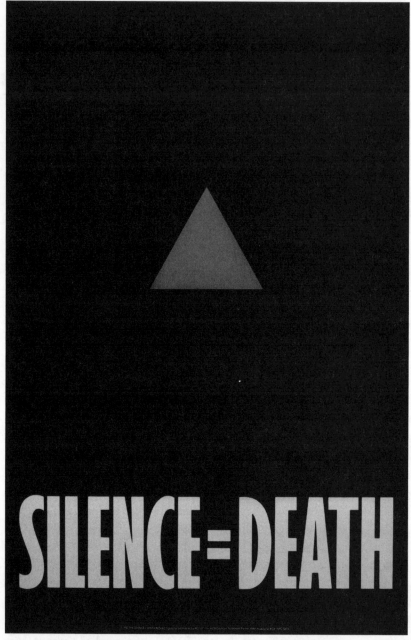

FIGURE 4.1 ACT UP New York's "Silence = Death" poster. (Held in the ACT UP/ NY Records, New York Public Library Digital Gallery.)

Kramer's 1987 letter caught the attention of the Lesbian and Gay Community Services Center in Manhattan, which invited him to be a guest speaker at a lecture series held that March. The firebrand struck a chord among his audience, as he captured their mounting frustrations over the government's sluggish response to fighting AIDS and failure to secure basic rights for gays and lesbians.[18] The audience showed immediate interest in holding another meeting to discuss what could be done about AIDS. Almost overnight, Kramer's speech hastened the formation of ACT UP. It did so by giving voice to a growing number of AIDS activists, most of them young, white, middle-class gay men, who were committed to displays of political anger and who refused to be silenced by the politics of respectability. Their first protest followed within weeks. On March 24, demonstrators gathered on New York's Wall Street in front of Trinity Church, where they demanded the faster release of experimental medications that could save the lives of people with AIDS and lower prices for existing AIDS drugs. Seventeen demonstrators were arrested, but ACT UP's protest had made a bold statement: AIDS was no less than a political issue, and activists frustrated by government and corporate neglect would stop at almost nothing to secure funding, drugs, and political rights for people affected by the epidemic.[19]

Members of ACT UP defined their movement as "a diverse, nonpartisan group of individuals united in anger and committed to direct action to end the AIDS crisis." In their "Working Document," they declared: "We protest and demonstrate [. . .] we meet with government and public health officials; we research and distribute the latest medical information; we are not silent."[20] ACT UP's organizational structure reflected members' commitment to progressive politics. In pointed contrast to GMHC's bureaucratic hierarchy, they attempted to foster an egalitarian, grassroots ethos that would allow all members' voices to be heard. Elected positions garnered no additional decision-making power, and all major decisions were brought to the floor for a vote. Floor meetings occurred on Monday nights and were open to the public. ACT UP members first met in the Lesbian and Gay Community Services Center in the West Village, but soon had to move their Monday night meetings, which could draw upwards of seven hundred members, to the Great Hall at Cooper Union. Membership was open and required only that interested parties attend three meetings before voting.[21]

ACT UP also sponsored smaller committee sessions, such as a fundraising committee and a coordinating committee, which set the agenda for the Monday meetings. Other committees addressed particular topics, such as Treatment and Action, which focused on medical issues, or Women's Action, which emphasized how HIV/AIDS affected women, a population often left out of both medical and political AIDS work.[22] Members could also start informal working or affinity groups, which fell outside the official banner of ACT UP. Members often formed such groups to carry out actions that they did not want to bring to the general floor for a vote, sometimes in order to avoid delay or controversy.[23] Finally, members could form caucuses, official groups within ACT UP that did not require a majority vote. Lesbians, Latino/a members, and Asian and Pacific Islanders formed separate caucuses, for instance, to confront issues insufficiently addressed by the larger, predominantly white male group.[24]

ACT UP deployed a variety of tactics in its activist endeavors. Some members pursued more traditional avenues of political work, such as researching drug and treatment issues and meeting with medical and political figures as well as representatives from major drug companies. But ACT UP became best known—or most notorious—in the 1980s and 1990s for its use of agitprop and street theater techniques. In its early work on medical issues regarding AIDS, ACT UP combined ostentatious acts of street theater with behind-the-scenes meetings with medical and public health professionals. This dual approach proved effective. Under pressure from activists, for instance, the Food and Drug Administration substantially reduced the timeline for its drug approval process and allowed people with HIV/AIDS early access to drugs still undergoing testing.[25] ACT UP also pressured the pharmaceutical company Burroughs Wellcome to lower the price of AZT, one of the first drugs approved for treatment.[26]

In these battles, ACT UP modeled itself in part after feminist and black civil rights movements and encouraged acts of civil disobedience. The organization's Civil Disobedience Training Manual opened with an apt quotation from the abolitionist leader Frederick Douglass:

> Those who profess to favor freedom, yet deprecate agitation, are men who want crops without plowing up the ground. They want rain without thunder and lightening. They want the ocean without the awful roar of its many waters. This struggle may be a moral one; or it may be a physical one; or it may be both moral and physical; but it must be a struggle. Power concedes nothing without a demand. It never did and it never will.[27]

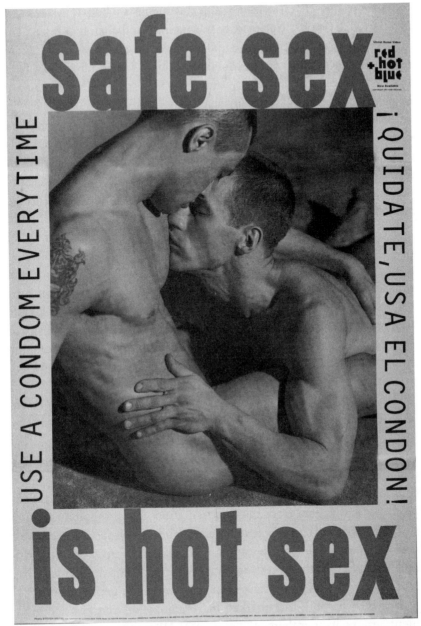

FIGURE 4.2 ACT UP New York's "Safe sex is hot sex" poster demonstrated the organization's sex-positive ethic. (Held in the ACT UP/NY Records, New York Public Library Digital Gallery.)

Here, Douglass characterized political struggle as both physical and moral. ACT UP's physical presence was intense, and often highly successful; its moral struggle, though subtler, proved just as significant. While ACT UP's successful ventures into the politics of medical treatment have attracted a good deal of scholarly attention, the organization's work with religious communities has been overlooked.[28]

Religion was not ACT UP's primary focus. But members' attempts to work with and against religious communities illustrated their awareness of the significance of religious power in the United States and its potential role—whether positive or negative—to shape the politics of public health, particularly in regard to the AIDS epidemic. ACT UP's protests against the Catholic Church represented the most striking example of this realization. These demonstrations also most clearly revealed ACT UP's own moral agenda: the dissemination of knowledge about HIV/AIDS that could save people's lives, including information about safe sex. This moral position was part of a broader commitment to a new ethics of safe sex that arose in gay, lesbian, and queer communities in response to the AIDS epidemic (Figure 4.2). Folded within this approach was an alternative moral stance regarding sex that privileged the sexual freedom of the individual and the public responsibility of state and local government to make available information about safe sex and access to health care.

Having Faith in ACT UP

ACT UP encountered religion in a number of ways, particularly through the backgrounds and practices of its members and through outreach to churches in minority communities. This background offers a portrait of ACT UP far different from the representation of anti-religious secularists painted by many of their opponents (and sometimes even by their own members). The demographic composition of ACT UP has garnered significant attention from members, critics, and academics alike. Most of these cases have focused on class, race, and gender diversity— or lack of diversity—that marked the organization and sparked arguments among its members.[29] Though ACT UP was democratic in ethos, racial minorities and women charged the larger group with various degrees of racism and sexism, from blatant discrimination to more subtle forms of prejudice. For instance, some women and people of color highlighted that white male members framed minority issues as distractions from what they took as the more important work of the group regarding AIDS treatment and activism.[30] The demographic close up: makeup of ACT UP reflected this imbalance.

Sociologist Gilbert Elbaz conducted a formal survey of over four hundred ACT UP members in the summer of 1989 that offers a useful demographic profile.[31] Whites accounted for a little less than 80% (324 members) of the respondents, and almost the same number were male (329 members). Women constituted 19.5% (80 members). African Americans accounted for 5.6% (23) of members, and 2.4% (10) identified as Hispanic.[32] As one might expect, the overwhelming majority identified as gay, lesbian, or homosexual; most were middle-class and had some college education. The racial, sexual, and class politics of ACT UP deserve the attention they have received, but the organization's religious makeup has received little notice. The religious demographics of ACT UP provide a snapshot of its membership only months before the Stop the Church demonstration.

The survey asked participants both for their religion of birth and their current religious preference.[33] Almost a third (32.4%, or 134 members) claimed to have been born and raised Catholic, 29.3% (121) Protestant, 17.2% (71) Jewish, and 7.7% (32) listed no religion. The current religious preferences of members illustrate a clear drop-off in the number who identified as religious, as 48% (201 members) cited no religious preference at all. But a significant portion of members did retain a religious affiliation: 23.5% (97) claimed they now had their own personal religion, 8.5% (35) identified as Jewish, and 6.5% (27) said they were Catholic. That a solid 38.5% (159 members) continued to identify as religious is important to point out for a group often represented as secular, if not hostile toward religion.[34] The relatively high percentage of respondents who indicated having a "personal religion" follows a broader historical trend in American society after the Second World War, and especially since the 1960s. Over these decades, Americans moved away from organized religions toward what they described as personal forms of spirituality, a shift captured in the commonly heard line "I'm spiritual but not religious." We might consider this shift not a decline in American religion, but a transformation in the way that religion was practiced and understood. Members of ACT UP very much mirrored this demographic shift, even if they also tended to identify as non-religious at higher rates than the broader American population.[35]

Beyond these demographic markers, several members of ACT UP recognized the importance of religion in American public life. Members of the Majority Action Committee, which was formed to address the specific needs of people of color, reached out to religious leaders in the African American community, visiting churches in Harlem to speak out about the AIDS epidemic. These churches provided a gateway to get their message across about HIV prevention and activism to much of the city's black population.[36] African American ACT UP member and legal scholar Kendall Thomas, who was raised in an evangelical household, recounted his work with the churches as one of his proudest moments with the organization:

> It was very moving to me, to be in a little church called the Philadelphia Baptist Church in Harlem, during ACT NOW—the Nine Days of AIDS Action. And to have been a facilitator—I guess that's a good term—of some of the first conversations in that little congregation, in which people felt that they could acknowledge that they either had AIDS, or that people in their family were sick, or that people in their family had died—so that people could name and acknowledge to one another, in that context, particularly, which, because of my autobiography, meant a lot to me.[37]

Kendall discussed the problems educators faced in convincing communities to acknowledge the prevalence of HIV/AIDS. His work in Harlem was "an early effort in that project," he stated:

> And it wasn't a typical ACT UP action. And, as I said, there was a very small group of people who were involved. I remember Maria Maggenti being one of the people who sort of stood in the corner, there, with the 1-in-61 poster that Gran Fury had developed. I think it may have been their first poster—certainly one of their first posters. And, that possibility—taking the resources within a predominantly white, well educated, if not well off, comfortable community and using those resources to do work in other communities meant more to me than anything else.[38]

The Majority Action Committee's work with churches in Harlem suggests ACT UP members' willingness to work with religious organizations, especially as a pragmatic method to disseminate information about HIV/AIDS. But ACT UP is still best known not for such cooperation, but for its opposition to the city's Catholic hierarchy.

Leading up to the December demonstration, AIDS activist Larry Kramer already had a run-in with Cardinal O'Connor. While giving a testimony before the hearings of the Presidential Commission on HIV in Washington, D.C., Kramer introduced himself as a co-founder of GMHC and ACT UP. The former was the first and largest AIDS organization up to that point, and the second a direct-action group, Kramer explained, "that pickets, among others, the White House, *The Saturday Evening Post*, St. Patrick's Cathedral, and is at this moment picketing outside this meeting itself."[39] In this testimony, Kramer decried the poor state of AIDS research and funding. He pleaded for the committee to include the participation of the gay community in its proposed solutions, asking them to "Let us help!"[40]

Kramer derided the committee's lack of credibility on AIDS. Most members, he accused, had been cited in the media "saying something offensive about gay people."[41] While expecting little from the commission, Kramer continued, "We pray this will be one of those rare and precious and God-inspired occasions," in which "the most unlikely heroes have emerged and triumphed over their perceived images." Kramer ended his speech in his typical, if controversial, style. "In closing," he continued, staring directly into Cardinal O'Connor's eyes:

> I would like to remind you of a few gay people who are part of your history, too. Leonardo Da Vinci, who painted *The Last Supper*. Michelangelo, who painted the Sistine Chapel and sculpted the most beloved *Pieta*. King James I, who undertook the most famous translation of the Bible. St. Augustine. Cardinal Newman. Cardinal Spellman. Pop Julius II. Pope Paul VI. Pope Benedict IX. Pope Sixtus IV. Pope John XXII. Pope Alexander VI. Pope Julius III. Joan of Arc. Thank you.[42]

Kramer's speech was an indictment—and of O'Connor most of all. But it was also a unique lesson (even if not quite historically accurate) for how we tell the history of the Catholic Church and homosexuality, one in which the two were not at odds. Kramer's closing thoughts betrayed a glimpse of optimism concerning the past and future relationship between homosexuality and religion. That glimmer of hope was dashed when the American bishops released "Called to Compassion," condemning discussion of contraception in any aspect of AIDS education, including both public programs and those sponsored by the Catholic Church. ACT UP's most memorable foray into religious politics would shortly follow. It would be staged not in Washington, D.C., but on New York's Fifth Avenue: O'Connor's home turf.

Stopping the Church

"Stop killing us! Stop killing us!" a protestor cried out. He held his hands up to his face to project his voice, straining as it pierced the stale silence of the cathedral.[43] He was standing in St. Patrick's Cathedral, a historic landmark in New York City. It was also the seat of one of the Catholic Church's most powerful prelates and the target of his imperative: Cardinal John J. O'Connor. It was December 10, 1989, the second week of Advent. Around 4,500 demonstrators had marched down Fifth Avenue earlier that morning holding signs reading "Condoms, not prayer," "Keep your church out of my crotch," and "Keep your rosaries off my ovaries!"[44]

While protesters amassed outside the cathedral, about one hundred activists entered St. Patrick's, where they passed out their own programs to parishioners explaining why they had come. O'Connor expected the demonstration, which ACT UP and WHAM! had announced in advance. Police stationed themselves inside and outside of the cathedral, and the cardinal made copies of his homily in advance, in case he would not be able to complete it from the pulpit. Along with other political leaders, the outgoing mayor, Ed Koch, a friend and ally of the cardinal, attended in a show of support.

The service proceeded without disruption until O'Connor began his homily. A couple minutes in, protesters started falling to the floor of the aisles. Their mass die-in symbolized the needless deaths from AIDS that continued in large measure, they maintained, because of the Catholic Church's opposition to condom use. Others began shouting to O'Connor from the pews, "You're murdering us!" and "Stop it! Stop it! Stop it!" Police started removing demonstrators. As one woman was carried out, she yelled out to the parishioners looking on: "We're fighting for your lives, too!"[45] In perhaps the most infamous act during the demonstration, at least one activist, a younger gay man and former altar boy, crumbled a Communion wafer and threw it to the floor. By the end of the service, police had arrested 111 activists, including 43 from within the cathedral, many of them carried out on orange stretchers as they remained, faithfully, dead.

Figuring Protest

The demonstration at St. Patrick's Cathedral was not an isolated incident, but part of a series of protests stretching into the early 1990s that challenged the Catholic Church's positions on condoms, homosexuality, and abortion. But even the first protest was not without precedent. O'Connor had proven a controversial religious and political figure almost immediately upon taking up his post as Archbishop of New York. Years before Stop the Church, gay activist Andrew Humm and members of the Coalition for Gay and Lesbian Rights had begun protesting outside St. Patrick's, criticizing O'Connor for stepping out of bounds by meddling in political affairs. The Lavender Hill Mob had also organized protests against O'Connor in the years leading up to the Stop the Church demonstration. Members took note of the cardinal's vocal support for the Vatican when it stripped Seattle's relatively gay-friendly Archbishop Raymond Hunthausen of his authority. The Mob also grew angry when O'Connor dismissed Charles Curran of his teaching duties at Catholic University, deeming his positions on sexuality and abortion too liberal. They staged a protest against O'Connor at the Alfred E. Smith Memorial Dinner held at the Waldorf-Astoria Hotel in New York. And following Cardinal Ratzinger's description of homosexuality as "an intrinsic moral evil" in his 1986 letter, the Mob held a demonstration at St. Patrick's Cathedral, in which nine members walked out, hand in hand, during O'Connor's homily.[46]

O'Connor's reputation within the gay and lesbian community only worsened when he stopped allowing the gay Catholic group Dignity to hold meetings at the cathedral.[47] In accordance with Ratzinger's 1986 letter, no groups supporting the practice of homosexual activity could use church property to hold meetings. To oppose this decision, some members of Dignity formed the Cathedral Project, a direct-action group that protested monthly outside of St. Patrick's. At his bequest, the city granted O'Connor an injunction to ban the protesters from the area immediately outside the church, forcing them to move across the street.[48]

Even more disappointing for many AIDS activists were two meetings held by the Catholic leadership in 1989 to discuss the church's response to the AIDS crisis. On November 13, 1989, O'Connor opened the Vatican's first meeting on AIDS by condemning the use of condoms and needle exchange programs as means to curb the spread of HIV.[49] The Vatican conference followed shortly after the Catholic bishops of the United States approved a statement urging chastity rather than the use of condoms in

HIV prevention. The statement, "Called to Compassion," departed from the previous, more moderate approach taken in "Many Faces of AIDS," which disapproved of the use of condoms but nonetheless allowed for education about prophylactics within the broader context of Catholic moral tradition.[50] O'Connor found himself among a growing cadre of conservative bishops who opposed the first statement for failing to adhere to what he considered traditional Catholic teachings on sexuality. As many gay activists understood it, the Catholic Church was not merely calling for a moratorium on condom use but was condemning any form of sexuality outside of monogamous, heterosexual marriage: in effect, attacking homosexuality and interfering with activists' efforts to save lives through HIV/AIDS prevention.

Alongside the Catholic Church's hardened public opposition to homosexual behavior and condom use, the American bishops renewed their opposition to abortion at their November 1989 meeting, providing yet another reason for protestors to organize. During the second day of the annual meeting of the National Council of Catholic Bishops—the same meeting in which "Called to Compassion" was approved—three hundred Catholic leaders engaged in an animated discussion of abortion. Cardinal Joseph Bernardin of Chicago, who chaired the anti-abortion activities committee, introduced a new anti-abortion resolution that easily passed. According to Bernardin, the bishops' long-term goal was to pass a human life amendment that would grant the fullest possible constitutional protection for the unborn child. Moreover, he noted, the statement defined life as starting with conception, using language "to counter the idea that a 'pro-choice' stance can be a responsible Catholic option."[51] The resolution upheld that "no Catholic can responsibly take a 'pro-choice' stand"—a controversial position given the number of Catholic politicians, particularly in the Democratic Party, who attempted to adhere to their faith while safeguarding constitutional protections for women's right to choose.[52] The new statement rumbled like thunder throughout New York, where O'Connor had already set the press and politicians on edge by making similar remarks a few years earlier. O'Connor ceded no gray area in Catholic theology regarding abortion and no opt-out clause for Catholic politicians who were either constitutionally or ideologically disposed to uphold pro-choice legislation. The cardinal had made his position quite clear when he insisted that Catholics "in good conscience cannot vote for a candidate who explicitly supports abortion."[53]

O'Connor sparked further controversy when he expressed his desire to join a protest with Operation Rescue. Founded in 1986, the pro-life organization received national attention after members began breaking laws to prevent women from gaining access to abortion procedures, including handcuffing themselves to clinic doors in order to block entry. In 1988, O'Connor praised Auxiliary Bishop Austin Vaughan of Orange County, New York for his participation in an Operation Rescue rally, during which he helped block the entrance to the Women's Suburban Clinic in Paoli, Pennsylvania.[54] In October of 1989, O'Connor replied to a query about how far he would go to shut down an abortion clinic: "I wish that I could go on a rescue." "I talked to my lawyers," he continued, "and their advice is that it would be inappropriate." O'Connor clarified his predicament: "What I have to weigh is if the value of my being arrested, and its visibility, would outweigh the possible jeopardy . . . of operations of the Archdiocese of New York."[55]

ACT UP member Vincent Gagliostro explained in an interview how O'Connor's support for Operation Rescue prompted him to co-organize the Stop the Church protest. That night, he was with his friend and fellow member Victor Mendolia in midtown Manhattan. "We are on the roof of his building, completely bombed out of our minds, screaming off the top," Gagliostro recalled, "because Cardinal O'Connor had just said some hideous thing about something—I think it was the abortion thing. We were like, we know what we have to do. We have to have an ACT UP demonstration against St. Patrick's. That's how it started."[56] Following their conversation, Gagliostro and Mendolia presented their idea to the floor at an ACT UP meeting. It drew few objections at first, but as they proceeded to explain possible plans for the demonstration, members began to worry about "the whole notion of offending" members of the religious community.[57]

Gagliostro, who grew up attending Catholic schools in New Jersey, admitted it was difficult to organize the demonstration because he had to communicate with gay Catholic members of Dignity: "I was sitting there totally respecting what they had to say but not understanding how they could participate in a religion that hates them." "When you are coming from that place, it's very difficult for someone like me to be concerned about offending people," Gagliostro explained, "because I'm offended." He noted that even Victor and he did not have to be talked out of protesting *inside* the cathedral, especially since the protest was never against the lay people in the church to begin with. In fact, the name of the protest—"Stop the Church"—first met with many objections. The other phrase under consideration was "Stop This Man." The demonstration, Gagliostro remarked, "was really a demonstration against Cardinal O'Connor much like a demonstration citing Koch as an enemy of Albany."[58] From the very beginning, ACT UP members acknowledged the potential controversy surrounding the protest and attempted to clarify its focus on the Catholic hierarchy and Cardinal O'Connor in particular.

Given O'Connor's recent comments regarding abortion, ACT UP members decided to co-organize the demonstration with WHAM! As Gagliostro explained, this was "kind of challenging for ACT UP because ACT UP is not an organization whose purpose is to deal with abortion rights." But, he continued, "it was kind of easily decided that you just couldn't have a demonstration against the Catholic Church if that wasn't an issue."[59] At meetings on the floor, members discussed the ramifications of the protest and placed it in historical perspective. One member recounted previous demonstrations at churches, explaining how in 1872 blacks were banned from a Catholic church in Connecticut and told to go to a Baptist service down the road. Not content with this, black Catholics protested the next Sunday and "stopped the church." Then at the turn of the century, she continued, women at Seneca Falls were banned from meeting in a church, so they protested during Communion. "People have been stopping the church for a long time," she pleaded—we're "not doing anything radical!"[60] Placing Stop the Church in a broader historical trajectory allowed this activist to script the demonstration as part of a longer struggle for civil rights and as a form of religious protest in itself.

According to Gagliostro, ACT UP officially only organized the protest outside the cathedral. Affinity groups led the demonstration inside. They included members who knew their actions "couldn't be brought to the floor of ACT UP because they would know that they were going to do them. It was like left up to the people who wanted to do what they wanted to do to just do it."[61] While ACT UP members did consider protesting within the cathedral, we had decided "we don't want to know about it."[62] Indeed, Gagliostro asserted, ACT UP never formally intended to disrupt the Mass, a point that his interviewer and fellow ACT UP member Sarah Schulman (who took part in the demonstration) had not even known until he mentioned it. In other words, ACT UP "officially" had nothing to do with the protests inside the cathedral, with one exception: ACT UP printed a facsimile of the church program that was handed out to parishioners as they entered the building.

An "Action Update" regarding Stop the Church supports Gagliostro's recollection. "OUR TARGETS," it stated, "are John Cardinal O'Connor and the Catholic church hierarchy," and the key issues are "safer sex education, condoms and needles, abortion, homophobia, and violence against gays and lesbians." "Our underlying issues," the update continued, "are freedom of choice, the right to control our own bodies, and the separation of church and state." The statement outlined the scenario for the demonstration, calling for participants to gather "in 'mass'" in front of the cathedral at 9:30am, with the protest culminating in a mass die-in *outside* the church. The update only then included a section for "Affinity Groups" that described actions that might take place inside the cathedral. It cautioned potential demonstrators to consider the political and legal ramifications of such actions, before suggesting the best time to begin their protest:

> It is recommended that affinity groups that wish to participate in civil disobedience inside the cathedral consider all the political ramifications of such an action as well as the legal situation around the cathedral. Affinity groups may wish to time their actions to coincide with the homily of the mass—the time when O'Connor gives his sermon. This will help to isolate O'Connor as the target of the action, as opposed to the people gathered for worship that day.[63]

The statement betrays ACT UP's expectation for some form of protest inside the cathedral, as it guided readers toward the proper time to perform their unnamed "actions." It emphasized that members of affinity groups should begin their acts of civil disobedience during O'Connor's homily to underscore to their protest against him, rather than the lay parishioners.[64]

ACT UP and WHAM! advertised widely in preparation for the demonstration. They sent out mailings to organizations sympathetic to their cause, placed advertisements in local newspapers like the *Village Voice*, *OutWeek*, and college newspapers, and wheat-pasted fliers throughout the city (see Figures 4.3 to 4.5). Organizers also sent press kits to local television stations and newspapers outlining their reasons for the protest.[65] In the month leading up to the event, ACT UP media coordinator Jay Blotcher released weekly media advisory updates and letters to the press.[66] In one letter, the organizers explained the purpose of their action was "to protest the Church's interference in city, state and federal AIDS and abortion policies." The demonstration "comes on the heels of the October [*sic*] meeting

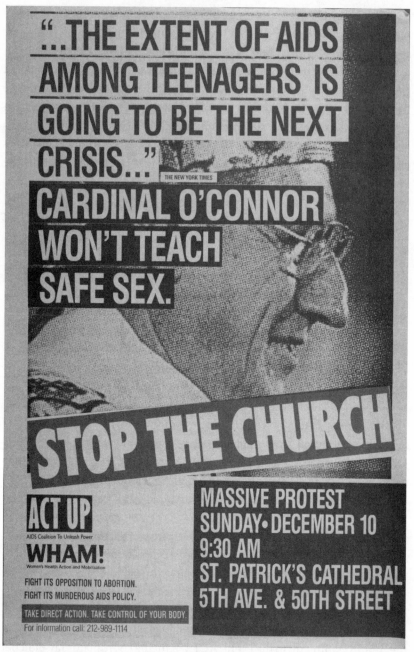

FIGURE 4.3 ACT UP New York's Stop the Church flier: "'The extent of AIDS among teenagers is going to be the next crisis': Cardinal O'Connor won't teach safe sex." (Held in the ACT UP/NY Records, New York Public Library Digital Gallery.)

in Baltimore," where the Bishops opposed education about condoms, and "the recent Vatican AIDS conference, where cardinals spent their time criticizing gays and IV drug users," they argued, "rather than concentrating on steps to educate people at risk and foster compassion for the sick." ACT UP and WHAM! have joined together, the letter proclaimed, "to send Cardinal O'Connor and the Church hierarchy a clear message: Stop peddling moralizing as legislature."[67]

A separate media advisory alert described the die-in planned outside the cathedral, which would be "complete with colorful placards and costumes." But this statement also noted that Operation Rescue, identified as the "radical anti-abortion group [that] has repeatedly defied a court injunction against its sit-ins at abortion clinics across the nation," had announced it would be present to challenge the Stop the Church demonstration. The report repeated the issues of concern, which it summarized as the "assault of gays and lesbians," the need for "education, not moralizing," and "a woman's right" to her own body. "We are marching on the Church to show the Cardinal and his fanatic followers that their religious bullying infringes on the personal rights of all Americans," read an update from one of the lead organizers, Victor Mendolia: "Moralizing is not a substitute for education and religious doctrine is not political policy."[68]

A week before the demonstration, ACT UP and WHAM! issued a letter to the parishioners of St. Patrick's Cathedral. "We are activist groups concerned about the rights of women, lesbian and gay people, and people with AIDS," it announced: "We are also concerned about education and healthcare as they pertain to all people." Activists anticipated the anxieties parishioners might have about the protest: "You may be wondering why we have chosen Saint Patrick's Cathedral as our focal point. It is after all, your place of worship." The letter acknowledged, "We are aware of this, and yet, we ask for your understanding and participation." It cited O'Connor's support for Operation Rescue and his encouragement that "all good Catholics" join these illegal pro-life protests. The letter to parishioners also recalled Saint Patrick's silence every year during the Gay Pride March. The annual march included two minutes of silence to commemorate people who had died of AIDS. To show their respect, churches throughout the city would break that silence by ringing their bells in unison. "Missing from that polyphony," ACT UP and WHAM! informed the parishioners, "are the bells of Saint Patrick's."[69]

The letter further expressed worry concerning the recent Vatican AIDS conference and the Catholic Church's stance against condoms, abortion, and euthanasia. Underlining these issues was Cardinal O'Connor's active role in city politics, the activists declared, including his threat to excommunicate Governor Cuomo for his pro-choice stance on abortion. The separation of church and state, the letter insisted, is best for everybody, including Catholics. "Religious freedom is dependent on a separation of church and state," it reasoned, since it would be impossible to allow one religion to be made into law without "undermining our entire system of government." "We oppose the punishment of Catholic people for having political beliefs that differ from those of the church hierarchy," the letter concluded, attempting to strike a patriotic chord of solidarity: "Separation of church and state is in all of our best interests."[70]

Following the protest, Gay Men's Health Crisis issued a statement applauding the protesters' impulse to act. "We are in complete sympathy with the rage and pain that motivated the protesters," it read, "and feel that the need for direct action has never been more urgent than now." But GMHC distanced itself from the specific actions that took place inside the cathedral, which "shifted public attention [away] from the real issues raised by Cardinal O'Connor's damaging positions and actions on AIDS." On the basis of this reason alone, the organization claimed, the protest was a "mistake." The bulk of GMHC's statement, however, focused on making an even stronger case against O'Connor. It underscored the cardinal's disregard for the "well-documented fact" that condoms help to prevent the transmission of HIV. "If the Cardinal cannot accept scientific facts about AIDS," GMHC warned, "he should stay out of the debate. And if he makes political statements, he must accept a political response."[71] The GMHC statement offered a somewhat different argument against O'Connor's participation in the AIDS debate than that offered by ACT UP. GMHC declared a new baseline for entering public discussion about HIV/AIDS, which was a common respect for scientific facts. In making this case, their statement drew a line between science and politics that many AIDS activists, including members of ACT UP, already considered not merely tenuous, but also impossible to sustain. For ACT UP, science was political: and in this case, so too was religion.

ACT UP tried to preempt negative media coverage by issuing a position statement. It explained that while O'Connor had presented himself as a hapless victim, ACT UP would not apologize for the actions of protesters against a religious institution that "limits the rights of all Americans to make personal decisions in their own lives." The statement affirmed the cardinal's right to his own personal religious beliefs and to teach those beliefs to members of his church, but it decried "'church leaders' oppressive public policies" that affected the broader community, including the rights of teenagers to receive comprehensive sex education (including AIDS education) as a component in the public school curriculum, access to condoms and birth control, and women's rights to their bodies.[72]

ACT UP also addressed the demonstration inside that church, which garnered the most mainstream media attention. "Individual ACT UP and WHAM members who chose to enter the church—a number of them Catholics and People With AIDS—were not trying to deny parishioners' right to worship," explained the position statement. Rather, it continued,

> these demonstrators felt so strongly about the issues that they needed to make this peaceful, non-violent political statement— some silently, some vocally—in the place where Cardinal O'Connor himself has made so many dangerous and misguided political statements. They entered peacefully, as members of the congregation, and were greeted by a sea of uniformed police officers.[73]

Reflecting on the protest years later, Gagliostro noted, "We had no idea that that many people were going to show up. And it's one of those demonstrations where I think, sitting here today, once again I can say, 'We were right.'"[74] Gagliostro and other members of ACT UP defended the righteous cause of their protest, but any victories may have been pyrrhic at best. The media storm that followed Stop the Church depicted a demonstration steeped not in the patriotic values of religious freedom and the promotion of sexual and women's rights, but one acted out in childish anger through acts of sacrilege and defined by extreme positions hardly recognizable as American at all.

Re-Presenting Protest in the Mainstream Media

ACT UP had gained a great deal of media experience from earlier protests and often proved skillful in gaining sympathetic coverage. Despite sending out media kits ahead of Stop the Church to explain their goals, however, activists found mainstream coverage of the demonstration siding against them. Organizers of the protest recorded a variety of common problems in media coverage of the event, like calling protesters "gay activists" instead of "AIDS activists," concentrating on the demonstrations inside the cathedral rather than the larger protest outside and the major issues that had brought them there, and interviewing mostly worshippers who opposed the activists' cause.[75] Their worries were well placed. While the protest made front-page news the next day in three of New York's daily papers, it was not received well.[76]

New York City's major newspapers framed the protest as an issue of religious freedom and focused on the disturbance of the service within the cathedral. They depicted the demonstration not merely as a political quarrel, but as an unreasonable act of sacrilege, a violation of personal freedom, and even a protest against religion itself. The editors of *New York Newsday* regretted that innocent parishioners "who came to St. Patrick's Cathedral to pray undisturbed and hear the sermon last Sunday never got a chance."[77] In "The Storming of St. Pat's," the liberal-leaning *New York Times* supported the right to peaceful protests outside the cathedral but remarked that "some of the demonstrators turned honorable dissent into dishonorable disruption." The editors tethered the "offensive" actions of the protestors to the very "ideas" behind the demonstration. "To deny clergy and laity alike the peaceful practice of religion," the editorial continued, "grossly violates decent regard for the rights of others, let alone the law. Far from inspiring sympathy, such a violation mainly offers another reason to reject both the offensive protesters and their ideas."[78] For the *Times*, the corruption of the messengers and of the message proved one and the same.

The often sensationalist *New York Post* depicted an "invasion" of St. Patrick's by activists who "seemed set on confirming every possible negative cliché about homosexual extremism." Its editorial described how activists carried signs with racy, sexualized slogans, while "many made the charge, striking in its falsity, that the Catholic Church is killing people." The editors upheld O'Connor's position on the moral limits of safe sex: "In a city plagued by soaring rates of illegitimate births and AIDS transmission, the cardinal's moral message has a powerful resonance; perhaps at no time in the city's history has such a message seemed more pertinent." The cardinal's slogan, "'Good medicine is good morality,'" the article quipped, "displays far more insight into human nature than 'Condoms, not prayer,'" as the signs of several protesters read.[79]

Coverage was no friendlier outside of New York. The *San Francisco Chronicle*'s initial coverage of the protest was mostly descriptive. But the following day the paper issued an editorial that declared the disruption of Catholic Church services, "whether by abortion rights activists or AIDS protesters," to be "despicable, intolerable acts." It described protestors as

AIDS "militants" targeting O'Connor and his church. While acknowledging the "well-intentioned sincerity of at least some of the demonstrators," the editorial concluded that such acts of protest would hurt the AIDS activist movement in the long run.[80] Randy Shilts, writing for the *San Francisco Chronicle*, also criticized the protest. He wondered whether the demonstration in New York, along with similar actions occurring about the same time in Los Angeles and San Francisco, were planned by "some diabolical reactionary group dedicated to discrediting the gay community."[81]

Shilts explained to readers why activists had gone after the Catholic Church. He cited the religious institution's opposition to condom use and gay rights, including its role in defeating San Francisco's domestic partnership bill the month before. "That, however, does not give gay protesters the prerogative to deny Catholics their rights," Shilts maintained, "including the right to worship and the right of their leaders to deliver whatever pronouncements they like without having to worry about the intimidation of vandals. It is not only morally wrong to violate these rights—it is strategically stupid." Finally, Shilts tied the protests to "a long, ugly tradition of anti-Catholic prejudice," the undercurrents of which "are certainly present in the rhetoric of some of the AIDS protesters."[82]

AIDS, Stop the Church, and Anti-Catholicism

The charge of anti-Catholicism resonated among Catholics in New York City. In his Editor's Report for *Catholic New York*, the weekly newspaper of the archdiocese, George Costello described the scene he witnessed upon arriving at St. Patrick's the morning of the demonstration. A crowd of almost a hundred members, mostly young men, paraded down 5th Avenue holding placards that carried "filthy" inscriptions he could not bring himself to repeat. "Just imagine the worst," he instructed his readers, "and you've pretty much got it." The protesters chanted demands that the Catholic Church "teach safe sex." "Based on what I saw and heard," Costello wrote, "I think that both their ability to hate and their preoccupation with sex must border on the limitless. It was hard to tell which they hated more, the Church or Cardinal O'Connor." The demonstrations outside the cathedral proved "vile," "disgusting," and "supremely insulting," yet "all that happened outside the Cathedral, gross as it might have been, was merely a preamble for the outrages committed inside." Because of their seating arrangements, he explained, most of the press was fortunate to be blocked from witnessing the worst of the demonstration inside. Less lucky was a man caught in the middle of the protest inside the cathedral, who described the anguish of the parishioners: "'We cried,' he told a priest friend of mine. 'Everybody around me was crying. How can this be going on?'" In a claim repeated in a few Catholic accounts, he continued, "The sacred host was violated at least seven times, not just once," as it had been reported elsewhere.[83] Costello framed the protest as a wholly unreasonable attack against the church, one that resulted not merely in a momentary disruption, but a scene too awful to detail. Moreover, he noted the distortions already occurring in media accounts, which downplayed the number of times the host was desecrated. Like ACT UP, some Catholics faulted the press for its unfair coverage, though they accused media of being pro-secular and blind to (if not colluding with) rampant acts of anti-Catholicism.

The same issue of *Catholic New York* ran a detailed story of the protest titled, "Unfair, Unjustified and Offensive," which included O'Connor's response. "I pray that this doesn't happen again," he stated, "but if it happens again and again and again, the Mass will go on or I will be dead . . . It would have to be over my dead body that the Mass will not go on." The cardinal refused to budge on his moral position: "No demonstration is going to bring about any kind of yielding on my part," he stated: "I'm the Archbishop of New York and I have to teach what the Church teaches." O'Connor felt "very sad" for the protesters themselves. "There was clearly so much hatred," he lamented: "I honestly feel deeply sad when people hate, whomever they hate and for whatever reason. It's not that they hate me. That's not the important part. But I think all hatred is destructive and it primarily destroys the hater, not the person hated."[84]

O'Connor recognized the intentions of the protesters, including their disagreement about the effectiveness of condoms. But he maintained that promoting condom use would be "irresponsible," since it would "worsen rather than lessen the epidemic." After his homily was drowned out by protesters, the cardinal stopped speaking and invited worshippers to stand and pray as he recited the prayers "Our Father," "Hail Mary," and "Glory Be to the Father," along with a decade of the Rosary. O'Connor concluded his response by placing the Catholic Church within the American tradition of religious freedom, a tradition flouted by the AIDS protestors. "One thing that is prized by the people of the United States," he explained, "is that every religious group is permitted to worship peacefully within its sanctuary."[85]

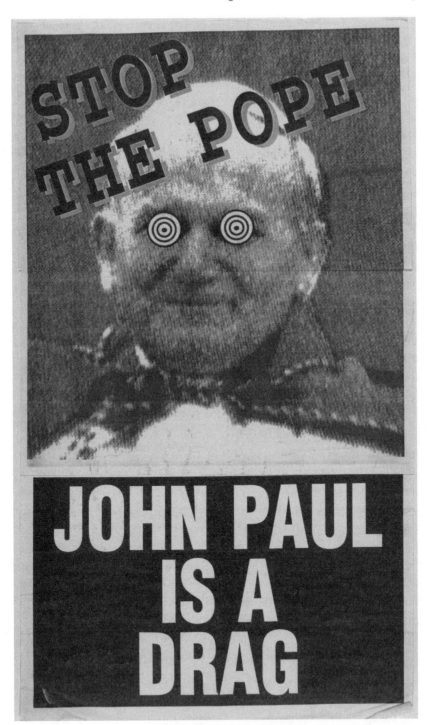

FIGURE 4.4 ACT UP New York's "Stop the Pope: John Paul is a drag" poster. (Held in the ACT UP/NY Records, New York Public Library Digital Gallery.)

Catholic New York also reported condemnations of the protest from other religious leaders. They too represented the demonstration as an offense against the practice of religious freedom by positioning limitless, anti-church gay activists against both religion and freedom. A statement by six major Jewish organizations stated: "The right to worship, unimpeded, is one of the most important freedoms enjoyed by all Americans ... (therefore) interference with worship services inside St. Patrick's Cathedral cannot be tolerated."[86] Rabbi Henry D. Michelman, executive president of the Synagogue Council of America, agreed. "This incursion into the church sanctuary, irrespective of the issues involved," he added, "violated other people's rights and was therefore unfair, unjustified and offensive." Richard F. Grein, Bishop of the Episcopal Diocese of New York, wrote a statement that other Christian leaders signed onto. "We are appalled by this singularly unacceptable extension of civil disobedience," it declared: "regardless of how we may feel about the reasons underlying the demonstrators' protest or about their right to exercise free speech, we cannot condone and must condemn this interruption of a service of worship, this denial of religious freedom."[87] For these religious leaders, the purposes for the protest were beside the point. In their accounts, nothing could be worse than the disruption of religious practice, which they understood as both a sacred act and a constitutional freedom. The demonstrators assaulted both.

But such condemnations did not arise only from religious groups. *Catholic New York* quoted members of the gay community who also opposed the demonstration. According to Andrew Humm, speaking on behalf of the Coalition for Lesbian and Gay Rights, "It was horrifying. We endorsed the demonstration outside the cathedral, but the point was lost by what happened inside. We condemn the acts of people who disrupt worship services."[88] Coverage of the protest continued the following week. Journalist Mary Ann Poust described it as "an unruly demonstration by homosexual and pro-abortion activists [who] disrupted Cardinal O'Connor's homily and caused general chaos."[89] She reported that at least three other AIDS activist and gay and lesbian rights groups had criticized the protest. Robert Pusilo, the head of Dignity, called the disruption of the Mass a "desecration." Other critics included Humm, cited the week before, and Timothy Sweeney, deputy director of Gay Men's Health Crisis. The Catholic paper suggested to its readers that ACT UP was little more than a radical, anti-religious fringe group. Even members of their own community condemned these acts, it reported: yet the demonstrators offered "no apologies."[90]

These discussions in *Catholic New York* simplified the gay response, though, since most gay rights groups did not offer a blanket criticism of the protest. They disapproved of only some of the actions that occurred inside of the cathedral that were—at least according to ACT UP—not part of the planned demonstration.[91] But in a larger sense, the damage had already been done. Articles such as "Unfair, Unjustified and Offensive" offered an important intervention in the history of the reception of Stop the Church. *Catholic New York* invoked the quintessential American ideal of religious freedom, which, as the paper demonstrated, was trampled by the protesters. It depicted the activists, by contrast, as anti-religious and un-American. Letters written by readers of *Catholic New York* suggest the widespread circulation of this interpretation of the protest and illustrate the historically informed sensitivity many Catholics had toward acts that could be construed as targeting their faith.[92]

Readers of the archdiocesan newspaper roundly condemned the protest and lamented the desecration of the Communion wafer.[93] Mariann Beals of Brooklyn wrote, "I was horrified and deeply grieved by the outrage committed in St. Patrick's Dec. 10 by so-called activists. Especially terrible was the direct insult to the Eucharist." She clarified, "this spells out what such people are doing: attacking God himself."[94] Barbara Braum, president of the Rockland County Coalition of Lay Catholics for Life in Nyack, New York, read about the sacrilege with "profound sorrow and dismay," calling it "a day that will go down in the annals of Church history as a day of shame and monstrous evil." She located the protest in the legacy of American anti-Catholicism. "We pray for an end to the bigotry and prejudice against the Church in America," she wrote: "We hope for fair treatment in the media of the Catholic Church, which has contributed so much to America."[95] Richard D. McKeon of Lake Peekskill added to this sentiment. He read the protest as part of a larger anti-Christian trend in the emerging culture wars. "There are many anti-Christian groups in this country with one purpose," he wrote: "to silence the edifying effects of our religion, aided and abetted by many Catholics with political aspirations who have watered down Catholicism to placate the secularists."[96] Edward Scully, writing from the Bronx, likewise interpreted the protest as yet another example of anti-Catholicism. "Something must be done!" he pleaded. "Remember the old days, when the Know-Nothings tried similar tricks?" Scully continued: "Archbishop Hughes organized his Irish immigrant congregation to drive them away. It succeeded!"[97]

Father Benedict J. Groeschel, C.F.R. offered one of the most developed readings of the protest in the pages of *Catholic New York*. He served as director of the Archdiocesan Office for Spiritual Development and was one of the founders of Courage, the Catholic Church's approved support group (and alternative to Dignity) for people with same-sex attractions who vowed to be celibate to conform to church teaching on homosexuality. Groeschel recounted his experience at two different protests. On December 9, he attended an "aborutary" in Englewood, New Jersey, and the next day he witnessed the Stop the Church protest at St. Patrick's.[98] At the first demonstration a group of women, including several nuns, blocked the entrance to a place "where the lives of unborn defenseless children are terminated." The police appeared uncomfortable handcuffing nuns and "prying grandmothers out of the crowd," but the mayor of the town maintained a smile on his face. Groeschel took this smile as a sign that the mayor enjoyed the task of breaking apart the protest as he directed his troops. He invoked the civil rights movement to characterize the first protest. "Shades of Jackson, Miss., in the 60s!" he exclaimed. At one point, a "frightened looking black girl" came into view, appearing "confused and embarrassed." An African American gospel choir sang "Were you there when you crucified my Lord?" as she darted past them to enter the building, where, Groeschel wrote, she would "choose death rather than life." But she was "also a victim," he explained, "as were the police officers and even the pro-abortion demonstrators who were as deceived as the crowds at the Nuremberg rallies," all "deceived into thinking that some human beings have no rights at all."[99]

Groeschel compared this scene to the protest at St. Patrick's, during which "demonstrators were dressed up as devils, satanic bishops with obscenities written on phony miters." He recounted in detail the now-infamous scene inside the cathedral. After the initial disturbance during the service had settled, he began to distribute Communion. Groeschel was "particularly moved" by the opportunity "to give the body of Christ to several members of Courage." Then suddenly "something very strange happened [. . .] an event both horrifying and pitiful," Groeschel continued: "A conservatively dressed man in his 20s took the sacred Host from me, lifted his hand and quietly said, 'This is what I think of your God,' and he crushed the Host allowing the particles to fall on to the floor." This young man, Groeschel urged, was himself "a victim of the evil." He was "deceived into choosing a curse rather than a blessing as the young woman in Englewood had been deceived into choosing death rather than life." Groeschel then asked his readers to consider their own passive roles in going along with "the moral decline of our country."[100] He placed complacent Catholics in the same potential trajectory of national moral decline as the poor black girl and the misguided man who desecrated the Communion wafer. Good Catholics, too, could be swept into the moral decline of the nation, if they were not careful to uphold the church's moral stances regarding abortion and sexuality, not only for themselves, but for all Americans.

A far more forceful renunciation of the demonstration appeared in the politically conservative *Fidelity Magazine* in J. Joseph Garvey's essay, "The Homofascist Invasion of St. Patrick's Cathedral."[101] Garvey served as executive secretary to the Ad Hoc Alliance to Defend the Fourth Commandment, a group dedicated to fighting Opus Dei, of which Garvey formerly was a member. This essay stood out even among the most conservative Catholic responses, but it warrants consideration. Garvey provided one of the most detailed analyses of the demonstration and its position in the history of anti-Catholicism. And his essay was archived by members of ACT UP, suggesting a sense of what activists hoped to counter through their actions.

Garvey opened with a quotation from Adolf Hitler describing the "'almost mathematical certainty'" that a political campaign drawing on "'spiritual terror'" would succeed, "'particularly [among] the middle class, which is neither mentally nor morally equal to such attacks.'" This campaign of spiritual terror would unleash "'a veritable barrage of lies and slanders against whatever adversary seems most dangerous, until the nerves of the attacked person break down.'" According to Garvey, this quotation "could have been written by almost anyone" in America in the 1980s. But in this context, he claimed, that spiritual terror was directed toward leaders of the Catholic hierarchy and other moral traditionalists, whose pro-life positions had been abandoned by members of the government who had "Kooped-out," by "jumping the prolife ship."[102] For Garvey, direct attacks on the Catholic Church best illustrated this point, as bishops "have been subjected to a barrage of lies and slander." They had become targets of spiritual terror in anti-Catholic attacks that were "so chillingly reminiscent of the brown-shirted hooliganism of another era."[103]

The main perpetrators, Garvey declared, were the pro-choice and AIDS activists who demonstrated at St. Patrick's. Garvey described the activists as "radical homosexuals who crawled out from the dark underbelly of the 'gay rights' movement and slouched up Fifth Avenue toward St. Patrick's

Cathedral." The gay and lesbian community—which "includes all sexual aberration: bestiality, pederasty, sadomasochism, necrophilia, etc."—was "lashing out irrationally at the prelate who has done more for New York AIDS victims than any other non-governmental figure."[104] Garvey narrated how the service proceeded as normal until O'Connor began the homily. At that point, he wrote, "the homofascists struck, charging down the aisle shouting insults and obscenities."[105] Garvey repeated other critics' claim that seven or eight protesters had broken the host and thrown it to the floor, though the "secular media reported over and over that only one such incident occurred."[106]

Garvey cast the entire protest as yet another episode in the long history of anti-Catholicism. He recalled one of historian Arthur Schlesinger's arguments about the role of religion in John F. Kennedy's presidential election campaign. Kennedy could only become a viable candidate if he assured Americans that his Catholicism would never obstruct his political duties. A presidential candidate's need to qualify his Catholic faith in such a way revealed for Garvey "the deepest bias in the history of the American people"—that "the most luxuriant, tenacious tradition of paranoiac agitation has been anti-Catholicism." Garvey compared Catholics to other minority groups in the United States. Whereas blacks, Jews, women, and gays are fully expected to follow their identity-based political agendas, he argued, Catholics "are expected to do the reverse on issues involving their identity." When Catholics vote based on their Catholic faith, "they are immediately perceived as genuine threats to the civil religion, the 'American Way,'" he wrote.[107] Garvey's suggestion that prejudice against Catholics ranked historically above racial or gender oppression—or that it constituted "the deepest bias" in American history—was grossly exaggerated. But his argument about the need for Catholicism to change in order to fit within the strictures of American democracy, lest it pose a threat to it, warrants attention.

Garvey's complaint foreshadowed more recent—and granted more nuanced—scholarly arguments that secular democracies like the United States presume an often unacknowledged Protestant bias in defining what constitutes proper religion and the exercise of religious freedom. This bias is rooted in the history of modern liberal notions of individual freedom that emerged alongside and through Protestant understandings of religion as a matter of belief. Taken together, they have rendered religion an issue of private conscience more than one of public or political practice. This liberal understanding of religion, which has become

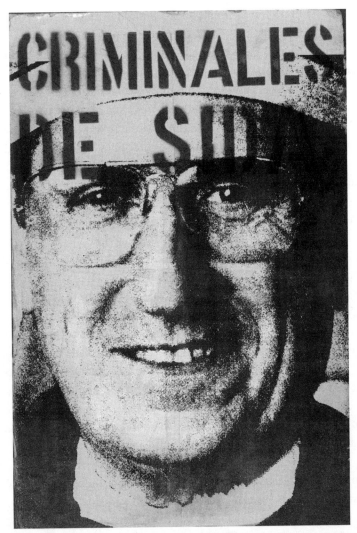

FIGURE 4.5 ACT UP New York's "Criminales de SIDA" poster featuring Cardinal O'Connor. (Held in the ACT UP/NY Records, New York Public Library Digital Gallery.)

commonsense for many Americans, also emerges from a longer history of exlusions. It arose in part from Enlightenment suspicions of emotional piety and church authority. The Scottish philosopher David Hume, for instance, famously derided the "enthusiasm" of some Protestant sects and the "superstition" of Catholics as "corruptions of true religion." The former were ruled by their passions, the later dependent upon the leaders of the church and their rituals. Enlightenment thinkers increasingly championed instead the importance of individual reason and personal autonomy. Religion deemed "good" in this understanding would be governed by rationality and restricted largely to personal belief—the path followed by modernist strains of Protestantism. These liberal assumptions about what constitutes "religion," and in turn "religious freedom," persist today, both in American law and in assumptions about the limited place of religion in the public sphere. They have even posed legal and cultural challenges for those who practice other models of religion, including some forms of Islam, Native American religions, evangelical Christianity, and Catholicism.[108]

Garvey saw this dynamic at work in pressures to keep the Catholic Church out of politics for the sake of democracy. "More widely understood by all Americans, but again never stated openly," Garvey contended, "is the fact that our Constitutional 'Doctrine' of the Separation of Church and State really means the segregation of the Catholic Church from real political influence." And worse, he continued, the "vast majority of American Catholics accept the American Arrangement," one that has allowed Catholics "political viability only if they stay in their assigned place, the back of the pluralistic bus."[109] Drawing on the liberal model, secular Americans, Protestants, and even some Catholics defined religion as private and nonpolitical and, thus, not a threat to the practice of secular democracy. To go against this model was to overstep an historically entrenched boundary. Garvey considered this boundary not merely unnecessary but a threat to Catholic tradition.

For Garvey, the politics of abortion epitomized this point. Pro-life groups like Operation Rescue "have become reprehensible to the establishment, not because of a disagreement on abortion," he argued, "but because they violate the truce so carefully fabricated by Catholic politicians [he mentions Mario Cuomo specifically] collaborating with those who hate the Church." Garvey collapsed the Stop the Church demonstrators into this larger mainstream as purveyors of anti-Catholic bias: "this country's Catholics were rudely reminded that the ball park we've all been playing in belongs to 'them,' and that 'they' are willing to stop at nothing to make their point."[110] Garvey viewed the protestors not as an aberration from the American norm because of their sexuality or political positions, but rather as part of the secular American mainstream. The protest at St. Patrick's was another manifestation of America's long battle against true Catholicism, and the protestors merely its latest foot soldiers.

This claim of anti-Catholicism also caught the attention of historian of religion Philip Jenkins. He pegged ACT UP's protest as one of the two the most "notorious examples" of the "new anti-Catholicism," which he considered "the most significant unconfronted prejudice in modern America."[111] Older forms of anti-Catholicism in American history have included Protestant attacks on Catholic theology, anti-immigration sentiment against Irish and German transplants, and classism. But the new anti-Catholicism, Jenkins maintains, grew out of the sexual revolution of the 1960s and focused on cultural issues concerning gender and sexuality, especially abortion and homosexuality. "In addition to feminists," he writes, "gay activists have been among the leading contemporary critics of Catholicism and the Church." Even more, "opposition to Catholicism has become a major component of gay political organization, a powerful symbol of 'what we are fighting for.'" No group within the gay community has been more outspoken in its virulent anti-Catholicism than ACT UP, he argued. And though not representative of the gay community as a whole, Jenkins contends, ACT UP has "provided a significant force in gay political and social organization."[112]

Taken together, the responses of the mainstream media, Cardinal O'Connor, and a variety of conservative-leaning Catholic writers and historians painted an overwhelmingly negative picture of the Stop the Church demonstration at St. Patrick's. They depicted the protestors not merely as political radicals and unreasonable trouble-mongers, but also as secularist gays and feminists bent on attacking the Catholic Church. No piece of evidence in this portrayal stood out more than the desecration of the Communion wafer, which came to symbolize the protestors' disregard for religious freedom.

Speaking Out: Gays and Lesbians Debate Stopping the Church

Coverage of the protest in the gay media reveals different narratives about activists' goals and their understanding of religious and sexual freedom. The weekly magazine *OutWeek*, operated by several members of ACT UP, provided members of the gay and lesbian community an alternative space to debate the protests against O'Connor and the Catholic Church.[113] Their responses disclose disagreement and sometimes ambivalence about the demonstration. Coverage in *OutWeek* underscored internal battles through which gays and lesbians weighed sexual rights, especially the right to be practicing homosexuals, alongside religious freedom, including the church's right to condemn homosexual behavior and abortion.

A week ahead of the Stop the Church demonstration, *OutWeek* ran an editorial that set the tone for the protest by listing the gay and lesbian community's grievances against the Catholic Church. "The 1986 Papal encyclical justifying violence against gays, the banning and harassment of the gay Catholic group Dignity, the recent Vatican conference on AIDS that an observer called 'three days of gay bashing,' the Pope's declaration that AIDS is caused by 'sexual misconduct,'" the editorial accused, "all illustrate the church's role as a font of homophobia." As a longtime foe of the gay community, it continued, "the Vatican has decided to declare open war on homosexuals."[114] The authors regretted that some people might "question the wisdom of open attacks on the church," which risked alienating moderate or sympathetic Catholics. But the problem, their statement contended, was that "Catholic condemnation of homosexuality is based on a supposedly 'holy' belief that our love is a sin and that we are inherently sinners." That Catholic opposition to homosexuals was grounded in divine law posed a potential bind for demonstrators. "Gays and lesbians may hesitate to challenge the spiritual views of others," the editorial reasoned: "but when those spiritual views oppress us we must challenge them, strongly and openly."[115]

The authors thus found themselves in a catch-22: how could they reconcile religious freedom with sexual freedom? They attempted to frame the protest against *politics*, particularly the politics of the church hierarchy. They therefore avoided protesting against "religion," understood implicitly as the private beliefs of parishioners, and targeted instead the specific *political* positions of the Catholic Church, which they deemed fair game for public action. But the lines between the two blurred—as the church's political views issued from "supposedly holy beliefs"—and actions involved in the protest sparked intense debate even among gays and lesbians.

Several members of the gay community supported the spirit of the protest but opposed the tactics that activists employed. Andrew Humm, whose comments were picked up by mainstream papers and *Catholic New York*, irritated many AIDS activists when he spoke out against the protest. In a letter to *OutWeek*, Humm attacked ACT UP's failure to condemn "the actions of a small splinter group that disrupted the religious service on Sunday at St. Pat's," which has "distracted the lesbian and gay community from the goal of limiting the influence of religious bigots such as John

O'Connor to focusing us on the issue of whether or not freedom of religion should be abridged in order to advance our goals."[116] Humm argued that O'Connor was already losing ground to gay and AIDS activists, even among mainstream leaders and the media. With the exception of the conservative *New York Post*, he claimed, editorials attacking the cardinal's positions on condoms and reproductive freedom appeared in all the major papers. Even health officials such as NYC Health Commissioner Steve Joseph publicly opposed O'Connor's positions, stating on a *Nightline* episode, "This policy will increase AIDS deaths in New York." Furthermore, he continued, O'Connor lost on the gay rights bill, and Mayor-elect Dinkins had pledged to prosecute Operation Rescue. Humm concluded that gay activists were winning, if slowly and unevenly, but their cause had been set back by the Stop the Church protest. "Stopping people from praying on Sundays is not going to advance our agenda," he complained. Even worse, it provided O'Connor's first chance at positive press in months, he wrote, as political leaders and writers came to his defense.[117]

Humm was not the only reader of *OutWeek* to contest the demonstration. Michael Flynn opposed the protest because of his Christian beliefs. "True," he admitted, "O'Connor is no friend of ours. He's authoritarian, rigid and remote." But "as a Christian," he argued, "I believe he deserves to be treated in the same way we demand to be treated—with respect and dignity. I also believe that a church service should never be a place to vent hatred." For Flynn, the church was by definition a place set apart from politics and hatred, and the protesters trampled over this important division. "To see unbalanced miscreants ridicule the faithfuls' beliefs, mock the churchgoers' feelings and desecrate the most sacred element of Catholic worship—a consecrated host," he wrote, "is sickening and repulsive."[118] Bob Johnston also opposed the protest, describing the desecration of the host as "a real offense to God." "It is one thing to attack O'Connor," he charged, "and another thing to attack Jesus Christ!"[119]

Ronald Najman, a member of a gay-affirming Lutheran congregation in Manhattan, considered the relationship between gay rights and religious freedom. He agreed that members of the gay community should challenge harmful religious policies but opposed some of the actions taken at the cathedral. While peacefully "picketing cathedrals" seemed reasonable, "blocking church entrances" and "disrupting services" were not acceptable, since they "deprive others of their Constitutional right to the free exercise of religion."[120] Najman thus distinguished the different levels of disrupting services. Some forms, such as standing quietly during a homily in protest, might be okay, while "aggressively trying to interrupt religious services" was "simply stated, wrong." He did not premise this point on the sanctity of the church, but on the need for religious freedom common to gays and nongays alike.

According to Najman, interrupting services was not merely bad form, but also illegal under New York State law—and for good reason. "This statute," he argued, "not incidentally, protects worshippers belonging to gay- and lesbian-positive denominations [. . .] from disruptive assaults by homophobes." He drew together the rights of gays and lesbians and those of religious practitioners:

> the right to worship is as fundamental as the most basic of gay rights—the right to express love, physically or otherwise, to the consenting adult for whom one feels that love, regardless of gender. Gay rights and freedom of religion are identical in one respect: they both depend on the guarantee of freedom of conscience.[121]

Najman refused to see gay and lesbian rights as antithetical to religious freedom. Because religious freedom also protected the rights of gay religious followers, any attack on such freedoms would go beyond attacking the Catholic Church: it would damage their own community as well. This reading also provided an important point of difference between Najman and some AIDS and gay activists. By reading sexual and religious rights together, Najman suggested both centrally concerned the "freedom of conscience"—they were matters of individuals' privately held beliefs. This position extended the liberal approach to religion to sexual identity and gay rights. But it left little room to understand the public dimensions of Catholic belief and political participation, as demonstrated by O'Connor's forays into the politics of abortion, sexuality, and AIDS work, or to understand the sexual politics advanced by gay and AIDS activists who demanded public recognition, civil rights, and government support.

Some members of ACT UP also vented their disapproval in the pages of *Out Week*. James Keenan, who described himself as a "proudly lapsed Catholic and longtime secular humanist" with little goodwill toward the Catholic Church or O'Connor, nonetheless called the protest an act of anti-Catholic bigotry.[122] He considered the destruction of the Communion wafer "the most dramatic example of this attitude," as it mocked Catholic beliefs. Even worse, it alienated "potential political allies," including lay Catholics. Keenan wanted to push ACT UP toward pragmatic forms of community building. "The church's anti-condom, anti-sex education position will only be defeated by a strategy of *subversion* or *outflanking*," he explained:

> Subversion in the sense that Catholic lay people and low level clergy will eventually be persuaded of the foolishness of the church's official position and will act accordingly (as they do with respect to birth control); outflanking in the sense that other religious and secular institutions will eventually be persuaded of the need to criticize the Catholic Church's position and to prevent it from adversely affecting public policy.[123]

Keenan thus opposed the ostentatious, theatrical style of the Stop the Church demonstration. Sounding much like Humm, he called instead for coalition building in order to render the church's positions ineffective. Some ACT UP members defended the protest against these charges.

Terry McGovern penned a response to Humm and others who were critical of the protest. McGovern was inside the cathedral on the day of the protest though not part of the disruption itself. In her letter to *OutWeek*, she bemoaned the "countless columns written by Irish Catholics who claim to be particularly pained by the horrific desecration of their cathedral built by their dirt poor Irish immigrant forefathers as a tribute to *their* Saint." She offered an alternative narrative. "I am an Irish Catholic," McGovern explained: "I describe myself as such because I have found it to be an inescapable phenomenon in my life." Her great grandparents had relied on the soup kitchens offered by St. Patrick's when they fled Ireland to resettle in Manhattan. And they received what little formal education they got from the cathedral, where one of her grandfathers had even served as an altar boy. According to McGovern, her grandfather taught her to be a proud Catholic and to "always remember that my family had always fought with their lives for that right," and "that persecution was not okay." McGovern encountered a different side of the Catholic Church while attending Catholic school and Georgetown Law School, a side that viewed women as "secondary at best and [taught] that sexuality was evil." These lessons filled her with "a finely honed sense of hypocrisy."[124] But her sense of pride also remained.

In response to Humm, McGovern countered, "My life has been consistently disrupted by the Catholic church," as have the lives of other gays and lesbians "who lived tortured childhoods trying to reconcile Catholic doctrine which they were being taught with their sexuality." Now with the

AIDS crisis, she continued, "Cardinal O'Connor is not simply worship-
ping his God. He is preaching the politics of our genocide from that
pulpit. We cannot be fooled by mainstream outrage—we are fighting for
our lives." Here, McGovern denied the idea that the church itself was off-
limits. O'Connor preached the politics of abstinence and opposed gay
rights and abortion rights directly from the pulpit, she asserted. The cardinal had already crossed any line intended to protect religion from politics. "As a descendant of the Irish who built that cathedral, and dedicated
that cathedral to new and better lives free of political persecution," Mc-
Govern concluded, "I thank those of you who disrupted that mass."[125] Mc-
Govern reinterpreted ACT UP's demonstration not as antithetical to
religion and religious practice, but as continuous with the spirit of religious and political freedom that she attached to her family's Irish Catholic
heritage and their entanglement with the history of St. Patrick's.

Dan Hunter and Servalan Erik wrote together in support of the protest
as well. They complained that the media focused on the "invasion" and
made O'Connor the victim, whereas the "main issue is the church's continuous interference in the political arena to impose their religious views
on everyone, religious or not. These views are outdated and interfere with
people that may or may not be Catholic."[126] They asserted that the goal of
the protest was threefold: to protect women's rights to abortion, to stop
church interference in AIDS education and the distribution of safe-sex
literature, and to stop the church from blocking gay and lesbian civil rights
legislation. "Regarding the interruption of services," they wrote, "we are
against interfering with the right to worship, but it had to be done under
the circumstances."[127] For these activists, the demonstration within the
cathedral was regrettable but justified. Like McGovern, they accused the
Catholic Church of crossing what they considered the proper boundaries
of politics and religion: by introducing politics into the pulpit, the church
leaders forewent any consideration of the sacred distinctiveness of the
cathedral.

Victor Mendolia, one of the organizers of Stop the Church, thanked
OutWeek for excellent coverage of the protest in light of what he considered the mainstream media's consistent misrepresentations. He also
pushed against Humm's criticism of the demonstration, claiming that
Humm had attempted to sabotage the protest by fostering dissent among
the activists, including members of Dignity and the Cathedral Project.
Mendolia pointed out that many Dignity and Cathedral Project members
could not take part in the protest—not because they opposed it, as Humm

suggested, but because of a previous injunction against them brought by O'Connor. Banned from church premises, they would have faced extra legal problems if arrested at the demonstration. Mendolia then addressed Dignity and its president, Robert Pusilo. "Never have I been more proud of Dignity, than as I read the stories in the papers in the days that followed the demonstration," he reported:

> Bob articulated the reasons for the demonstration impeccably and made it clear, while they did not approve of the action inside the cathedral, they supported the reasons for the action inside the cathedral. I salute the brave women and men of the Cathedral Project and Dignity who for almost three years have opposed through direct action, the hypocritical hierarchy . . . Dignity is surely a friend in the struggle to stop church interference in our lives.[128]

Recalling the protest, Mendolia affirmed, "We have sent a message, not only to the religious community, which is killing us with their fake morality, but also the political community. The message is NO MORE BUSINESS AS USUAL!"[129]

Though Dignity disapproved of the disruptions within the cathedral, some members countered the argument that the crumbling of the wafer resulted in an act of desecration.[130] According to Pusilo, Dignity board members held a theological discussion after the demonstration. Seven out of eleven members thought that crumbling the wafer was not an act of desecration because the wafer had not been properly consecrated. The wafer only becomes the body of Christ after the priest consecrates it, they reasoned. However, the protests within the cathedral had already begun when the crumbling occurred, which meant that O'Connor would have become enraged. "He carried that anger to the consecration," explained Pusilo, but "Christ cannot be consecrated in anger."[131] This gesture suggested the theological stakes involved in the protest for members of Dignity and their support for ACT UP.

Dignity member John Calve voiced his support for the demonstration in a letter to *OutWeek* condemning the Catholic Church's resistance to safe-sex education. "The bottom line on safe sex," Calve wrote: "it saves lives."[132] The "real reason" O'Connor opposed safe-sex education in the gay community was because it "encourage[d] 'immoral' homosexual behavior." Calve considered untenable the church's simultaneous intolerance of gays and promotion of AIDS treatment. "For example," he explained, "Cardinal

O'Connor favors the 'fair treatment of AIDS patients' but fails to realize that his position—that gays are sick and abnormal—helps to create the unfair and abusive treatment received by gay AIDS patients." This logic made no sense to Calve. "How can you have sympathy for GAY AIDS patients and total condemnation of GAYS?" he exclaimed.[133]

Two letters that appeared in *OutWeek* homed in on the issue of religious freedom. Paul Guzzardo took a strong secularist position against religion, one predicated on the limited role of faith in modern times. "As we approach the millennium in the years from now," he predicted, "the religious foundations of western civilization as well as other religious foundations of non-western civilizations will finally be challenged by modern man."[134] To him, one demonstrator's now-infamous act of crumbling the Communion wafer represented perhaps the first act in modern history "to shake the foundations of today's religious beliefs." But Guzzardo was not completely opposed to religion. He offered a way for religion and the modern future to coexist: "Unfortunately all religious institutions are anti-gay, anti-female and this must change in order for religion as we know it today to survive in the next millennia." Guzzardo backtracked here from his secularist stance, criticizing not "religion," but rather sexism and homophobia in religious institutions.

In "Freedom from Religion," Tom Shultz expressed his frustration that the media portrayed the protest as "sacrilegious and disgraceful."[135] "The media laments about how we attacked freedom of religion," he wrote—but "I'm much more concerned with freedom FROM religion."[136] Shultz decried what he saw as hypocritical coverage in the mainstream press:

> Where were the editorials of outrage when O'Connor publicly stated that he wanted to get arrested with Operation Rescue, an organization that violates the law by blocking entrances to abortion clinics thus interfering with women's health care, not to mention the violent verbal abuse these women are subjected to by these fanatics.[137]

Despite his anger toward the Catholic Church, and toward O'Connor in particular, Shultz concluded his letter by drawing an analogy between the Stop the Church demonstration and the revolutionary spirit of Jesus. "According to Christian mythology," he explained, "Jesus Christ walked into the temple of God with a whip and drove the money-changers out! I think we did something comparable last Sunday when we entered and protested at the cathedral." Though ACT UP has been marginalized from mainstream society, he continued, "there can be no doubt of the righteousness of our cause."[138] Shultz's letter demonstrated the very complexity the protest presented, even for activists, as they attempted to negotiate their righteous anger with the freedom of religion. While his initial argument called for freedom *from* religion, by the end Schultz presented one of the most religious interpretations of the demonstration in its wake: that Stop the Church was "something comparable" to an act of religious protest itself.

Sexual Freedom, Religious Freedom, and the Politics of Jesus Camp

Very few accounts of Stop the Church have remembered it as an act of religious or even Catholic protest. Much the opposite has been the case. How did depictions of Stop the Church as anti-religious succeed in mainstream and Catholic news coverage, while ACT UP's efforts to characterize their actions as part of the American tradition that separated church and state fell short? Part of the answer no doubt rests in the representation of the Catholic Church as the victim of an aggressive attack, one that did not merely target O'Connor and the church hierarchy, as activists maintained, but that also interrupted the Sunday Mass for thousands of regular parishioners and resulted in the desecration the host. For many, the charges against O'Connor could not justify stomping on the rights of these bystanders, the lay religious who were portrayed as innocent not only by Catholics and mainstream media, but also by AIDS activists themselves.

This representation of the protest also reveals a number of historical assumptions about American Catholicism, secularism, and religious freedom that we might parse out. In order to frame the church as a victim and parishioners as innocent, Catholic and mainstream accounts posited activists as aggressively and unreasonably attacking religious freedom, if not religion itself. They made this rhetorical point in part by emphasizing activists' sexuality, drawing an implicit contrast between their own cherished religious values versus activists' call for a version of sexual freedom that fell outside the bounds of good moral citizenship. Both the Catholic press and mainstream papers such as the *New York Times* chastised the "homosexual" activists—repeatedly using this term, rather than "AIDS" activists—for carrying "racy" or "filthy" signs, for committing "despicable, intolerable acts," and for attacking the constitutional guarantee of religious freedom.

Most discussions of the protest, including those in *Catholic New York* and *OutWeek*, defined religious freedom in liberal terms—as the freedom for individuals to hold specific religious beliefs and to worship in peace. This way of thinking removed religion from the realm of politics and relocated it within the private domain of individuals and the church: that is, distinct from the political sphere, separated from the public, and off-limits to protest. Approaching religion in this way meant that critics of the protest framed it as an attack on the religious rights of individual Catholics or upon Catholicism as a whole, rather than as a protest against the political policies advocated by Cardinal O'Connor and the church hierarchy, as activists specified. To maintain this position, critiques of ACT UP that appeared in the mainstream press and in *Catholic New York* sidelined discussions of O'Connor's involvement with city politics and with the politics of public health, despite the fact that the cardinal's powerful voice in these debates was itself the instance of boundary crossing that prompted activists to demand a separation of church and state and to storm the cathedral. Given the cultural saturation of liberal approaches to thinking about religion, it was hard for most commenters—including many Catholics and AIDS activists—to see Catholic political positions as religious, rather than as interruptions to or distractions from "real" religion. In the end, within the limitations of this rhetoric, Stop the Church was cast as a secular protest against religion.

But Stop the Church challenges this interpretation, especially if we take seriously Schultz's suggestion that the demonstration was something like an act of religious protest. To be sure, a number of activists spurned Catholicism and even "religion" on strongly secularist grounds. But Terry McGovern and Tom Schultz, writing in *OutWeek*, were not alone in recognizing the religious elements of the protest. While some activists engaged in a secular, political protest against an oppressive church hierarchy, others, including many members of Dignity, understood the demonstration precisely as religious protest. If we take religion and secularism not as opposites, but rather as overlapping practices, as Talal Asad has suggested, then new readings of this demonstration become possible.[139]

O'Connor's article "A Sacrilege Recalled" in *Catholic New York* offers one alternative. Perhaps no act gained more attention in coverage of the protest than the crumbling of the Communion wafer. Mainstream and Catholic accounts repeatedly described it as an act of anti-Catholic hatred and an attack on religion. O'Connor denounced it as a particularly vicious assault, an attack on that most sacred aspect of religion that must be preserved from politics. As he noted, protesting the church hierarchy was one thing, but attacking the consecrated host was a direct assault on Christ himself, an act of "sacrilege." Later in the piece O'Connor writes that the act bordered on "demonic." These namings are suggestive.

The word *sacrilege* combines two Latin terms: *sacer*, or sacred, and *legĕre*, to gather or steal. An older meaning of sacrilege referred to the act of stealing something consecrated to God, or sacred.[140] What if we take O'Connor at his word and consider the protestor's act not as a secular assault upon religion, but as an act of theft or a denial of ownership? We might read the desecration of the host as a gesture of religious protest against the church's failure to regard what the young man considered the true meaning of Christ's life or the true site of Christ's presence. Granted this reading is only suggestive, and the young man's act would have had little power if he did not regard the Eucharist as meaningful in some way, if not sacred. Revisiting Groeschel's description of the demonstrator in the pages of *Catholic New York* fills in some of these gaps.

The Franciscan priest recalled the man's appearance, which he found even more surprising than the crumbling of the host. He looked "sad and confused" and uttered his words—"this is what I think of your God"—very softly, the way people talk "when they go to confession." Groeschel could not square this solemn manner with the act of desecration. "Blasphemy," he wrote, "is seldom pronounced in a reverent tone."[141] So what to make of this protester? Despite his surprise, Groeschel interprets the young man's act as anti-religious blasphemy and as evidence for the "the moral decline of our country." I want to suggest that, if we stay within the Catholic vocabulary of sacrilege that O'Connor suggested, we might also read it as a ritual of protest, a theft by a former altar boy, a devout—even Catholic—demonstration against the church hierarchy. The young man would hardly be the first in history—or even the first Catholic—to commit such an act.[142] The visual history of ACT UP extends this reading. It suggests that Stop the Church was not only a battle between secular activists and the Catholic Church but also a struggle over competing claims to the true message of Jesus Christ. It demonstrates not one moral vision that is in decline, but two different religious and moral visions coming into conflict.

Two Stop the Church posters depict Jesus as an ACT UP protestor. In the first (Figure 4.6), he wears the symbolic Silence = Death pin and drives a stake into O'Connor, while exclaiming, "Let me demonstrate!" The poster is jarring, both for the depiction of Jesus as an ACT UP member

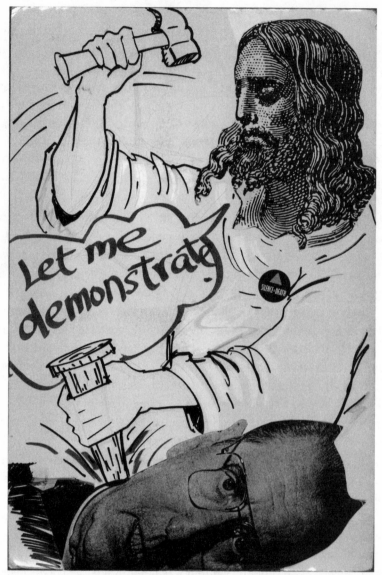

FIGURE 4.6 ACT UP New York's "Let me demonstrate" poster featuring Jesus Christ hammering a stake into Cardinal O'Connor's neck. (Held in the ACT UP/NY Records, New York Public Library Digital Gallery.)

and for the scene of violence. But looking closer, the representation of O'Connor is also important. The top of the cardinal's head is cropped, which has the effect of giving him horns. The poster constructs a battle between good and evil, Jesus and the devil. It slots the son of God on the side of ACT UP. The second poster (Figure 4.7) also features Jesus. This

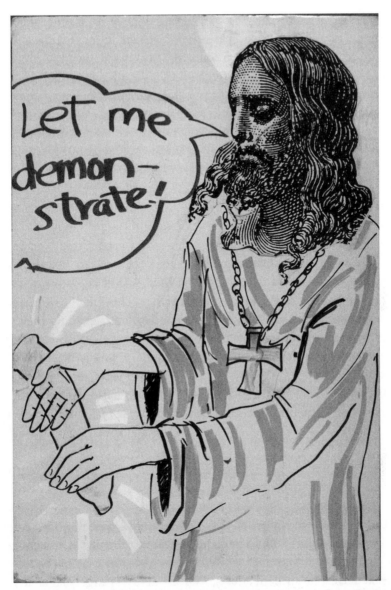

FIGURE 4.7 ACT UP New York's "Let me demonstrate" poster, featuring Jesus Christ holding a condom and wearing a cross. (Held in the ACT UP/NY Records, New York Public Library Digital Gallery.)

time he dons a cross and holds out a condom, as he again states, "Let me demonstrate!" The poster playfully represents Jesus as a sex educator, and one who clearly favors education about condom use. He again sides with ACT UP. Read alongside these images, the act of crumbling the wafer might be interpreted not as an attack on Jesus, but rather as a refusal of the Catholic Church's power to own and to define Jesus, visually or bodily. Stealing Jesus to their side, these AIDS activists re-scripted the secular versus religious narrative to formulate their own protest religion. The leadership of the Catholic Church and ACT UP offered distinct moral visions concerning AIDS and sexuality, to be sure; but in both cases their visions were as political as they were religious.

True to ACT UP's legacy, Stop the Church was nothing if not promiscuous in its religious and political significance. The protest was political and secular, but it was also religious, perhaps even in some respects Catholic, as the distinction between these categories was blurred and at times refused by activists themselves. Representations of the demonstration have resisted these multiple, even conflicting meanings, as media coverage and historical narratives alike have instead constructed a battle between secular gay activists and the sacred church. In notable ways, Catholics and AIDS activists alike operated within and against liberal logics regarding sexual and religious freedom. The Catholic Church and its supporters steadfastly promoted moral positions regarding what constituted healthy, proper forms of sex. Sex ought to be kept within the private sphere of the home, and it should be monogamous and heterosexual. Sex education, moreover, ought to teach basic values of abstinence and fidelity. Importantly, the Catholic hierarchy advanced its morality of sex not only among Catholics but also in citywide and even national political and legal debates. What was good for the Catholic Church was good for all Americans.

Activists within ACT UP and WHAM! also politicized sex. They promoted an alternative ethics of sexual freedom that included individual rights to education about condoms and birth control, legal access to abortion, and civil rights for gays and lesbians. Moreover, they urged, these sexual rights should be kept free from religious encroachment. In their view, it was not sex but rather religion that needed to be checked. Despite strident efforts, ACT UP activists largely failed to convince the broader public of their cause—including their argument that Catholic leaders overstepped the boundaries of church and state by promoting a religious and moral politics that endangered women, gays and lesbians, people with HIV/AIDS, and everyone denied comprehensive sex education. Media accounts of the protest sacrificed activists' arguments for sexual freedom for a different vision of freedom, for religious freedom. In a battle posed between sexual rights and religious freedom, the latter won the sympathies of historical representation.

The Catholic vision, at least when running up against that of gay and lesbian AIDS activists, was embraced as the moral vision for the nation. As religious freedom—with its presumption of religion as generally private, innocent, and good—was upheld, the activists' moral vision of sexual freedom became lost in the fray.

Afterword

"When I think about those soldiers or airmen or Marines or sailors who are out there fighting on my behalf and yet feel constrained, even now that 'don't ask, don't tell' is gone, because they are not able to commit themselves in a marriage, at a certain point I've just concluded that for me personally it is important [. . .] to go ahead and affirm that I think same sex couples should be able to get married."

—PRESIDENT BARACK OBAMA, ABC News interview with Robin Roberts

"I simply do not see why the nation has to have an official sexuality."

—LAUREN BERLANT, *The Queen of America Goes to Washington City*

"The time has come to think about sex."

—GAYLE RUBIN, "Thinking Sex: Notes for a Radical Theory of the Politics of Sexuality"

"AND EVERYTHING HAD changed," author and activist Paul Monette explained in his 1994 memoir *Last Watch of the Night*, assessing his life twelve years into the AIDS crisis. Religion found itself at the top of his list. "Not surprisingly, my rabid contempt for official religions, the Orwellian lies and the Kapos," he wrote, "had only deepened over time." For Monette, as for many gay AIDS activists, "religion" had come to signify organized hatred and militancy. "It's clear now that the fundamentalists' agenda of lies and hate grows daily," Monette continued: "and it's Protestant and it's Catholic and it's Muslim and it's Jewish." In his view, it seemed "that the hatred of queers was at the top of the list for most religions."[1] Rafael Campo, an AIDS activist, poet, and medical researcher, would agree. "Religion," he wrote for a 1995 compilation of writing about the epidemic, "still implies AIDS is a punishment, meted out by an unloving, unforgiving, and unimaginable God, intent with wrath."[2]

Monette and Campo expressed the anger toward organized religion that a number of gay and AIDS activists shared. It was the same frustration displayed in ACT UP's Stop the Church demonstration a few years earlier. Religious hostility toward gay men, lesbians, and people with AIDS had come to a head by the late 1980s and early 1990s. It was not only Christian Right leaders like Jerry Falwell, but even more moderate evangelicals such as Billy Graham and Ron Sider, who questioned whether AIDS was God's judgment or perhaps a divine warning that homosexuality was immoral.[3] National opinion was hardly more sympathetic. With the arrival of the "gay plague" and the ascendance of culture wars conservatism, the number of Americans who considered homosexual relations "always wrong" rose from 73% in 1980 to an all-time high of 78% by 1987.[4] Americans were afraid of this new disease that doctors seemed to know so little about and which the media did little more than sensationalize. Following many of America's religious leaders, they linked AIDS to sexual immorality.

By the 1990s, opposition to gay rights had become one of the Christian Right's most galvanizing political and cultural issues. And it achieved some success, particularly in the passage of the Defense of Marriage Act (DOMA). This legislation would allow states to refuse to recognize same-sex marriages performed legally in other states and effectively barred same-sex couples from receiving any of the federal benefits attached to heterosexual marriage. The law passed both houses of Congress by large margins and was signed into law by President Bill Clinton, a Democrat, in September 1996. Gay AIDS activists like Monette and Campo, it seemed, had good reason to castigate "religion." Their impression of religious hostility towards homosexuality and the AIDS epidemic has been reproduced in most historical and journalistic accounts of this episode in American history. *After the Wrath of God* does not deny this impression of religious hostility but complicates it.

This book has examined the importance of religion to the history and politics of the AIDS crisis in the United States. When histories of the epidemic have included religion, they have emphasized conservative religious opposition to AIDS and safe sex programming as well as fulminations against homosexuals. I have surveyed instead the attempts of a broader range of religious actors to forge compassionate responses to people with

HIV/AIDS and to combat, to varying degrees, charges that AIDS was a divine punishment. Since the 1980s, Catholics, Jews, and mainstream liberal and evangelical Protestants have formed the largest response to AIDS outside of the grassroots efforts of gays and lesbians and public efforts organized by the state. They have issued denominational statements, authored pastoral manuals on how to care for people with AIDS, and founded thousands of AIDS ministry programs throughout the United States. Religious leaders from varied denominational and political backgrounds have shaped popular understandings of AIDS as well as public policies regarding the disease at local, national, and even international levels. These efforts have ranged from mainline Protestant denominations that called for government support for AIDS research to conservative evangelicals and Catholics who lobbied for the allocation of government funding for abstinence education in George W. Bush's President's Emergency Plan for AIDS Relief. Taken as a whole, this history recovers the diversity of American Christians engaged with AIDS work in the 1980s and early 1990s, moving well beyond voices issuing from the Christian Right. This history also suggests the power of Christian rhetoric in the modern United States by demonstrating the ability of Christian knowledge workers to shape the sexual and moral construction of the AIDS epidemic, including the formation of AIDS relief work and public health policy.

Religious, and particularly Christian, voices have been especially influential in positing the moral construction of the AIDS epidemic and in advancing public health initiatives based in particular moral approaches to sexual behavior. Granted, a number of liberal and mainline Christians and Jews followed secular public health experts in defining AIDS as a biomedical issue. They provided care and compassion for those people affected by the disease and called for an end to discrimination, often not only against people with HIV/AIDS but also against gay men and lesbians. Though more politically progressive Christians often stopped short of condoning homosexual practice, they nonetheless attempted to disarticulate homosexual sinfulness from the new disease. Their moral vision more often equated people with AIDS to Jesus' category of the poor or the oppressed and downplayed sexuality—including sexual blame—when possible.

American evangelicals and Catholic leaders often advanced a different approach. They tethered HIV and AIDS to sexual immorality and prescribed biblically or morally based approaches to sexuality to curb their spread. Here, HIV/AIDS was not merely a biomedical phenomenon, but also, in its constitution, a moral one. For a number of evangelical and Catholic leaders, immoral sexual behavior did not just spread infection; it occupied a central role in the etiology of the disease itself. AIDS was recast as both a moral epidemic and a medical one. Medicine and morality did not simply go hand in hand in these accounts: they were equivalent. Of course, this approach was ultimately not limited to evangelicals or the Catholic leadership. It overlapped with mainline approaches and resonated with the broader American public.[5]

In the United States, religious discussions of the epidemic have long drawn a close relationship between AIDS and the moral status of sexuality, particularly homosexuality. Michael Warner has described the special role morality has played in the formation of queer identity and politics. "Unlike other identity movements," he has observed, "queerness has always been defined centrally by discourses of morality." To be sure, he continued, moral prescriptions have a long history of governing gender, race, and class as well. But in these cases, Warner explained, they have focused on *how* to be a proper woman or man, or a good worker, or a civilized person, "but not whether to be one." "Queerness," in contrast, "bears a different relation to liberal logics of choice and will as well as to moral languages of leadership and community, in ways that continually pose problems both in everyday life and in contexts of civil rights."[6]

Religion adds another layer to this story. Queerness also bears a different relation to theological notions of proper moral behavior that have shaped debates regarding sexuality and the AIDS epidemic. For many evangelicals and Catholic leaders, moral discipline could teach proper forms of sexuality and provide the salve for both queer identity and HIV/AIDS. Evangelicals such as Rick and Kay Warren, Ron Sider, and C. Everett Koop granted that comprehensive sex education might prove pragmatic, but only a "return" to biblical sexual mores could stop the spread of AIDS. In their understanding, this meant abstinence before marriage and fidelity within heterosexual marriage. For some members of the Catholic hierarchy, not even comprehensive sex education could be condoned: marriage and celibacy were the church's solutions.[7] In this understanding, the epidemic could be ended only by disciplining subjects through these moral lessons, by making their sexual behaviors align with biblical or traditional teachings about sexual morality. These lessons were not directed only at fellow Christians.

The AIDS epidemic provided Christians a new site through which to elaborate a broader sexual morality for the American public—a particular understanding of sexual behavior that has shaped proper moral citizenship. Of course American Christians discussed sex before the epidemic, but AIDS changed their rhetoric in two significant ways. First, because medical and media discourses defined AIDS as a sexually transmitted disease, and one metonymically tied to homosexuality, AIDS provided American Christians a sturdy platform from which to proclaim biblical and traditional mores concerning sex. The epidemic added fuel to the moral jeremiads issued from the Christian Right concerning the wages of sin, especially sexual sin. The fruits of this movement can be seen in DOMA and in the passage of constitutional amendments banning same-sex marriage in a number of states in the late 1990s and 2000s.[8]

Yet the AIDS epidemic also effected a shift in Christian rhetoric about sexuality. Countering the perceived excesses of the sexual revolution of the 1960s and 1970s, leaders in the Christian Right pronounced a largely negative politics of sexuality, one marked by fulminations against pornography, divorce, extramarital sex, and homosexuality. At the same time, though, a number of American Christians shifted toward a more positive discourse of sexual morality.[9] Their discussions of AIDS prevention focused less on attacking sexual sins than on promoting a new program for having moral sex, which was defined through abstinence before marriage and monogamy.[10] This is not to say that the negative, anti-sex discourse was not also "productive"—that is, that it did not have effects that went beyond saying "no."[11] The Christian Right's focus on matters of abortion and homosexuality also contributed to the proliferation of national discussions of sex. But whereas much of their rhetoric focused on what not to do, the AIDS epidemic prompted an increasing number of religious leaders to promote a positive prescription for sex, one more readily taken up in both public health endeavors and high school sex education curricula.

Evangelicals and Catholics promoted their view of sexual morality through ministry programs, denominational statements, pastoral documents, and popular writing. This morality was also translated into secular terms and extended to the American public, not least through Surgeon General Koop's national AIDS campaign. Koop admitted the importance of comprehensive sex education and condom use but repeatedly emphasized abstinence and monogamy. His pamphlet *Understanding AIDS* also targeted and re-imagined its mainstream American reader: the married heterosexual couple who likely knew little about AIDS yet had much to fear should their sexual practices stray from the moral norm. Homosexuality was conspicuous through its absence in this national campaign, as gay men and lesbians lived at the margins of moral citizenship.

To be sure, this moral approach was not uncontested. Among Christians, voices differed over the status of homosexuality, the morality of condom use, and the necessity and content of sex education. Members of the Christian Right, for instance, slammed Koop's call for sex education, as they promoted anti-sex campaigns declaiming the sinfulness of homosexuality and trumpeted Victorian sexual morals. But a new movement was already under way, an effort to provide sex education that would instruct Americans in the healthful and moral benefits of abstinence and monogamy. Sex need not be dangerous, the message rang, so long as it followed the proper moral design. And as Obama would later suggest, so long as sexuality and spirituality were united.

AIDS activists voiced quite different views about the AIDS epidemic and sexual practice. Though rarely adopting explicitly the language of "the moral," AIDS and gay and lesbian activists promoted an ethic of sexual freedom that celebrated homosexuality and privileged safe sex, monogamous or otherwise. Yet this sexual ethic was often posited against conservative religious values. When the two have gone head to head, as they did following the Stop the Church demonstration, religious freedom has trumped sexual freedom. But this ethic also found little resonance outside of America's gay enclaves or among a select set of gay and AIDS activists. Indeed, by the early 1990s, even the gay community had shifted the focus of its political struggles away from championing individual rights, the politics of safe sex, and sexual exploration toward promoting what historian George Chauncey has called a "new ethic of monogamy"—an ethic that has bolstered arguments for legal marriage.[12]

Gay Marriage, HIV/AIDS, and the Demands of Moral Citizenship

In *Why Marriage?* Chauncey argues that the AIDS crisis, along with the lesbian baby boom of the 1980s, provided the foundation for the gay marriage movement. AIDS in particular introduced gay men and their lesbian allies to the realities of death and made them all too aware of the fragile legal status of their relationships.[13] During this period, AIDS also prompted some gay men to challenge the promiscuous sexual ethos of the earlier generation. A new conservative gay political movement, led by writers such as Andrew Sullivan and Jonathan Rauch, championed marriage as the next step for gays and lesbians to achieve cultural respectability—that is, to enter the privileged circle of American moral citizenship.[14]

This interpretation, already glimpsed in Randy Shilts' famous *And the Band Played On* and in Larry Kramer's *The Normal Heart*, reads the AIDS epidemic as a reality check for the excessive promiscuity of a previous generation of gay men. AIDS, in this account, provided a wake-up call for gay men to mature into adults and to realize the innate value of intimate, monogamous relationships. The American mainstream has been open to this narrative, as the fight for gay marriage rights has gained a number of successes since the 1990s. One of the most significant was the repeal of DOMA in 2013. The achievements of the gay marriage movement—which are at the time of this writing, however, still incomplete—signify a shift in the boundaries of moral citizenship as I have described them. Over time, the focus on abstinence and heterosexual monogamy has allowed for the inclusion of same-sex monogamy as well. But such gains in gay rights have also come at some cost, which is only sometimes recognized by national gay rights leaders. The gay marriage movement has foregrounded intimate, happy (usually white and middle class) same-sex couples in long-term relationships. Whether pragmatic or not, this strategy has overlooked or whitewashed the history of the gay liberation movement and the development of sexual practices, including safe but sometimes non-monogamous sex, championed by an earlier generation of gay and AIDS activists.[15] They have, in other words, bent the normative ideals of gay relationships, including gay sex, toward those demanded by the terms of moral citizenship. This moral—even moralizing—approach to gay sex continues not only to define gay marriage debates but also to inform the politics of HIV prevention. Two examples are particularly salient.

The continuing criminalization of HIV demonstrates the devastating legal and social consequences that follow from failing to adhere to the normative model of gay monogamy. In 1990, the passage of the Ryan White CARE Act required states that wanted to receive federal funding to fight HIV/AIDS to criminalize the purposeful transmission of HIV. Over thirty states eventually passed laws extending this mandate—criminalizing not only purposeful transmission, but also the failure to disclose one's positive status in sexual encounters. These laws often do not take into account whether HIV is actually transmitted. Merely the threat of transmission can result in charges of attempted manslaughter or murder, a position that recalls the American bishops' worry that the mere "semblance" of support for homosexuality or condom use could lead to grave danger. In one of the most public cases of such a law taking effect, Nick Rhoades was arrested in Iowa in 2008 after failing to disclose his status during a one-time hookup. At the time, Rhoades was on anti-retroviral treatment and had an undetectable viral load, and he wore a condom during anal sex. His sexual partner learned about Rhoades' status and rushed to the hospital for testing. Rhoades was later charged with a class B felony in Iowa, found guilty, and sentenced to twenty-five years in jail. Activists began campaigning on his behalf and, after eleven months, his sentence was reduced to time served, plus five years of supervised probation and registration as a sex offender for the rest of his life.[16] The sexual panic glimpsed in this case and others like it became a moral and legal panic over gay promiscuity and, by association, over the transmission (or mere semblance of transmission) of HIV. Disciplining gay sex was another means to prevent disease.

In addition to criminalization, gay marriage has also become a strategy to prevent the spread of HIV. Aubrey Loots and Danny Leclair made history during the 2014 Tournament of Roses Parade in Pasadena, California. They became the first gay couple to wed during the New Year's parade, as they processed down the street on a wedding cake float. This marriage, other than being gay, probably would not have raised many eyebrows among queer and AIDS activists, except for the importance of the float they were on—the one sponsored by the AIDS Healthcare Foundation, the largest community HIV/AIDS healthcare organization in the United States. The theme for their parade float was "Living the Dream: Love Is the Best Protection," making explicit their effort to connect gay marriage to HIV prevention. Their marriage quickly became a symbol bringing together the history of AIDS and the history of the struggle for gay marriage. In other words, it symbolized one of the many public health arguments mobilized to support same-sex marriage—that gay marriage, by promoting monogamy, could be a key tool in the fight against HIV/AIDS.[17]

The overlap here between gay marriage and the normative ideal of monogamy is important. The link between monogamy and HIV prevention—so reminiscent of the arguments made by Koop, Rick and Kay Warren, the Catholic bishops, and many others—becomes clear in discussions about a new biomedical effort to prevent the spread of HIV. On May 14, 2014, the U.S. Public Health Service released a set of clinical practice guidelines for the use of pre-exposure prophylaxis (PrEP). This approach repurposes two medications commonly used to treat HIV infection as a form of prevention for people who are HIV negative. In 2012, the Food and Drug Administration approved the anti-retroviral Truvada, made by Gilead Sciences, to be used for prevention purposes. This pill quickly became for men who sleep with men what the birth control pill has been for women who sleep with men: a biomedical step toward sexual free-dom.[18] And like the birth control pill, PrEP has animated new anxieties about sexual promiscuity and immorality.

Christian responses to the use of PrEP have only begun to emerge, mostly from Catholic leaders and conservative evangelicals. Following the 20th International AIDS Conference, held in Melbourne, Australia, in July 2014, Monsignor Robert Vitillo expressed reservations about PrEP. Vitillo has served as a special adviser on HIV and AIDS for Caritas Inter-nationalis, a collection of Catholic relief and social service organizations, and previously served as president of the National Catholic AIDS Network Board of Directors. Speaking to Catholic reporters, Vitillo lamented the continued stigma and discrimination that people with HIV and AIDS faced, especially in the United States and other "high-income countries," where people assume the problem is more or less solved. This denial about HIV becomes even more worrisome with the advent of PrEP: "With PrEP people can develop a sense that they don't have to worry about infec-tion anymore. So they can have all the sexual encounters they want, or inject all the drugs they want, with a perception that they're protected from HIV." Although Vitillo agreed with a number of developments in the treatment of HIV and AIDS, he decided not to sign the "Melbourne Dec-laration," which affirmed the importance of nondiscrimination in the battle against HIV/AIDS. The declaration emphasized the need to combat sexism, homophobia, and transphobia and called for the decriminaliza-tion of HIV, which would include promoting legal equality for at-risk pop-ulations. Vitillo worried that the statement promoted "activities or behaviors which aren't in agreement with Catholic teaching."[19]

Linda Harvey, the founder of Mission: America, a nonprofit organiza-tion dedicated to educating conservative Christians about a host of culture wars issues, penned an article for the biblically oriented blog Barbwire. Harvey worries about the new health guidelines concerning PrEP, which she calls a "promiscuity pill." The pill could replace what she and many other Christians consider the already alarming use of condoms as a new form of sex education and HIV prevention taught in public schools. Ac-cording to Harvey, the main causes of the AIDS epidemic remain "anal sex between men" and "primarily promiscuous heterosexual sex or intra-venous drug use." Yet "none of these behaviors," she argues, "are essential to human happiness and productivity." Like condoms, PrEP enables people to do things they ought not do in the first place. Harvey offers an alternative solution: "launch a nationwide campaign that is pro-marriage (the authentic man/woman kind)."[20]

Save for the caveat about "authentic" marriage, Harvey's statement does not sound that different from the positions taken by some AIDS activists. Leading up to the Rose Bowl Parade, Ged Kenslea, spokesman for the AIDS Healthcare Foundation, said his organization champions same-sex marriage precisely because it encourages the kind of behavior that prevents the spread of HIV. "We believe that marriage saves lives," he explained.[21] This emphasis on marriage as a primary form of HIV prevention overlapped with statements made by the Foundation's president, Michael Weinstein, who called Truvada a "party drug." "There's an element of the gay community that espouses 'anything goes,' that is for sexual freedom and not giving an inch," he continued: "but demonizing me or AHF isn't going to shut us up." His comments set off a debate among activists and public health leaders. A number of men using PrEP had experienced what they have called the "'Truvada whore' syndrome"—judgments for being promiscuous or being "seen as a slut."[22] It seemed that Weinstein was adding to such attacks. The always outspoken gay AIDS activist Larry Kramer also jumped into the fray. In an interview with the *New York Times*, Kramer stated, "there's something to me cowardly about taking Truvada instead of using a condom."[23]

Both Weinstein and Kramer insist that using condoms should be privileged over a new medicine whose side effects, they note, remained a deterrent to daily adherence and therefore a threat to their success. They worried that gay men taking PrEP would forego condoms, but Kramer also registered his nostalgia for the broader kind of protest politics seen in the 1980s with groups like ACT UP. Activists of that generation were far more critical of biomedicine and pharmaceutical companies than gay men are today, even as they insisted upon the need for ongoing research. Kramer makes a good point. There has been strikingly little resistance to or even acknowledgment of the medicalization of safe sex, which has become the business of biomedical researchers and pharmaceutical companies rather than grassroots activists—and PrEP is no exception. But these important criticisms are blunted by the emphasis on gay marriage as the solution, which is visible not only in the AIDS Healthcare Foundation's stance but also in Kramer's work.

The occasion for his interview with the *Times* was the much-heralded release of the HBO movie *The Normal Heart*, directed by Ryan Murphy (the creator of the hit television show *Glee*) and starring a handful of Hollywood's leading men. Nominated for sixteen Emmy Awards, and winning in the category of "Outstanding Television Movie," the film was adapted from Kramer's 1985 play of the same title. It is an autobiographical depiction of his early work with Gay Men's Health Crisis in New York City. First performed at the Public Theater in Manhattan, the play captured the panic and fear that many gay men in the city faced in the early years of the AIDS crisis. But it also introduced one of the central debates dividing gay and lesbian activists in this period: the place of queer sex amid a life-threatening epidemic.

Kramer joined the choir of voices admonishing gay men to limit sexual encounters. In *The Normal Heart*, he recast this call in medical terms. Consider this exchange from the play. "Why aren't you telling them, bluntly, stop!" chided Emma Brookner, a medical doctor during the first years of the AIDS crisis, who thought community leaders were not doing enough to tell gay men to stop having sex. "Every day you don't tell them," she faults Ned Weeks (Kramer's surrogate), "more people infect each other." Kramer's play ends with Weeks wedding his lover, who is dying from AIDS. Emma officiates. "We are gathered here in the sight of God to join together these two men," she says: "I can see no objection. This is my hospital, my church." And so it proceeds. The wedding should be read alongside Weeks' earlier remark to a friend: "The gay leaders who created this sexual-liberation philosophy in the first place have been the death of us. Mickey, why didn't you guys fight for the right to get married instead of the right to legitimize promiscuity?"[24] While Murphy's film leaves out this last statement, it magnifies and sentimentalizes the wedding scene, which now must be read against the more recent successes of the gay marriage movement. It is a wistful look back at an earlier phase in gay life, before gay men grew up.

There are many good reasons to support gay marriage. But we might ask why it is that the gay marriage movement has become so attached to the narrative of romantic sexual monogamy as the normative model for queer life and how this vision has become the salvific hope for ending HIV/AIDS.[25] To criticize this narrative is not necessarily to criticize gay marriage. But I want to resist this conservative plot that would have AIDS prompt gay men to grow into sexual adulthood defined by monogamy and marriage. And I want to augment Chauncey's interpretation by suggesting another affective basis for the gay marriage movement, which is the force of a powerful American sexual morality and the social pressure and desire for national citizenship that demand comportment with this ideal. If, as Chauncey suggests, the very formation of a conservative gay movement marked the growing acceptance of gays and lesbians in American society, it also signaled their moral assimilation to the powerful rhetoric of American sexual morality—a moral creed that continues to define gay marriage debates and HIV/AIDS prevention policy.

After the Wrath of God argues that through the AIDS epidemic, American Christians helped build a national movement for sexual reform, one that sought to correct the purported moral declension witnessed in the 1960s and 1970s. If AIDS did not spark the creation of this moral rhetoric, it did quicken efforts to advance a larger moral agenda regarding sex. This new program succeeded precisely because it denied that AIDS was God's wrath on homosexuals. It suggested instead that the epidemic provided divine evidence for God's sexual morality. Christian or not, and for better or for worse, we live with that morality today.

Notes

INTRODUCTION

1. Grant Wacker, "Billy Graham's America," *Church History* 78, no. 3 (September 2009), 492, 490. Since Gallup first started polling Americans on which men and women they most admired in the world, the evangelist has made the list of "top ten" a remarkable fifty-seven times, more than any other figure in history. This covers polls conducted between 1946 and 2013. The next highest contender is Ronald Reagan, who has made the top ten list thirty-one times. Graham has never been named number one—which has usually gone to sitting presidents—but has been named the second most admired man numerous times. Jeffrey M. Jones, "Obama, Clinton Continue Reign as Most Admired," *Gallup Politics*, December 30, 2013, http://www.gallup.com/poll/166646/obama-clinton-continue-reign-admired-man-woman.aspx.

2. Associated Press, "Graham Apologizes for Speech Calling AIDS a Payback for Sin," *Chicago Tribune*, Oct. 10, 1993, 6.

3. Thomas H. Stahel, "Of Many Things," *America*, June 21, 1986, n.p.; Stahel, "Christ, Come Quickly," *America*, July 31, 2006, http://americamagazine.org/issue/579/faith-focus/christ-come-quickly; Jerry Falwell, "AIDS: The Judgment of God," *Liberty Report*, April 1987, 5.

4. Stahel, "Of Many Things."

5. A number of scholarly studies have illuminated the influence of the Christian Right on the history of AIDS, sexuality, and gay and lesbian activism, including Ashley Ruth Lierman, "The Plague Wars: Encounters between Gay and Lesbian Activism and the Christian Right in the Age of AIDS" (Ph.D. dissertation, Drew University, 2009); Tina Fetner, *How the Religious Right Shaped Lesbian and Gay Activism* (Minneapolis: University of Minnesota Press, 2008); Dagmar Herzog, "Missionary Positions," *Sex in Crisis: The New Sexual Revolution and the Future of American Politics* (New York: Basic Books, 2008), 127–162; recent

journalistic accounts include Esther Kaplan, *With God on Their Side: George W. Bush and the Christian Right* (New York: New Press, 2005) and Michelle Goldberg, *Kingdom Coming: The Rise of Christian Nationalism* (New York: W.W. Norton, 2007). According to sociologist Susan Chambré, the faith community provided the second major community response to the AIDS crisis, after the earliest grassroots efforts by the lesbian and gay community, which have garnered more historical attention. Susan M. Chambré, "The Changing Nature of 'Faith' in Faith-Based Organizations: Secularization and Ecumenism in Four AIDS Organizations in New York City," *Social Service Review* 75, no. 3 (Sept. 2001), 440, and *Fighting For Our Lives: New York's AIDS Community and the Politics of Disease* (New Brunswick, NJ: Rutgers University Press, 2006). As will become clear, religious communities and the lesbian and gay community also overlap in this history.

6. Actor Rock Hudson's death from AIDS-related complications in 1985, and NBA star Earvin "Magic" Johnson's public announcement in 1991 that he was HIV-positive, were two important moments during which national attention was drawn to the epidemic.

7. The benefits of the AIDS cocktail, also known as Highly Active Antiretroviral Therapy (HAART), were presented at the 11th International Conference on AIDS in Vancouver, British Columbia in 1996 and, following a series of publications in medical journals shortly thereafter, sparked this turning point in the treatment of HIV. For the longer history of treatment and research, see Mark Mascolini, "HAART, Hubris and Humility," *The Body*, September 2006, http://www.thebody.com/content/art40378.html; for criticism of media efforts to reduce the advent of the AIDS cocktail to a single team, rather than a complex history of collaboration, see Martin Delaney's oral presentation, "History of HAART: The True Story of How Effective Multidrug Therapy Was Developed for Treatment of HIV Diseases," *Retrovirology* (Suppl 1) 2006, S6, http://www.retrovirology.com/content/3/S1/S6.

8. Elizabeth Fee and Daniel M. Fox, eds., *AIDS: The Making of a Chronic Disease* (Berkeley: University of California Press, 1991) locate this shift from AIDS being considered a plague to a chronic condition earlier. I do not necessarily contest this observation, but would note that the shift itself was both uneven and not final. HAART most certainly revolutionized medical treatment in the mid-1990s, but even if we date the biggest shift to the mid-1990s, we must understand that many people, even if acting on a lack of information, continue to fear AIDS (or fear contracting HIV) and consider it a death sentence. And many others do not have access to the medical care that has enabled AIDS to become chronic.

9. An emerging body of scholarship on the history of the evangelical Left and of religious liberalism and mainline Christianity also suggests new ways of narrating this history. See David R. Swartz, *Moral Minority: The Evangelical Left in*

an Age of Conservatism (Philadelphia: University of Pennsylvania, 2012); Brantley W. Gasaway, *Progressive Evangelicals and the Pursuit of Social Justice* (Chapel Hill: University of North Carolina, 2014); Matthew Hedstrom, *The Rise of Liberal Religion: Book Culture and American Spirituality in the Twentieth Century* (New York: Oxford University Press, 2013); Elesha J. Coffman, *The Christian Century and the Rise of the Protestant Mainline* (New York: Oxford University Press, 2013); Leigh E. Schmidt and Sally M. Promey, eds, *American Religious Liberalism* (Bloomington: Indiana University Press, 2012); Leigh E. Schmidt, *Restless Souls: The Making of American Spirituality* (New York: HarperCollins, 2005); Pamela Klassen, *Spirits of Protestantism: Medicine, Healing, and Liberal Christianity* (Berkeley: University of California Press, 2011); Courtney Bender, *The New Metaphysicals: Spirituality and the American Religious Imagination* (Chicago: University of Chicago Press, 2010); David A. Hollinger, *After Cloven Tongues of Fire: Protestant Liberalism in Modern American History* (Princeton, NJ: Princeton University Press, 2013); and Jason S. Lantzer, *Mainline Christianity: The Past and Future of America's Majority Faith* (New York: NYU Press, 2012).

10. My work builds upon pioneering scholarship on religion and the AIDS crisis. J. Gordon Melton published an early collection of denominational statements in *The Churches Speak On: AIDS: Official Statements from Religious Bodies and Ecumenical Organizations* (Detroit: Gale Research Inc., 1989). On American Catholics, see Richard L. Smith, *AIDS, Gays, and the American Catholic Church* (Cleveland, OH: Pilgrim Press, 1994) and Mark R. Kowalewski, *All Things to All People: The Catholic Church Confronts the AIDS Crisis* (Albany, NY: SUNY Press, 1994). On Jewish responses, see Moshe Shokeid, "'We Are an Extended Family': Confronting the Rampage of an Epidemic," *A Gay Synagogue in New York* (Philadelphia: University of Pennsylvania Press, 2002), 216–231, and Gad Freudenthal, ed., *AIDS in Jewish Thought and Law* (Hoboken, NJ: Ktav Publishing, 1998). On African American churches, see Angelique Harris, *AIDS, Sexuality, and the Black Church: Making the Wounded Whole* (New York: Peter Lang, 2010); Dan Royles, "'Don't We Die Too': The Political Culture of African American AIDS Activism" (Ph.D. dissertation, Temple University, 2014), especially 127–172; Sandra L. Barnes, *Live Long and Prosper: How Black Megachurches Address HIV/AIDS and Poverty in the Age of Prosperity Theology* (New York: Fordham University Press, 2013); and Ronald Jeffrey Weatherford and Carole Boston Weatherford, *Somebody's Knocking on Your Door: AIDS and the African American Church* (New York: Haworth Press, 1999). On AIDS and its religious metaphors, see Susan Palmer, *AIDS as an Apocalyptic Metaphor in North America* (Toronto: University of Toronto Press, 1997), who details responses to HIV/AIDS from a variety of minority religious communities, and Thomas L. Long, *AIDS and American Apocalypticism: The Cultural Semiotics of an Epidemic* (Albany: State University of New York Press, 2005), who links the rhetoric of

apocalypse across Christian discourses and AIDS and gay activist cultural productions. On Islam, see Farid Esack and Sarah Chiddy, *Islam and AIDS: Between Scorn, Pity and Justice* (Oxford: Oneworld Publications, 2009). On Buddhism, see Wendy Cadge, "Lesbian, Gay, and Bisexual Buddhist Practitioners," in Scott Thumma and Edward R. Gray, eds., *Gay Religion* (Walnut Creek, CA: Altamira, 2004), 139–152; José Ignacio Cabezón, "Homosexuality and Buddhism," in Arlene Swidler, ed., *Homosexuality and World Religions* (Valley Forge, PA: Trinity Press International, 1993), 81–102. On Native American responses, see Irene S. Vernon, *Killing Us Quietly: Native Americans and HIV/AIDS* (Lincoln: University of Nebraska, 2001). On the porous boundaries between religious and secular AIDS work, see Courtney Bender, *Heaven's Kitchen: Living Religion at God's Love We Deliver* (Chicago: University of Chicago Press, 2003).

11. These arguments are indebted to a rich body of scholarship on religion and sexuality and on secularism, including Lynne Gerber, *Seeking the Straight and Narrow: Weight Loss and Sexual Reorientation in Evangelical America* (Chicago: University of Chicago Press, 2011); Mark D. Jordan, *Recruiting Young Love: How Christians Talk about Homosexuality* (Chicago: University of Chicago Press, 2011); Kathryn Lofton, "Queering Fundamentalism: John Balcom Shaw and the Sexuality of a Protestant Orthodoxy," *Journal of the History of Sexuality* 17, no. 3 (September 2008), 439–468, and *Oprah: The Gospel of an Icon* (Berkeley: University of California Press, 2011); Tracy Fessenden, *Culture and Redemption: Religion, the Secular, and American Literature* (Princeton: Princeton University Press, 2006); Talal Asad, *Formations of the Secular* (Palo Alto, CA: Stanford University Press, 2003); and Janet R. Jakobsen and Ann Pellegrini, *Love the Sin: Sexual Regulation and the Limits of Religious Tolerance* (New York: NYU Press, 2003) and "Introduction: Times Like These," *Secularisms* (Durham, NC: Duke University Press, 2008), 1–38.

12. This translation into secular speech occurs even as Christian writers have themselves repurposed such ostensibly secular languages of public health, biomedicine, and sexual identity in making their claims.

13. Gerber, *Seeking the Straight and Narrow*, 54. Also see Jonathan M. Metzl and Anna Kirkland, editors, *Against Health: How Health Became the New Morality* (New York: NYU Press, 2010).

14. In the modern period, what has been deemed "good" religion is religion that is "moral," that is, where the focus is more on being a good person than on gaining salvation—it is, usually, a variant of liberal Protestant Christianity. This history of the moral arose in part through racist and colonialist assumptions about human progression and civilization that stretch back at least to the European Enlightenment. My point is that this genealogy of the moral remains with us. See Robert A. Orsi, "Snakes Alive: Religious Studies between Heaven and Earth," *Between Heaven and Earth: The Religious Worlds People Make and the*

Scholars Who Study Them (Princeton, NJ: Princeton University Press, 2005), 177–204. Also see the literature cited in note 25.

15. My thanks to Wallace Best for prompting me to see this aspect of my project and to Leslie Ribovich for pushing me toward clarity.

16. I do not want to overstate the distinction between morality and moral language; to be sure, the ways people talk about morality, including the languages they use, also constitute morality. While I focus mostly on spoken and written texts in this study, moral language could be broadened to include a wider range of practices in addition to speech and writing. A full discussion of Kantian and Aristotelian views of morality and ethics, especially as taken up by scholars like Michel Foucault and Saba Mahmood, falls beyond the scope of this project. I will note, in following Foucault's model, that by "morality" I mean codes of conduct, norms, values, or injunctions. I use the language of "ethics" to mark a subset of practices that constitute ethical or moral subjects. For an excellent account of this distinction, see Saba Mahmood, *The Politics of Piety: The Islamic Revival and the Feminist Subject* (Princeton, NJ: Princeton University Press, 2005), 25–34. Jarrett Zigon adopts a similar approach, though he also draws on Deleuze and Gautari to theorize what he calls "moral assemblages" in his work on HIV/AIDS and the Russian Orthodox Church. Zigon defines "the moral" as three different but often related components: institutional morality (governments, organized religion), the public discourse of morality (media outlets, public protest, art and literature), and morality as embodied dispositions, akin to what Marcel Mauss called habitus. He defines ethics as the conscious and intentional effort to cultivate a moral habitus. Zigon, *"HIV Is God's Blessing": Rehabilitating Morality in Neoliberal Russia* (Berkeley: University of California Press, 2010), especially 62–72, and Zigon, *Morality: An Anthropological Perspective* (Oxford and New York: Berg Publishers, 2008).

17. Jakobsen and Pellegrini describe this translation as the secularization of Christian discourse into social relations, in "Introduction," 1–38.

18. Michel Foucault, *Security, Territory, Population: Lectures at the College de France, 1977—1978*, trans. Graham Burchell (New York: Picador, 2009), especially lectures one through three. These are forms of what Foucault calls biopower. He first distinguishes discipline from security or regulation in the final lecture in his 1975–1976 series, *"Society Must Be Defended": Lectures at the College de France 1975–1976*, trans. David Macy (New York: Picador, 2003), 239–264. He oscillates between the language of security and of regulation, focusing on the former term in the 1977–1978 lectures, while emphasizing the latter in *The History of Sexuality, Vol. 1: An Introduction*, trans. Robert Hurley (New York: Vintage, 1990). Also see Thomas Lemke, *Biopolitics: An Advanced Introduction*, trans. Eric Frederick Trump (New York: NYU Press, 2011), especially 33–52.

19. Foucault calls the former process *normation*, while he terms the mechanism of regulation or security *normalization*. He argues that the tactics of security/

regulation increasingly modified or displaced disciplinary tactics, as the science of population became dominant in modern society: "mankind," he puts it at one point, eventually gave way to "the human species." Foucault, *Security, Territory, Population,* 56–57, 63; also see Foucault, *The History of Sexuality,* especially 133–160.

20. On the moral construction of medicine, see Byron Good, *Medicine, Rationality, and Experience: An Anthropological Perspective* (Cambridge, UK: Cambridge University Press, 1994) and Arther Kleinman, *The Illness Narratives: Suffering, Healing, and the Human Condition* (New York: Basic Books, 1988). Good argues, "it is precisely the conjoining of the physiological and the soteriological that is central to the constitution of medicine as a modern institution" (86).

21. Historians often write about morality or moral arguments, but there is little consensus about what "morality" is. The term often becomes an empty form— to be filled in with variegated conservative religious or cultural arguments—or sometimes even shorthand for claims that seem vaguely religious. It would be obvious to say, simply, that AIDS was a "moral" epidemic. And the AIDS epidemic did not, of course, provide American Christians their first occasion to engage in moral debate. I hope this book allows us to think more critically and concretely about *how* AIDS in the United States emerged as a moral epidemic, what the content of this morality was, and what work this morality did in public and political debate, including among religious leaders, regarding AIDS and sexuality. I hope my elaboration of moral arguments about AIDS and sexuality in this period will contribute to studies of morality, and especially Christian morality regarding sex, in other periods and cases, including the history of social hygiene, germ panics, body image, marriage, sex education, abortion, and pornography debates, to name only a few possibilities. Instructive studies include Jeffrey P. Moran, *Teaching Sex: The Shaping of Adolescence in the 20th Century* (Cambridge: Harvard University Press, 2002); Leslie Woodstock Tentler, *Catholics and Contraception: An American History* (Ithaca, NY: Cornell University Press, 2004); Allan Brandt, *No Magic Bullet: A Social History of Venereal Disease in the United States since 1880* (New York: Oxford University Press, 1987); R. Marie Griffith, *Born Again Bodies: Flesh and Spirit in American Christianity* (Berkeley: University of California Press, 2004); Rebecca L. Davis, *More Perfect Unions: The American Search for Marital Bliss* (Cambridge, MA: Harvard University Press, 2010); Nancy Tomes, *The Gospel of Germs: Men, Women, and the Microbe in American Life* (Cambridge, MA: Harvard University Press, 1998); and Whitney Strub, *Perversion for Profit: The Politics of Pornography and the Rise of the New Right* (New York: Columbia University Press, 2010). I also do not want to suggest that the AIDS crisis was wholly unique in the history of Christian responses to disease. For a longer, comparative history of Christianity, sexuality, and disease (including an excellent chapter on the AIDS crisis), see Peter Lewis Allen, *The Wages of Sin: Sex and Disease, Past and*

Present (Chicago: University of Chicago Press, 2000). What I do find different about the AIDS epidemic in this history is the convergence in the 1980s and 1990s of Christian political influence and Reaganite conservatism with the emergence of regulatory forms of biopower.

22. Will Kymlicka and Wayne Normal, "Return of the Citizen: A Survey of Recent Work on Citizenship Theory," in Ronald Beiner, ed., *Theorizing Citizenship* (Albany, NY: SUNY Press, 1995), 283–322. Margot Canaday, *The Straight State: Sexuality and Citizenship in Twentieth Century America* (Princeton, NJ: Princeton University Press, 2009), 7–10, offers a very helpful historiographical account of this distinction and an elaboration on the idea of citizenship as a status.

23. Lauren Berlant, "Citizenship," in Bruce Burgett and Glenn Hendler, eds., *Keywords in American Cultural Studies* (New York and London: NYU Press, 2007), 37–42; on sexual citizenship, see Canaday, *The Straight State*; Robert O. Self, *All in the Family: The Realignment of American Democracy since the 1960s* (New York: Hill and Wang, 2012), 75–100; and Nancy Cott, *Public Vows: A History of Marriage and the Nation* (Cambridge, MA: Harvard University Press, 2000).

24. Benedict Anderson, *Imagined Communities: Reflections on the Origin and Spread of Nationalism* (London and New York: Verso, 1991 [1983]), remains the best starting point for thinking about the nation as an "imagined community."

25. Historians have amply documented this point, showing how often religion, race, and sexuality have informed one another in naming who counts as a person. See Evelyn Brooks Higginbotham, "African-American Women's History and the Metalanguage of Race," *Signs* 17, no. 2 (Winter 1992), 251–274; Merril D. Smith, ed., *Sex and Sexuality in Early America* (New York and London: NYU Press, 1998); Martha Hodes, *White Women, Black Men: Illicit Sex in the Nineteenth-Century South* (New Haven, CT: Yale University Press, 1997); Robert Orsi, *The Madonna of 115th Street* (New Haven, CT: Yale University Press, 3rd ed., 2010); Sally Engle Merry, *Colonizing Hawai'i: The Cultural Power of Law* (Princeton, NJ: Princeton University Press, 2000).

26. On Reagan-era conservatism, see Andrew E. Busch, *Reagan's Victory: The Presidential Election of 1980 and the Rise of the Right* (Lawrence: University Press of Kansas, 2005); Sean Wilentz, *The Age of Reagan: A History, 1974–2008* (New York: HarperCollins, 2008); Daniel K. Williams, *God's Own Party: The Making of the Christian Right* (Oxford and New York: Oxford University Press, 2010); Daniel Rodgers, *The Age of Fracture* (Cambridge, MA: Harvard University Press, 2011); Self, *All in the Family*.

27. Lauren Berlant, *The Queen of America Goes to Washington City: Essays on Sex and Citizenship* (Durham, NC: Duke University Press, 1997), 3. I call this a "reemergence" because, as Berlant has shown, we can trace this genealogy of the sentimental national sphere back to the nineteenth century. Berlant, *The Female Complaint: The Unfinished Business of Sentimentality in American Culture* (Durham, NC: Duke University Press, 2008).

28. Self, *All in the Family*, 6.

29. For an incisive analysis of both the contingency and the importance of "family values" to this history, see Seth Dowland, "'Family Values' and the Formation of a Christian Right Agenda," *Church History* 78, no. 3 (September 2009), 606–631. In his excellent analysis of gender and sexuality politics since 1960s, *All in the Family*, Self insists upon reading cultural issues of gender and sexuality alongside and as co-constitutive of economic ones, including the rise of neoliberalism. For an instructive analysis along these lines, see Bethany Moreton, *To Serve God and Wal-Mart: The Making of Christian Free Enterprise* (Cambridge, MA: Harvard University Press, 2009). On the importance of race to the history of postwar conservatism and the anti–gay rights movements, including the Christian Right, see Dan Carter, *The Politics of Rage: George Wallace, the Origins of New Conservatism, and the Transformation of American Politics* (New York: Simon and Schuster, 1995); Gillian Frank, "'The Civil Rights of Parents': Race and Conservative Politics in Anita Bryant's Campaign against Gay Rights in 1970s Florida," *Journal of the History of Sexuality* 22, no. 1 (January 2013), 126–160; and Randall Balmer, *Thy Kingdom Come: How the Religious Right Distorts Faith and Threatens the Nation* (New York: Basic Books, 2006), 1–34.

30. Berlant, *Queen of America*, 3.

31. Berlant, *Queen of America*, 15.

32. Thomas Yingling, *AIDS and the National Body*, Robyn Wiegman, ed. (Durham, NC: Duke University Press, 1997), 43.

33. Scholars of religion might hear the undertones of Durkheimian sociology, especially as this tradition has been extended by Mary Douglas, Robert Bellah, and James Davison Hunter, in my discussion of the social body and its mapping onto American nationhood through moral rhetoric. I am indebted to this tradition but also hope to depart from its tendency to underscore social stability and the formation of the social group rather than the conflicts through which that social group's margins become formed and outsiders produced.

34. The historiography of the AIDS crisis in the United States in the period under study here is immense, but see Allan Brandt, "'Plagues and Peoples': The AIDS Epidemic," *No Magic Bullet*, 183–204; Elizabeth Fee and Daniel M. Fox, eds., *AIDS: The Burdens of History* (Berkeley: University of California Press, 1988); Ronald Bayer, *Private Acts, Social Consequences: AIDS and the Politics of Public Health* (New Brunswick, NJ: Rutgers University Press, 1991); Virginia Berridge and Philip Strong, eds., *AIDS and Contemporary History* (Cambridge, MA: Cambridge University Press, 1993); Mirko D. Grmek, *History of AIDS: Emergence and Origin of a Modern Epidemic* (Princeton, NJ: Princeton University Press, 1993); John-Manuel Andriote, *Victory Deferred: How AIDS Changed Gay Life in America* (Chicago: University of Chicago Press, 1999); Jonathan Engel, *The Epidemic: A Global History of AIDS* (New York: Smithsonian Books/ Collins, 2006); Deborah B. Gould, *Moving Politics: Emotion and ACT UP's Fight*

against AIDS (Chicago: University of Chicago Press, 2009); and especially Jennifer Brier, *Infectious Ideas: U.S. Political Responses to the AIDS Crisis* (Chapel Hill: University of North Carolina, 2009). For cultural studies accounts, see Simon Watney, *Policing Desire: Pornography, AIDS, and the Media* (Minneapolis: University of Minnesota Press, 1987); Douglas Crimp, ed., *AIDS: Cultural Analysis, Cultural Activism* (Cambridge, MA: MIT Press, 1988) and Crimp, *Melancholia and Moralism: Essays on AIDS and Queer Politics* (Cambridge, MA: MIT Press, 2004); Erica Carter and Simon Watney, eds., *Taking Liberties: AIDS and Cultural Politics* (London: Serpent's Tail, 1989); Cindy Patton, *Inventing AIDS* (New York: Routledge, 1990) and *Globalizing AIDS* (Minneapolis: University of Minnesota Press, 2002); and Paula A. Treichler, *How to Have Theory in an Epidemic* (Durham, NC: Duke University Press, 1999).

35. Cindy Patton, *Sex and Germs: The Politics of AIDS* (Boston: South End Press, 1985); Dennis Altman, *AIDS in the Mind of America* (Garden City, NY: Anchor/Doubleday Press, 1986); Randy Shilts, *And the Band Played On: Politics, People, and the AIDS Epidemic* (New York: St. Martin's Press, 1987). Positive evaluations of sexual practices that proliferated in the wake of gay liberation include Eric E. Rofes, *Reviving the Tribe: Regenerating Gay Men's Sexuality and Culture in the Ongoing Epidemic* (New York: Routledge, 1995); Patrick Moore, *Beyond Shame: Reclaiming the Abandoned History of Radical Gay Sexuality* (Boston: Beacon Press, 2004); and Michael Warner, *The Trouble with Normal: Sex, Politics, and the Ethics of Queer Life* (Cambridge: Harvard University Press, 1999).

36. It is possible that Dugas, like many gay men, understood the attempt to stop gay men from having sex as another effort by the perceived homophobic scientific establishment and conservative government to limit their freedom. Shilts, *And the Band Played On*, 21–23, 136, 138, 147, 165. My discussion is indebted to Timothy Murphy, *Ethics in an Epidemic: AIDS, Morality, and Culture* (Berkeley: University of California Press, 1994) and Douglas Crimp, "How to Have Promiscuity in an Epidemic," October, vol. 43 (Winter 1987), 237–271. For more recent assessments, see Phil Tiemeyer, *Plane Queer: Labor, Sexuality, and AIDS in the History of Male Flight Attendants* (Berkeley: University of California Press, 2013), 136–193, and Richard A. McKay, "'Patient Zero': The Absence of a Patient's View of the Early North American AIDS Epidemic," *Bull. Hist. Med.* (Spring 2014), 161–194.

37. Murphy, *Ethics in an Epidemic*, 14–15; also see Crimp, "How to Have Promiscuity," 237–271.

38. Shilts' depiction was further popularized in the 1993 HBO film version of *And the Band Played On*, directed by Robert Spottiswoode, which if anything amplified the moralism of this narrative.

39. Engel, *The Epidemic*, 13–14.

40. Indeed, AIDS activists and gay men did support many public health recommendations, including education about safe sex practices and the distribution

of condoms. And most public health leaders stopped short of calling for mandatory testing and reporting. For a more balanced treatment of the debate between public health measures and individual civil rights, see Bayer, *Private Acts, Social Consequences*, especially chapter 2.

41. Engel, *The Epidemic*, 39–40, emphasis mine.

42. Narratives of drug use are similarly fraught, as when writers label IV drug users as "drug abusers."

43. Patton, *Sex and Germs*; Altman, *AIDS in the Mind of America*; also see Simon Watney, *Policing Desire*; to my mind, the best recent account of the political history of the HIV/AIDS epidemic is Brier, *Infectious Ideas*.

44. On this last point, see Altman, *AIDS in the Mind of America*, 160.

45. Different ways of narrating debates about whether to close gay bathhouses illustrate this line of analysis. See Altman, *AIDS in the Mind of America*, 147–155.

46. We should distinguish *morality* from *moralism*, a term often used in a pejorative sense. Following historian Erling Jorstad, *The Politics of Moralism: The New Christian Right in American Life* (Minneapolis, MN: Augsburg Publishing House, 1981), 8–10, morality can be defined as the question of whether instances of human behavior can be deemed right or wrong. The important point here is that the definition of rightness and wrongness is always contested. In contrast, *moralism* distinguishes right from wrong, but posits the correct moral action in any situation because authority is found within an uncompromising or absolutist religious or moral tradition. On Christian moralism, also see Susan F. Harding, "American Protestant Moralism and the Secular Imagination: From Temperance to the Moral Majority," *Social Research* 76, no. 4 (Winter 2009), 1277–1306.

47. A similar opposition is repeated in writing on religion and sexuality, which frequently constructs homosexual and religious identities as mutually exclusive. On the long "Puritan" shadow cast over American sexual conduct, see Tracy Fessenden, Magdalena J. Zaborowska, and Nicholas F. Radel, eds., *The Puritan Origins of American Sex: Religion, Sexuality, and National Identity in American Literature* (New York: Routledge, 2001). For important early scholarly efforts to move beyond this impasse, see Melissa Wilcox, *Coming Out in Christianity: Religion, Identity, and Community* (Bloomington: Indiana University Press, 2003) and Dawne Moon, *God, Sex, and Politics: Homosexuality and Everyday Theologies* (Chicago: University of Chicago Press, 2004).

48. Important revisions to this history include Heather Rachelle White, "Homosexuality, Gay Communities, and American Churches: A History of a Changing Religious Ethics, 1946–1977" (Ph.D. dissertation, Princeton University, 2007) and Jordan, *Recruiting Young Love*.

49. See, for instance, the treatment of religion in Susan Hunter's otherwise quite trenchant, popular account, *AIDS in America* (New York: Palgrave, 2006).

50. See footnote 10 for suggestions.

51. I try to take seriously here anthropologist Talal Asad's argument that the religious and the secular are not a mutually exclusive binary, but rather (often) overlapping discursive terrains. See Asad, *Formations of the Secular*, especially 1–20.

52. David Bebbington, *Evangelicalism in Modern Britain: A History from the 1730s to the 1980s* (London: Unwin Hyman, 1989), 3. For a history of liberal Protestantism and the mainline denominations, see William Hutchison, *The Modernist Impulse in American Protestantism* (Durham, NC: Duke University Press, 1992); Peter J. Thuesen, "The Logic of Mainline Churchliness: Historical Background since the Reformation," in Robert Wuthnow and John H. Evans, eds., *The Quiet Hand of God: Faith-Based Activism and the Public Role of Mainline Protestantism* (Berkeley: University of California Press, 2002). On homosexuality and the mainline tradition, see Anthony M. Petro, "Mainline Protestants and Homosexuality," in *LGBTQ America Today: An Encyclopedia*, ed. John C. Hawley (Westport, CT: Greenwood, 2008), 943–949.

53. Dowland, "'Family Values,'" offers a useful guide.

54. George Marsden, *Understanding Fundamentalism and Evangelicalism* (Grand Rapids, MI: Wm. B. Eerdmans Publishing Co, 1991), 1.

55. On the emergence of the term "gay" in popular usage, see George Chauncey, *Gay New York: Gender, Urban Culture, and the Making of the Gay Male World, 1890–1940* (New York: Basic Books, 1994), 12–23; Jeremy W. Peters, "The Decline and Fall of the 'H' Word," *New York Times*, March 21, 2014, http://www.nytimes.com/2014/03/23/fashion/gays-lesbians-the-term-homosexual.html. For a critique of the MSM (and WSW) designation, see Rebecca M. Young and Ilan H. Meyer, "The Trouble with 'MSM' and 'WSW': Erasure of the Sexual Minority Person in Public Health Discourse," *American Journal of Public Health* 95, no. 7 (July 2005), 1144–1149. For an excellent cultural analysis of sexual politics, black men, and the "down low," including their relationship to the AIDS crisis, see Jeffrey Q. McCune, Jr., *Sexual Discretion: Black Masculinity and the Politics of Passing* (Chicago: University of Chicago Press, 2014).

56. Before 2000, and especially in the late 1980s, medical professionals also employed the term ARC (AIDS-Related Complex) to describe people with HIV expressing mild symptoms of illness. Also, keeping with the terminology of the period, I use STD (sexually transmitted disease) rather than STI (sexually transmitted infection), which is now preferred by most health professionals.

57. On the naming of HIV and AIDS, see Patton, *Inventing AIDS*. The People with AIDS movement emerged in the early 1980s and established the Denver Principles in 1983, in which they argued against the use of the term "victim." See Advisory Committee for People with AIDS, "Denver Principles" (1983), www.actupny.org/documents/Denver.html.

58. Not that such approaches would be unwelcome. For the sake of focus, I have sought to emphasize here the powerful rhetoric of AIDS and its Christian history.

I also would not want to position my narrative here against scholarship on "lived religion," if we understand lived religion not merely to point to moments of religious creativity and agency (understood all too often as something we "like" or as another form of "good religion") as opposed to negotiations of power and forms of subjection that often lead to pain, suffering, and oppression. In this sense, I am especially influenced by Orsi, *Between Heaven and Earth*; R. Marie Griffith, *Born Again Bodies: Flesh and Spirit in American Christianity* (Berkeley: University of California Press, 2004); and Mahmood, *Politics of Piety*.

CHAPTER I

1. Timothy C. Morgan, "'No world leader has done more for global health than President George Bush,'" *Christianity Today Liveblog*, Nov. 30, 2008, blog.christianitytoday.com; "President George W. Bush Receives 'International Medal of PEACE' That Coincides with PEPFAR Milestone on World AIDS Day," *AIDS Weekly*, Dec. 15, 2008, 63. Also see www.pepfar.gov.

2. "President George W. Bush," *AIDS Weekly*, 63.

3. Faith-based initiatives initially arose as a part of President Clinton's 1996 Welfare Reform bill called "Charitable Choice," but were expanded by Bush into a far more prominent federal program. See Rebecca Sager, *Faith, Politics, and Power: The Politics of Faith-Based Initiatives* (New York: Oxford University Press, 2010).

4. The percentage has increased gradually since 2003, but PEPFAR eventually required that one-third of all prevention funding be devoted to abstinence education. Herzog, *Sex in Crisis*, 127–162.

5. Cited in "False Choices Plague Anti-AIDS Fight," *Christian Century*, Dec. 26, 2006, 12–13. On the prospects for Obama's faith-based presidency, see Winnifred Fallers Sullivan, "You Gotta Have Faith-Based Politics," *Religion Dispatches*, Feb. 10, 2009, www.religiondispatches.org.

6. "False Choices Plague Anti-AIDS Fight," *Christian Century*, 12–13; Williams, *God's Own Party*, 269–270.

7. Jeff Zeleny and David D. Kirkpatrick, "Obama's Choice of Pastor Creates Furor," *New York Times*, Dec. 19, 2008, A19.

8. Hunter, *Culture Wars*, 43–44. See also Hunter and Alan Wolfe, *Is There a Culture War? A Dialogue on Values and American Public Life* (Washington, D.C.: Brookings Institute Press, 2006). For a useful analysis of how the culture wars developed in mainstream news media, see Diane Winston, "Back to the Future: Religion, Politics, and the Media," *American Quarterly* 59 no. 3 (Sept 2007): 969–989.

9. Catholic responses receive fuller treatment in chapters three and four.

10. "Met with Standing Ovation, Threats Minister Gives Condoms at AIDS Sermon," *Los Angeles Times*, Feb. 9, 1987, 13.

11. "Met with Standing Ovation, Threats Minister Gives Condoms at AIDS Sermon," 13 (grammar error in the original).

12. CDC, "*Pneumocystis Pneumonia–Los Angeles*," *Morbidity and Mortality Weekly Review*, 30, no. 1 (June 5, 1981): 1.

13. Molaghan, J. B., "The New 'Gay Diseases': Concern, not Panic," *Gay Community News*, Jan. 9, 1982, 3.

14. Brandt, *No Magic Bullet*, 183–204, locates AIDS within the longer history of nineteenth- and twentieth-century venereal diseases; Epstein, *Impure Science*, and Patton, *Inventing AIDS*, offer the best sociological and cultural studies accounts of this emergence; Shilts, *And the Band Played On*, offers a thorough, if at times problematic, account of the first years of medical work on the epidemic.

15. Patton, *Sex and Germs*; and Altman, *AIDS in the Mind of America*.

16. "Now No One Is Safe from AIDS," *Life* 2, no. 1 (July 1985), cover; James Kinsella, *Covering the Plague: AIDS and the American Media* (New Brunswick, NJ: Rutgers University Press: 1992); and Treichler, *How to Have Theory in an Epidemic*, especially 127–148, ably detail the sensationalism of media coverage.

17. On the history of conservative evangelicals and of the Christian Right, see especially William Martin, *With God on Our Side: The Rise of the Religious Right in America* (New York: Broadway Books, 1996); Clyde Wilcox and Carin Larson, *Onward Christian Soldiers: The Religious Right in American Politics* (Bloomington: Indiana University Press, 2006); Lisa McGirr, *Suburban Warriors: The Origins of the New American Right* (Princeton, NJ: Princeton University Press, 2001); Williams, *God's Own Party*; Darren Dochuck, *From Bible Belt to Sunbelt: Plain-Folk Religion, Grassroots Politics, and the Rise of Evangelical Conservatism* (New York: W. W. Norton, 2010); Molly Worthen, *Apostles of Reason: The Crisis of Authority in American Evangelicalism* (Oxford and New York: Oxford University Press, 2014), 198–240.

18. Quoted in Hans Johnson and William Eskridge, "The Legacy of Falwell's Bully Pulpit," *Washington Post*, May 19, 2007, A17; also see Susan Friend Harding, *The Book of Jerry Falwell: Fundamentalist Language and Politics* (Princeton, NJ: Princeton University Press, 2001), 156–160. For excellent accounts of this apocalyptic rhetoric, see Palmer, *AIDS as an Apocalyptic Metaphor*, 39–43 and Long, *AIDS and American Apocalypticism*, 1–28. Both authors show how the rhetoric of apocalypse extended beyond the Christian Right, including among other religious minority communities (in Palmer) and in the writing and performance of many queer and AIDS activists and artists (in Long).

19. "Report on Sexual Orientation Discrimination," prepared by Eileen Gillis, San Francisco AIDS Foundation Papers, Carton 4, Executive Director, Folder 1984–1985, 6–11, AIDS History Project Archive Collection, University of California, San Francisco.

20. "Impact AIDS: Revision of Brochure," San Francisco AIDS Foundation Papers, Carton 18: Education, F1991, AIDS History Project Archive Collection, University of California, San Francisco.

21. On the influence of the Religious Right on gay politics, see Fetner, *How the Religious Right Shaped Lesbian and Gay Activism.*

22. Diane Winston, "News Coverage of Religion, Sexuality, and AIDS," in *The Oxford Handbook of Religion and the American News Media* (New York: Oxford University Press, 2012), 377–384.

23. As Jason Bivins notes, "political fear is thus always pedagogical." See Jason Bivins, *Religion of Fear: The Politics of Horror in American Evangelicalism* (New York: Oxford, 2008), 10–11; 27.

24. Epstein, *Impure Science*; Michelle Cochrane, *When AIDS Began: San Francisco and the Making of an Epidemic* (New York: Routledge, 2004), especially 169–186.

25. According to *Special Report*, the Summit Ministries Resource Center has been publishing on the topic of homosexuality since 1977. The back page lists the educational affiliations of each author, including graduate and doctoral degrees (for Lutton and Cameron at secular state schools). David A. Noebel, Wayne C. Lutton, and Paul Cameron, *AIDS: Acquired Immune Deficiency Syndrome: A Special Report* (Manitou Spring, CO: Summit Ministries Research Center, 1986 [revised editions released later in 1986 and in 1987]); Cameron, *Exposing the AIDS Scandal* (Lafayette, LA: Huntington House, 1988); Gene Antonio, *The AIDS Cover-Up? The Real and Alarming Facts about AIDS* (San Francisco: Ignatius Press, 1986).

26. As Fredric Jameson reminds us, "pastiche is blank parody, parody that has lost its humor." Jameson, "Postmodernism and Consumer Society," in Hal Foster, ed., *The Anti-Aesthetic: Essays on Postmodern Culture* (Port Townsend, WA: Bay Press, 1983), 114.

27. Jordan, *Recruiting Young Love*, 174–176.

28. Didi Herman, *The Antigay Agenda* (Chicago: University of Chicago Press, 1998), 61.

29. Enrique T. Rueda and Michael Schwartz, *Gays, AIDS, and You* (Old Greenwich, CT: Devin-Adair Co., 1987), 3, ix. This text pulls substantially from Rueda's earlier work, *The Homosexual Network: Private Lives and Public Policy* (Old Greenwich, CT: Devin-Adair Co., 1982), which, Herman writes, he penned at the request of Paul Weyrich, one of the architects of the New Right (*Antigay Agenda*, 62).

30. David Chilton, *The Power in the Blood: A Christian Response to AIDS* (Brentwood, TN: Wolgemuth and Hyatt, 1987).

31. Chilton, *The Power in the Blood*, 15–16.

32. Chilton, *The Power in the Blood*, 207.

33. Rueda and Schwartz, *AIDS, Gays, and You*, 91. The original is in italics.

34. Herman, *Antigay Agenda*, discusses links between the threats of homosexuality and communism in the mid-twentieth century.

35. Billy Graham, "AIDS, Herpes, Sex, and the Bible," Tallahassee, Florida, Nov. 6, 1986. Collections 265, Records of the BGEA: Montreat Office: Billy Graham—Papers, Part I: Crusade Sermon Notebooks, Box 15, Folder 69; Ser.# 2163. The words "judgment of God" and "warning" are underlined in the notes for this speech.

36. Glenn Collins, "Facing the Emotional Anguish of AIDS," *New York Times*, May 30, 1983: 1, 14; Joseph Berger, "AIDS Patients Pose Difficult New Test for Clergy," *New York Times*, Jan. 19, 1986, A14; John Balzar, "American Views of Gays: Disapproval, Sympathy," *Los Angeles Times*, December 20, 1985; also see Diane Winston, "News Coverage," 382.

37. John Leo, "The New Scarlet Letter," *Time*, August 1982, http://content.time.com/time/magazine/article/0,9171,1715020,00.html.

38. Billy Graham, "Herpes, Sex and the Bible," Orlando, April 11, 1983. Collections 285, Records of the BGEA: Montreat Office: Billy Graham—Papers, Part I: Crusade Sermon Notebooks, Box 11, Folder 90. The words "judgment of God" and "warning from God" are underlined in the notes for this speech.

39. Sacvan Berkovitch, *The American Jeremiad* (Madison: University of Wisconsin Press, 1978), remains the best study of the jeremiad in the American tradition. Thomas Long demonstrates the power of the jeremiad in gay AIDS cultural production as well, especially in the work of Larry Kramer, in *AIDS and American Apocalypticism*, 63–106. I am most grateful to Mark Jordan for this insight that Christian discourse about AIDS and homosexuality is a discourse about sodomy.

40. My reading has focused on David Wilkerson, *The Vision* (Old Tappan, NJ: Revell, 1974); David Noebel, *The Homosexual Revolution* (Tulsa, OK: American Christian College Press, 1977); Tim LaHaye, *The Unhappy Gays* (Wheaton, IL: Tyndale House, 1978); Ruedo, *Homosexual Network*; and Randy Alcorn, *Christians in the Wake of Sexual Revolution: Recovering Our Sexual Sanity* (Portland, OR: Multnomah Press, 1985). A number of the theological and rhetorical tropes developed in these texts persist in Chuck and Donna McIlhenny's *When the Wicked Seize a City*, written with Frank York (Lafayette, LA: Huntington House, 1993 [republished by Authors Choice Press with an new addendum in 2000]). This book narrates the McIlhennys' battles against gay rights (and AIDS) in San Francisco, where Chuck McIlhenny served as pastor at First Orthodox Presbyterian Church. The McIlhennys' story is recounted in Hunter, *Culture Wars*, 3–30.

41. Alcorn, *Christians in the Wake*, 34. Alcorn would later write several works of nonfiction and fiction. He received the 2002 Gold Medallion Book Award for Fiction from the Evangelical Christian Publishers Association for his novel *Safely Home*. Omri Elisha, in "Moral Ambitions of Grace: The Paradox of Compassion

and Accountability in Evangelical Faith-Based Activism," *Cultural Anthropology* 23:1 (2008): 173–174, aptly calls this evangelical reconstruction of America's past, though in a slightly different context, "nationalist nostalgia."

42. Timothy LaHaye and Beverly LaHaye, *The Act of Marriage: The Beauty of Sexual Love* (Grand Rapids. MI: Zondervan, 1976).

43. LaHaye, *Unhappy Gays*, 13–17; Alcorn, *Christians in the Wake*, 33–41, 74–75; Alcorn also cites the philosophical sources of this new immorality, which include Naturalism, Relativism, Pluralism, and Hedonism.

44. LaHaye, *Unhappy Gays*, 8, 20. In *AIDS and American Apocalypticism*, Long recounts an earlier description of the "homosexual epidemic." In 1973, evangelist David Wilkerson detailed a prophecy about the future of the United States in his book *The Vision*. A decade earlier, he had gained enormous success with *The Cross and the Switchblade*. Adapted to the 1970 film of the same name starring Pat Boone and Erik Estrada, this book told the story Wilkerson's move to New York City to form his ministry and established him as a leading figure in the evangelical movement. In *The Vision*, Wilkerson elaborated his warning from God of five calamities, one of which included the sin of Sodom, which would be repeated in his day. In a separate section devoted to "The Homosexual Epidemic," Wilkerson warned that only two forces held homosexuals at bay—their rejection by society and their repudiation in church teachings—but both were at dire risk of being "swept away" (5–6).

45. Noebel, *Homosexual Revolution*, 20.

46. All of the conservative Christian texts I describe here explicitly connect homosexuality to the sin of sodomy, citing passages from the Bible, including Genesis 19, Romans 1, and 1 Corinthians 6, among others. My goal here is to demonstrate the resonance of older theological and political understandings of the story of Sodom in these modern accounts.

47. Gerber, *Seeking the Straight and Narrow*, especially 52–78, provides an excellent account of the psychological and medical sources used in the evangelical ex-gay movement, for instance. Heather White, *Reforming Sodom: Protestants and the Rise of Gay Rights* (Chapel Hill: University of North Carolina Press, forthcoming 2015) offers a novel account of the "homosexualization" of American Protestantism in the mid-twentieth century. She demonstrates how what now passes as commonsense in teachings about what the Bible says about homosexuality was invented over this century. Liberal Protestants, who were convinced of the efficacy of scientific investigation for religious insight, produced a "modern synthesis of morality and medicine," which included adding "the homosexual" into new translations of the Bible starting in the 1940s in place of a far more diverse array of sexual and other practices mentioned in the text before. In 1973, the New International Version, which quickly emerged as one of the most popular Bible translations among American evangelicals, likewise became "homosexualized." My thanks to Heather White for sharing this work with me.

48. Foucault, *History of Sexuality*, especially 36–49, and Jonathan Ned Katz, *The Invention of Heterosexuality* (Chicago: University of Chicago Press, 2007).

49. Mark Jordan makes this point most convincingly and provides the grounding for my discussion here: "the 'Homosexual' remains a theological artifact because Christian rhetorics of identity enforcement were infused into the category from the very beginning—in ways Foucault does and does not admit." The homosexual, then, appears as a variation "on the much older theological category of the sexualized sin-identity." Jordan, *The Ethics of Sex* (Oxford, UK and Malden, MA: Wiley-Blackwell, 2002), 95, and *The Invention of Sodomy* (Chicago: University of Chicago Press, 1997).

50. Jordan, *Invention of Sodomy*, 29; *Ethics of Sex*, 82–83.

51. Jordan, *Ethics of Sex*, 79–80.

52. Jordan, *Ethics of Sex*, 82–83.

53. Jordan, *Ethics of Sex*, 92.

54. Noebel, *Homosexual Revolution*, 155.

55. Noebel, *Homosexual Revolution*, 109. Noebel described homosexuals as a long-known threat to national security, especially through what he calls the Communist-oriented global conspiracy organization, "Homosexual International." Noebel, Lutton, and Cameron, in *Special Report*, 128–129, also mention homosexual threats to national security; Jordan, *Recruiting Young Love*, 175.

56. Cited in LaHaye, *Unhappy Gays*, 204; Noebel, *Homosexual Revolution*, 134.

57. LaHaye, *Unhappy Gays*, 110, 179. LaHaye's dating of 1957 was incorrect. That was the year that the Wolfenden Report (the Report of the Departmental Committee of Homosexual Offenses and Prostitution), which recommended the decriminalization of homosexuality, was published. Actual legal changes followed (unevenly so) some years later. The United Kingdom decriminalized homosexual sex in 1967. Scotland and Northern Ireland followed in 1980 and 1982, respectively.

58. Alcorn, *Christians in the Wake*, 160; Noebel, *Homosexual Revolution*, 141.

59. Jordan, *Recruiting Young Love*, 173–176, demonstrates as much in his reading of Cameron.

60. Harding, *Book of Jerry Falwell*, especially chapter one, 33–60.

61. "Diseases that Plague Gays," *Gay Synagogue News*, February 1982, and "Gay Diseases Symposium," *Gay Synagogue News*, April 1982, Congregation Beth Simchat Torah Collection, Box 4, Folder 1982, National Archive of Lesbian, Gay, Bisexual, and Transgender History, New York City. See also Shokeid, *A Gay Synagogue in New York*, 218–219.

62. Patricia Ward Biederman, "Lifestyles in Gay Community Tempered by Threat of AIDS," *Los Angeles Times*, June 16, 1985, 4; Biederman, Patricia Ward, "AIDS-Stricken Pastor of Homosexual Sect Clings to His Faith," *Los Angeles Times*, Oct. 13, 1985, 12.

63. A. Stephen Pieters, *"I'm Still Dancing!" A Gay Man's Health Experience* (Gaithersburg, MD: Chi Rho Press, 1991); Pieters, "Spiritual Strength for Survival"

and "HIV/AIDS: Is It God's Judgment? A Christian View of Faith, Hope and Love," http://www.thebody.com/content/art39714.html.

64. John Godges, "Religious Groups Meet the San Francisco AIDS Challenge," *The Christian Century*, Sept. 10–17, 1986, 771–775.

65. Godges, "Religious Groups Meet the San Francisco AIDS Challenge," 771.

66. Godges, "Religious Groups Meet the San Francisco AIDS Challenge," 772.

67. Revon Kyle Banneker, "Rev. Carl Bean: Perhaps the Most Important Black Gay Activist in the Entire World," Interview with Carl Bean, *BLK*, July 1989: 8–17; 10; Lynn Simross, "The 'Rev.' Responds to Calling Reaching Out to Minority AIDS Victims," *Los Angeles Times*, August 15, 1985, 1. Also see Bean's autobiography, Bean, with David Ritz, *I Was Born This Way: A Gay Preacher's Journey through Gospel Music, Disco Stardom, and a Ministry in Christ* (New York: Simon and Schuster, 2010).

68. Weatherford and Weatherford, *Somebody's Knocking on Your Door*; Dorie Gilbert, "*Focus on Solutions*: Black Churches Respond to AIDS: Interview with Pernessa Seale, Founder and CEO of The Balm in Gilead," in *African American Women and HIV/AIDS: Critical Responses* (Westport, CT: Praeger, 2003): 153–158; Yvette Flunder, Interview for the Lesbian, Gay, Bisexual and Transgender Religious Archives Network, conducted by Monique Moultrie, February 28, 2011, lgbtran.org/Interview.aspx?ID=25. On African American religious responses to AIDS, also see Cathy Cohen, *The Boundaries of Blackness: AIDS and the Breakdown of Black Politics* (Chicago: University of Chicago Press, 1999), especially 276–288; Harris, *AIDS, Sexuality, and the Black Church*; Royles, "'Don't We Die Too,'" 127–172; Stephen J. Inrig, *North Carolina and the Problem of AIDS* (Chapel Hill: University of North Carolina Press, 2012); and Jacob Levenson, *The Secret Epidemic: The Story of AIDS and Black America* (New York: Pantheon, 2004).

69. Mark I. Pinsky, "First Orange County Mass Set for AIDS Victims," *Los Angeles Times*, June 8, 1986, 8; Chandler, Russell, "20 Catholic Bishops Hit AIDS Ballot Proposition," *Los Angeles Times*, Sept. 16, 1986, 3.

70. Bruce Buursma, "AIDS May Be Church's Ministry of the '80s," *Chicago Tribune*, Nov. 16, 1985, 8.

71. Melton, *Churches Speak On: AIDS*, and "Religion and Religious Groups," *The Social Impact of AIDS in the United States*, ed. Albert R. Jonsen and Jeff Stryker, *Report on the Committee on AIDS Research and Behavior, Social, and Statistical Sciences*, National Research Council (Washington, D.C.: National Academy Press, 1993).

72. National Council of Churches of Christ in the U.S.A., "Resolution on Acquired Immune Deficiency Syndrome," and Presbyterian Church (U.S.A.), "Resolution on Acquired Immune Deficiency Syndrome," in Melton, *Churches Speak On: AIDS*, 115; 122.

73. Nick Bamforth, *AIDS and the Healer Within* (New York and London: Amethyst Books, 1987); Louise L. Hay, *The AIDS Book: Creating a Positive Approach* (Santa Monica, CA: Hay House Press, 1988).

74. See, e.g., John Fortunato, *AIDS: The Spiritual Dilemma* (San Francisco: Harper and Row, 1987); J. Michael Clark, *Defying the Darkness: Gay Theology in the Shadows* (Cleveland, OH: Pilgrim Press, 1997); Ronald E. Long, J. Michael Clark, and Michael J. North, *AIDS, God, and Faith: Continuing the Dialogue on Constructive Gay Theology* (Las Colinas, TX: Monument Press, 1992); and Letty M. Russell, ed., *The Church with AIDS: Renewal in the Midst of Crisis*, (Louisville, KY: Westminster/John Knox Press, 1990). For ealier Catholic considerations, see Eileen P. Flynn, *AIDS: A Catholic Call for Compassion* (Kansas City, MO: Sheed and Ward, 1985); Kenneth R. Overberg, SJ, ed., *AIDS, Ethics, and Religion: Embracing a World of Suffering* (Maryknoll, NY: Orbis, 1994); and former Jesuit priest Robert Goss's activist take, *Jesus Acted Up: A Gay and Lesbian Manifesto* (San Francisco: HarperSanFrancisco, 1993).

75. They later co-founded the Foundation for Interfaith Research and Ministry, which in 2000 became Interfaith CarePartners, a nonprofit organization that addresses the health care needs of people with AIDS or with Alzheimer's, children, and the elderly. See www.interfaithcarepartners.org.

76. Earl E. Shelp and Ronald H. Sunderland, "AIDS and the Church," *The Christian Century*, Sept. 11–18, 1985, 797–800.

77. Shelp and Sunderland, "AIDS and the Church," 799.

78. Earl E. Shelp, Ronald H. Sunderland, and Peter W.A. Mansell, M.D., *AIDS: Personal Stories in Pastoral Perspective* (New York: Pilgrim Press, 1986); Earl E. Shelp and Ronald H. Sunderland, *AIDS: A Manual for Pastoral Care* (Philadelphia: Westminster Press, 1987); Earl E. Shelp and Ronald H. Sunderland, *AIDS and the Church* (Philadelphia: Westminster Press, 1987 [second edition in 1992]); Shelp and Sunderland move toward an interfaith model for caregiving outlined in *Handle with Care: An Outline for Care Teams Serving People with AIDS* (Nashville, TN: Abingdon Press, 1990).

79. The category of "gay men" often becomes marked in popular media and general cultural reference as designating middle-class white American men in particular. It is worth noting that from the first years of their work, Shelp and Sunderland identified black gay men with HIV/AIDS as well.

80. Shelp and Sunderland, *AIDS: A Manual for Pastoral Care*, 38.

81. Shelp and Sunderland, *AIDS: Personal Stories*, 11; see also Shelp and Sunderland, "God and the Poor," *AIDS and the Church*, 77–90.

82. Shelp and Sunderland, *AIDS: Personal Stories*, 12–13.

83. Shelp and Sunderland, *AIDS and the Church*, 89.

84. Shelp and Sunderland, *AIDS and the Church*, 89.

85. Advisory Committee of People with AIDS, "The Denver Principles," adopted at the National Lesbian and Gay Health Conference, 1983, www.actupny.org/documents/Denver.html.

86. Shelp and Sunderland, "AIDS and the Church," 798.

87. It would be too reductive—not to mention inaccurate—to suggest that evangelicals have cared only about prevention, or that their efforts have been motivated solely by a desire to convert. I do not wish to suggest that here. But the *form* of evangelical ministry programs has led to a greater devotion to prevention, at least in their public discussions of AIDS relief.

88. The heading from this subsection is from "Getting Evangelical about AIDS," *Christian Century*, Feb. 22, 2003, 6; National Association of Evangelicals, "Statement on AIDS," in Melton, *Churches Speak on: AIDS*, 114.

89. National Association of Evangelicals, "Statement on AIDS," 114.

90. Southern Baptist Convention, "On AIDS (1987)," International Pentecostal Church of Christ, "Statement on AIDS (1987)," and Independent Fundamental Churches of America, "Resolution on AIDS-Abstinence-Condoms-Safe Sex (1988)," in Melton, *Churches Speak on: AIDS*, 129; 89; 89.

91. Cindy Patton, *Fatal Advice: How Safe-Sex Went Wrong* (Durham, NC: Duke University Press, 1996), and Bayer, *Private Acts, Social Consequences*, especially chapter two, "Sex and the Bathhouses: The Politics of Privacy."

92. C. Everett Koop and Timothy Johnson, "AIDS," in *Let's Talk: An Honest Conversation on Critical Issues: Abortion, Euthanasia, AIDS, Health Care* (Grand Rapids, MI: Zondervan, 1992): 61–84. I discuss Koop further in chapter two.

93. Koop, *Let's Talk*, 63.

94. "Churches Urged to Lead the Way in AIDS Care," *Christianity Today*, June 17, 1988, 58.

95. On evangelical activism and sex education, see Janice M. Irvine, *Talk about Sex: The Battles Over Sex Education in the United States* (Berkeley: University of California Press, 2002), and Christine J. Gardner, *Making Chastity Sexy: The Rhetoric of Evangelical Abstinence Campaigns* (Berkeley: University of California Press, 2011). One of the first extended articles on abstinence-only education appeared in *Christianity Today* in 1999 and detailed the efforts of Cathi Woods to institute such a program in Tennessee. See Gary Thomas, "Where True Love Waits: How One Woman Dramatically Changed the Teen Pregnancy Rate in Rhea County, Tennessee," *Christianity Today*, March 1, 1999, 40–45.

96. Ron Sider, "AIDS: An Evangelical Perspective," *Christian Century*, Jan. 6–13, 1988, 11. On Sider's role in the evangelical left, see Swartz, *Moral Minority*, 153–169, and Gasaway, *Progressive Evangelicals*, 163–190.

97. Sider, "AIDS: An Evangelical Perspective," 12–13. He further insists "on the right [. . .] to shape public policy in ways consistent with that belief without being called a bigot."

98. Sider, "AIDS: An Evangelical Perspective," 11–12.

99. Sider, "AIDS: An Evangelical Perspective," 14.

100. Dan Wooding, *He Intends Victory* (Irvine, CA: Village Books, 1994), 127–142, includes the story of Sonnenberg's AIDS ministry.

101. I do not want to imply here that sexuality was a new topic for evangelicals. My point is that homosexual sex was a relatively new subject matter and unseemly to most evangelicals, and indeed to most Americans, at the time.

102. Jimmy Allen, *Burden of a Secret* (New York: Random House, 1995).

103. Winston, "News Coverage," 377–378; Patton, *Inventing AIDS*, 77–97, and *Globalizing AIDS*; Treichler, *How to Have Theory in an Epidemic*, especially 205–234.

104. Cited in Rebecca Barnes, "The Church Awakens: Christians Make AIDS Fight a High Priority," *Christianity Today*, Jan. 2005, 22–23. For one of the first articles on AIDS in Africa in this magazine, see Timothy C. Morgan, "Have We Become Too Busy with Death," *Christianity Today*, Feb. 7, 2000, 36–44.

105. This also included a publishing boom for evangelical approaches to AIDS, including: Tetsunao Yamamori, David Dageforde, and Tina Bruner, *The Hope Factor: Engaging the Church in the HIV/AIDS Crisis* (Waynesboro, GA: Authentic Media; Federal Way, WA: World Vision, 2003); Jenny Eaton and Kate Etue, eds., *The aWAKE Project: Uniting Against the African AIDS Crisis* (Nashville, TN: Thomas, 2002); Jyl Hall, World Vision, et. al., *A Guide to Acting on AIDS: Understanding the Global AIDS Pandemic and Responding Through Faith and Action* (Tyrone, GA: Authentic in partnership with World Vision Resources, 2006); Dale Hanson Bourke, *The Skeptic's Guide to the Global AIDS Crisis: Tough Questions, Direct Answers* (Waynesboro, GA: Authentic Media 2004); Deborah Dortzbach and W. Meredith Long, *The AIDS Crisis: What We Can Do* (Downers Grove, IL: Intervarsity Press, 2006).

106. "Killing a Pandemic: The Church May Be Best Equipped to Deal HIV/AIDS a Crippling Blow," *Christianity Today*, Nov. 18, 2002, 40–41. See also, Mark Stricherz, "ABC vs. HIV: Christians Back Abstinence Fidelity Plan Against Deadly Virus," *Christianity Today*, April 2004, 30. For an important new study on black megachurches and HIV/AIDS, see Barnes, *Live Long and Prosper*, 99–142.

107. Kay Warren, *Dangerous Surrender: What Happens When You Say Yes to God* (Grand Rapids, MI: Zondervan, 2007), 18; a new edition was published as *Say Yes to God: A Call to Courageous Surrender* (Grand Rapids, MI: Zondervan, 2010); Kay Warren, "Wiping Out HIV," *Christianity Today*, April 2008, 64.

108. Ann Douglas, *The Feminization of American Culture* (New York: Knopf, 1977); Jane Tompkins, *Sensational Designs: The Cultural Work of American Fiction, 1790–1860* (New York: Oxford University Press, 1986), 123. Of course, sentimentality, and affect more broadly, are not unique to evangelicals or to their discussions of AIDS. Since the 1980s, mainline Protestants have also offered sentimental calls for care and compassion for people with AIDS. And efforts to

commemorate lives lost to the epidemic, such the AIDS Quilt, documented in Jeffrey Friedman and Rob Epstein, directors, *Common Threads: Stories from the Quilt* (New York: New Yorker Video, 2004), display powerful affective attempts to sort through suffering and loss at the hands of a devastating disease. Activists within ACT UP, described in chapter four, often drew upon public anger, or to sentimentality's close neighbors, kitsch and camp, to articulate their criticisms of government and church responses to AIDS. On sentimentality and American evangelicalism today, see Todd M. Brenneman, *Homespun Gospel: The Triumph of Sentimentality in Contemporary American Evangelicalism* (New York: Oxford University Press, 2013).

109. See, for instance, Kaplan, *With God on Their Side*. My point is not that Rick Warren or Graham resist this sentimental turn, but that they are taken more seriously as public figures in part because they are not read as being as sentimental as leaders like Kay Warren.

110. Melani McAlister, "What Is Your Heart For?: Affect and Internationalism in the Evangelical Public Sphere," *American Literary History* 20, no. 4 (2008): 878–879; Berlant, *Female Complaint*; Sara Ahmed, "Affective Economies," *Social Text* 22.2 (2004): 117–139.

111. McAlister, "What Is Your Heart For?" 870.

112. Such appeals also raise a number of concerns. As Berlant, *Female Complaint*, 6, explains, "a white universalist paternalism, sometimes dressed as maternalism" has historically been "embedded in the often sweetly motivated and solidaristic activity" of sentimental reform. Second, the rise of such intimate public spheres has led to the privatization of politics, in which the structural effects of racial oppression, class disparity, or patriarchy are often reduced to personal narratives of private pain and suffering. Indeed, we can see through their mass-produced memoirs and copyrighted ministry kits that American evangelicals have contributed to the commercialization of AIDS work, and their approaches often eclipse or downplay structural histories of poverty, colonialism, and sexism that have fostered health disparities and the spread of HIV/AIDS. Evangelicals have emphasized instead the importance of developing a personal relationship with Jesus Christ, through which one finds the strength to battle HIV.

113. Cited in Timothy C. Morgan, "Q&A: Kay Warren," *Christianity Today*, November 2, 2007, 19.

114. Rick Warren, "The P.E.A.C.E. Plan," HIV/AIDS Initiative Care Team Training Package, 2007. In the current version presented online, "P" has been updated to read "Promote reconciliation." Also see www.thepeaceplan.com (last accessed March 20, 2010). My thanks to Allison Schnable for sharing some of these materials with me and for her comments on an earlier version of this chapter.

115. Warren, "The P.E.A.C.E. Plan," HIV/AIDS Initiative Care Team Training Package.

116. Warren, "The P.E.A.C.E. Plan," HIV/AIDS Initiative Care Team Training Package. The Great Commandment can be found in Matthew 22:37-40 and the Great Commission in Matthew 28:16-20. Much of this information appeared earlier in Warren's *The Purpose Driven Church: Every Church Is Big in God's Eyes* (Grand Rapids, MI: Zondervan, 1995), though this book does not mention the AIDS crisis, which had not yet registered as an issue for Warren or for most American evangelicals.

117. "S.L.O.W. or S.T.O.P.?" HIV/AIDS Initiative Care Team Training Package, 2007; Interview with Kay Warren, "HIV/AIDS: S.L.O.W. It Down, Or S.T.O.P. It?" *Christianity Today*, November 2, 2007, http://www.christianitytoday.com/51236?start=1.

118. Kay Warren, "Learn a Church Based Strategy: Six Ways Your C.H.U.R.C.H. Can Minister to Those with HIV/AIDS," (emphasis in original), Saddleback: Care Team Training, 2006.

119. Amy DeRogatis nicely outlines this history in "What Would Jesus Do? Sexuality and Salvation in Protestant Evangelical Sex Manuals, 1950s–Present," *Church History* 74, no. 1 (March 2005): 97–137.

120. Tanya Erzen, *Straight to Jesus: Sexual and Christian Conversions in the Ex-Gay Movement* (Berkeley: University of California Press, 2006); Gerber, *Seeking the Straight and Narrow*. In "The Opposite of Gay: Nature, Creation, and Queerish Ex-gay Experiments," *Novo Religio* 11, no. 4 (May 2008): 8–30, Lynne Gerber observes the "queerish" tendencies of evangelicals. In a perhaps surprising anticipation of some of the arguments of queer theory, conservative evangelicals assumed the culturally constructed character of homosexuality and bisexuality, understanding these not as essential or natural identities, but as the result of social conditioning. On Saddleback's approach to ex-gay ministry, see the websites for the program Celebrate Recovery, saddleback.com/connect/ministry/celebrate-recovery and www.celebraterecovery.com.

121. Granted, of course, he would disagree about the precise content of that spirituality.

CHAPTER 2

1. Kaplan's quotation in the epigraph is cited in both Chilton, *Power in the Blood*, 17, and Antonio, *AIDS Cover-Up?*, 9; Koop's quotation is from M.B., "What the Doctor Ordered," *Moody Monthly*, October 1988, Box 55 Folder 7, C. Everett Koop Papers (hereafter, "Koop Papers"), National Library of Medicine; and Stowe's quotation is from "Stow to Koop," Box 94, Folder 18, Koop Papers, National Library of Medicine. Much of the Koop collection (though not, to my knowledge, these two items) is available at http://profiles.nlm.nih.gov/QQ/. James Fletcher, "Homosexuality: Kick and Kickback," *Southern Medical Journal* 77:2 (Feb 1984) 149–150. He quotes Romans 1 at length.

2. Fletcher, "Homosexuality," 149–150.

3. Fletcher, "Homosexuality," 149–150.

4. Foucault, *History of Sexuality*; Katz, *Invention of Heterosexuality*. Of course, moral condemnations of sodomy have a much longer history, as described in Jordan, *Invention of Sodomy*.

5. John Duffy, *The Sanitarians: A History of American Public Health* (Chicago: University of Illinois Press, 1992); George Rosen, *A History of Public Health* (Baltimore: Johns Hopkins Press, 1993 [1958]); Dorothy Porter, *Health, Civilization and the State: A History of Public Health from Ancient to Modern Times* (London: Routledge, 1999); Paul Starr, *The Social Transformation of American Medicine* (New York: Basic Books, 1984). I am not drawing a sharp divide here between the practices of medicine and of public health, though of course further analysis of this distinction could prove fruitful. Given the history of the AIDS epidemic, both as a new disease—thus initially lacking specialists—and as a constant "public threat," and given the major role played by the CDC and the public dissemination of information about AIDS, this line appears quite blurry.

6. Secular conservatives and religious progressives of course also entered this debate, but their positions were often eclipsed as public discourse surrounding sex education collapsed the various positions into the binary terms of the culture wars (pitting religious conservatives against secular progressives).

7. Despite the breadth of Koop's AIDS education campaign, as well as the extent of its circulation, it has received relatively little attention by historians of sexuality, religion, public health, or the AIDS epidemic. Historians of American religion have recently begun to address issues of religion and public health. Instructive studies include Claire Hoertz Badaracco, *Prescribing Faith: Medicine, Media, and Religion in American Culture* (Waco, TX: Baylor University Press, 2007); Linda L. Barnes and Susan S. Sered, eds., *Religion and Healing in America* (Oxford and New York: Oxford University Press, 2004); Heather D. Curtis, *Faith in the Great Physician: Suffering and Divine Healing in American Culture, 1860–1900* (Baltimore: Johns Hopkins Press, 2007); Klassen, *Spirits of Protestantism*; and Candy Gunther Brown, *The Healing Gods: Complementary and Alternative Medicine in Christian America* (Oxford and New York: Oxford University Press, 2013).

8. Historians of medicine have demonstrated the imbrication of medical and scientific claims in social and political history. My point, more specifically, is that they have underestimated the strength of religious claims on medical practice. See Charles E. Rosenberg, *The Cholera Years* (Chicago: University of Chicago Press, 1987); "Disease in History: Frames and Framers," *The Milbank Quarterly* 67 (1989): 1–15; and *No Other Gods: On Science and American Social Thought* (Baltimore: Johns Hopkins University Press, 1997); Brandt, *No Magic Bullet*, especially 51; Brandt and Martha Gardner, "Antagonism and Accommodation:

Interpreting the Relationship between Public Health and Medicine in the United States during the 20th Century," *American Journal of Public Health* 90, no. 5 (May 2000): 707–715; and Brandt and Paul Rozin, eds., *Morality and Health* (New York: Routledge, 1997).

9. For an inside history of Tenth Presbyterian, see Philip Graham Ryken, ed., with Allen G. Guelzo, William S. Barker, and Paul S. Jones, *Tenth Presbyterian Church of Philadelphia: 175 Years of Thinking and Acting Biblically* (Phillipsburg, NJ: P&R Publishing, 2004).

10. Koop, "The Word of God Applied to Me," in *Christ for the Nations*, founded by Gordon Lindsay, November 1986, 7, Box 100, Folder 11/1986, Koop Papers, National Library of Medicine.

11. On the history of American Presbyterianism and of the Reformed tradition, see D. G. Hart and John R. Muether, *Seeking a Better Country: 300 Years of American Presbyterianism* (Phillipsburg, NJ: P&R Publishing, 2007); Bradley J. Longfield, *Presbyterians and American Culture: A History* (Louisville, KY: Westminster John Knox Press, 2013); Hart, *Calvinism: A History* (New Haven, CT: Yale University Press, 2013); on the intellectual history of evangelicalism in this period, see Worthen, *Apostles of Reason*.

12. C. Everett Koop, *The Right to Live: The Right to Die* (Fort Collins, CO: Life Cycle Books, 1981); also mentioned in Koop, *The Memoirs of America's Family Doctor* (New York: HarperCollins, 1993 [1991]), 335.

13. Koop, *Memoirs*, 337. Also see Koop's epistolary discussion with ABC News' medical editor Timothy Johnson, in Koop and Johnson, "Abortion," *Let's Talk: An Honest Conversation on Critical Issues: Abortion, Euthanasia, AIDS, Healthcare* (Grand Rapids, MI: Zondervan, 1992), 15–38.

14. Francis Schaeffer, *A Christian Manifesto* (Wheaton: Crossway Books, 2005 [1981]); Barry Hankins, *Francis Schaeffer and the Shaping of Evangelical America* (Grand Rapids, MI: Eerdmans Publishing Company, 2008) offers a thorough account of Schaeffer's work; on his partnership with Koop, see 160–191.

15. Koop, *Memoirs*, 337–338.

16. Schaeffer and Koop, *Whatever Happened to the Human Race?* (Wheaton, IL: Crossway Books, 1983 [1979]) and *Whatever Happened to the Human Race?* DVD (Muskegon, MI: Gospel Communications, 2007 [1979 on VHS]).

17. Allen, *Wages of Sin*, 128.

18. The scholarly starting point for this shift is Robert Wuthnow's groundbreaking *The Restructuring of American Religion* (Princeton, NJ: Princeton University Press, 1988) and Hunter's *Culture Wars*. On Reagan's election, see Busch, *Reagan's Victory*; Wilentz, *Age of Reagan*, 73–126; Randall Balmer, *Redeemer: The Life of Jimmy Carter* (New York: Basic Books, 2014), especially 93–158; J. Brooks Flippen, *Jimmy Carter, The Politics of the Family, and the Rise of the Religious Right* (Athens: University of Georgia Press, 2011), 245–320.

19. "Koop Is Mentioned for the Surgeon General Slot," *Christianity Today*, January 2, 1981, 54. Also see William Shuster's report on Koop's official nomination, which came around the same time as the announcement that executive director of the Moral Majority Robert Billings would be named assistant secretary of education for nonpublic education. Shuster called this "a tremendous victory for the religious right wing." Shuster, "Koop for Surgeon General, Billing in at Education," *Christianity Today*, March 13, 1981, 58.

20. The AMA officially maintained that they did not oppose Koop specifically, but favored another candidate. In Koop's account, the executive vice president of the AMA James Sammons later admitted to him that their opposition came from Koop's position on abortion. Koop, *Memoirs*, 168–169.

21. Quoted in Bernard Weintraub, "Reagan Nominee for Surgeon General Runs into Obstacles on Capitol Hill," *New York Times*, April 7, 1981.

22. Weintraub, "Reagan Nominee for Surgeon General Runs into Obstacles on Capitol Hill." Also see Alexandra M. Lord, "Telling It Like It Is, 1981–1988," in *Condom Nation: The U.S. Government's Sex Education Campaign from World War I to the Internet* (Baltimore: Johns Hopkins, 2009), 138–161.

23. "Dr. Unqualified," *New York Times*, April 9, 1981, A22. Congress later overturned the age requirement so Koop could serve.

24. Margaret Carlson, "A Doctor Prescribes Hard Truth," *Time*, April 24, 1989, 82, Box 148, Folder 43, Koop Papers, National Library of Medicine.

25. See Koop's announcement, "Release of 1982 Report on Health Consequences of Smoking," Box 103, Folder 45, Koop Papers, National Library of Medicine. This specific quotation was not part of Koop's formal presentation but is recounted in Koop, *Memoirs*, 211. Luther Terry released the first Surgeon General's Report on Smoking and Health in 1964, and Congress quickly thereafter mandated an annual report on the *Health Consequences of Smoking*.

26. Koop, *Memoirs*, 211. On the anti-tobacco campaigns, see Martha Derthick, *Up in Smoke: From Legislation to Litigation in Tobacco Politics*, 2nd ed. (Washington, D.C.: CQ Press, 2004), especially 93–118.

27. David Bird, "U.S. Role in 'Baby Doe' Case Defended by Surgeon General," *New York Times*, Nov. 7, 1983, B4; Marcia Chambers, "Initiator of 'Baby Doe' Case Unshaken," *New York Times*, Nov. 13, 1983, A45; "Infant Handicaps Test the Meaning of Mercy," *New York Times*, Nov. 13, 1983, A8; Robert Spear, "Accord is Reached on Rules for Care in 'Baby Doe' Cases," *New York Times*, July 4, 1984, A1; and Koop, "Baby Doe and the Rights of Handicapped Children," in *Memoirs*, 304–331.

28. Koop, *Memoirs*, 304–331.

29. Epidemiologists were the first to study AIDS but soon gave way to these more "prestigious" fields within the scientific community. The status of epidemiology might be compared to that of applied research versus pure theory. This is not to say that scientific research on AIDS had been superb up to this point.

Arguably, it had been nowhere close. Fighting within the NIH and between the NIH and the CDC, lack of federal funding, and lack of interest among researchers who saw little prestige to be found working on a disease that affected homosexuals and drug users were all factors that slowed research considerably. Even the public announcement of the virus that caused AIDS, which would eventually be called HIV, was precipitated by a political struggle, as American scientist Robert Gallo likely stole his research findings from French researcher Luc Montagnier. Debate about who would own the copyright for HIV held up research as French and American governments sought a political solution. My point here is merely that virology and immunology had only very recently reached a point at which the complexities of HIV could be understood scientifically. For cultural and sociological analyses of this history, see Patton, *Inventing AIDS*, 51–76, and Epstein, *Impure Science.*

30. Treichler, *How to Have Theory*, especially 127–148; Kinsella, *Covering the Plague.*
31. Winston, "News Coverage of Religion, Sexuality, and AIDS," 386–387.
32. Winston, "News Coverage of Religion, Sexuality, and AIDS," 386–387. The federal program was the Ryan White Comprehensive AIDS Resources Emergency Act, or the Ryan White CARE Act. It is notable, of course, that the first major federal program of this nature was named for one of the "innocent victims" of AIDS, rather than for a gay person.
33. Patton, *Inventing AIDS*, especially 25–49, and Patton, *Fatal Advice.* On the history of organizing in New York City, see Chambré, *Fighting for Our Lives.*
34. Koop, *Memoirs*, 248.
35. William B. Turner, "Mirror Images: Lesbian/Gay Civil Rights in the Carter and Reagan Administrations," in John D'Emilio, William B. Turner, and Urvashi Vaid, eds., *Creating Change: Sexuality, Public Policy, and Civil Rights* (New York: St. Martin's Press, 2000): 3–28; Brier, *Infectious Ideas*, 78–121; Engel, *The Epidemic*, 69–102. My discussion in the following paragraphs is indebted to these works.
36. Turner, "Mirror Images," 21.
37. Brier, *Infectious Ideas*, 82–83. Goodwin is quoted in Brier, 83.
38. Brier, *Infectious Ideas*, 83–84.
39. Quoted in Brier, *Infectious Ideas*, 85.
40. Brier, *Infectious Ideas*, 86.
41. Quoted in Brier, *Infectious Ideas*, 87; also see Engel, *The Epidemic*, 77.
42. Koop, *Memoirs*, 255–258.
43. Koop, *Memoirs*, 260–261.
44. C. Everett Koop, "Surgeon General's Report on Acquired Immune Deficiency Syndrome," United States Public Health Service, October 22, 1986, 6, http://profiles.nlm.nih.gov/ps/retrieve/ResourceMetadata/QQBDRM.
45. Koop, "Surgeon General's Report on Acquired Immune Deficiency Syndrome," 31.

46. See "Dr. Koop's Decent AIDS Dissent," *New York Times*, October 25, 1986, A26, and "A Doctor's Good Advice," *Washington Post*, October 24, 1986, A26, in Scrapbooks 84, Koop Papers, National Library of Medicine.

47. Marlene Cimons, "Koop Urges AIDS Sex Course in Grade School," *Los Angeles Times*, Oct. 22, 1986, OC1.

48. "Gil Gerald to Koop," October 24, 1986, Scrapbook 84, Koop Papers, National Library of Medicine.

49. Jennie McKnight, "Can Koop Go Beyond His Report? Surgeon General Praised for Youth Sex Ed Push," *Gay Community News*, November 9–15, 1986, 1, 3.

50. Gordon Gottlieb, "Koop Defends Gov't AIDS Policies," *Gay Community News*, February 15–21, 1987, 1, 6; Self, *All in the Family*, 390.

51. Christian A. Brahmstedt, "A Shot of Morals," *The Washington Post*, October 28, 1986, A14; William F. Buckley, Jr., "Reservations about Dr. Koop's Advice . . ." *Unidentified Newspaper*, 1986, Scrapbook 84, Koop Papers, National Library of Medicine; and Rowland Evans and Robert Novak, "AIDS: What Should Children Know?" *Washington Post*, January 26, 1987, A11; and Koop, *Memoirs*, 276–277.

52. Koop, *Memoirs*, 273–274.

53. "Koop to Rev. Pat Robertson," March 2, 1987, Box 148, Folder 37, Koop Papers, National Library of Medicine.

54. Noebel, Lutton, and Cameron, *Special Report*, 148–173; passaged cited from 150–151; 169; 172. Also see Chilton, *Power in the Blood*, 49–50.

55. Cited in Carlson, "A Doctor Prescribes Hard Truth," 84.

56. Ronald Reagan, speaking on February 2, 1987, quoted in Steve Rivo, writer and producer, "ACT UP" segment for "Caught on Camera," *MSNBC*, November 2013, http://vimeo.com/91004429.

57. Quoted in Brier, *Infectious Ideas*, 90.

58. William J. Bennett, Secretary, United States Department of Education, "AIDS and the Education of Our Teachers: A Guide for Parents and Teachers," Office of Education Research and Improvement, October 1987, 17 (page 9 of the pamphlet itself), available from Education Resources Information Center (ERIC), http://files.eric.ed.gov/fulltext/ED284161.pdf.

59. Moran, *Teaching Sex*, 23–76.

60. The document is described and quoted in Brier, *Infectious Ideas*, 92.

61. *Congressional Record*, October 14, 1987, pp. S14202-S14220. Douglas Crimp presents an indispensable discussion of the amendment and the hearings leading up to it in "How to Have Promiscuity in an Epidemic," 237–271.

62. Pub. L. No. 100–202, 101 Stat. 1329–265 (1987) and 133 *Congressional Record*, Dec. 22, 1987 (Part II); Mary Harris Veeder, "Authorial Voice, Implied Audiences and the Drafting of the 1988 AIDS National Mailing," *Risk: Issues in Health & Safety* 4 (1993), 287; Brier, *Infectious Ideas*, 99.

63. Veeder, "Authorial Voice," and Barbara Gerbert and Bryan Maguire, "Public Acceptance of the Surgeon General's Brochure on AIDS," *U.S. Department of Health and Human Services; Public Health Reports*, 104 (April 1989), 130–133.

64. Health and Human Services, *Understanding AIDS*, Publication No. (CDC) HHS-88–8404 (U.S. Government Printing Office, 1988).

65. Brier, *Infectious Ideas*, 100.

66. Gerbert and Maguire, "Public Acceptance," and Lambert, "Flood of Phone Calls on AIDS Tied to Mailing," *New York Times*, July 3, 1988, A12.

67. Of course, public sex education and prevention campaigns for venereal disease were not new. Moran, *Teaching Sex*; Brandt, *No Magic Bullet*; Lord, *Condom Nation*.

68. Brier, *Infectious Ideas*, 88. Brier mentions Koop's Christian background and his contention that it informed his AIDS work. In the footnote to this passage, she explains that some people who worked with Koop came to view him as "'the antithesis' of social conservatism."

69. Engel, *The Epidemic*, 80; Self, *All in the Family*, 388; also see Turner, "Mirror Images."

70. Koop, *Memoirs*, 287.

71. On the limitations of traditional Christian versus secular humanist arguments about homosexuality, see Mark Jordan, "'Traditional' Christianity vs. 'Liberals'? It's Not That Simple," *Religion Dispatches*, January 8, 2010, religiondispatches.org.

72. While it is often understood as pejorative to call someone "moralistic," this is not my intent. Rather, I hope to show that AIDS work was inspired by a number of moral positions and that we can parse these moral positions more specifically than historians have so far.

73. C. Everett Koop, "Interview: Addressing the AIDS Threat," *Christianity Today*, 29:17, November 22, 1985, 52. This same issue included an article about evangelical efforts to provide compassionate support for gay men with HIV/AIDS, alongside another declaring gay marriage unchristian. "The Church's Response to AIDS," *Christianity Today*, November 22, 1985, 50–51; John R. W. Stott, "Homosexual Marriage: Why Same-Sex Partnerships Are Not a Christian Option," *Christianity Today*, November 22, 1985, 21–28.

74. Koop, "Interview," 52.

75. Koop, *Memoirs*, 264–265.

76. Koop, *Memoirs*, 264–265.

77. Other groups included The National Hemophilia Foundation, United States Conference of Local Health Officials, National Association of County Health Officials, American Medical Association, AIDS Action Council, American Red Cross, American Dental Association, Health Insurance Institute, American Council of Life Insurance, Washington Business Group on Health, Association of State and Territorial Health Officials, American Nurse Association, National

Minority AIDS Council, National Association of Secondary School Principals, National Association of Elementary School Principals, National Association of State Boards of Education, American Federation of Teachers, National Educational Association, and American Osteopathic Association.

78. "Henry D. Michelman to Koop," September 5, 1986, Scrapbook 85, Koop Papers, National Library of Medicine.

79. Koop, "Introduction to the AIDS Archive," Reminiscence, 2003, Koop Papers, National Library of Medicine.

80. "Larry Braidfoot to Koop," September 5, 1986, Scrapbook 85, Koop Papers, National Library of Medicine.

81. See, for instance, National Association of Evangelicals, "Statement on AIDS (1988)," reprinted in Melton, *Churches Speak On: AIDS,* 114.

82. "Charles McIlhenny to Koop," March 24, 1987, Box 94, Folder 18, Koop Papers, National Library of Medicine.

83. "Koop to McIlhenny," May 28, 1987, Box 94, Folder 18, Koop Papers, National Library of Medicine.

84. Koop, "Address at Liberty University," Reminiscence, 2003, Box 105, Folder 65, Koop Papers, National Library of Medicine.

85. Koop, "Address at Liberty University," January 19, 1987, Box 105, Folder 65, Koop Papers, National Library of Medicine.

86. Koop, "Address Presented to the Annual Meeting of the National School Boards Association," San Francisco, CA, April 4, 1987, Box 105, Folder 89, 26, Koop Papers, National Library of Medicine.

87. Self, *All in the Family,* 332; R. Marie Griffith, "The Religious Encounters of Alfred C. Kinsey," *Journal of American History,* 2, no. 95 (September 2008), 349–377; Beth Bailey, *Sex in the Heartland* (Cambridge, MA: Harvard University Press, 2002); Andrea Tone, *Devices and Desires: A History of Contraceptives in America* (New York: Hill and Wang, 2002); and John D'Emilio and Estelle B. Freedman, *Intimate Matters: A History of Sexuality in America* (Chicago: University of Chicago Press, 1988), especially parts three and four.

88. Flippen, *Jimmy Carter,* 117; National Religious Broadcasters, "History," available at http://nrb.org/about/history/.

89. Koop, "Address Presented to the National Religious Broadcasters, Washington, D.C.," February 2, 1987, Box 105, Folder 70, Koop Papers, National Library of Medicine.

90. Koop, "Address Presented to the National Religious Broadcasters, Washington, D.C.," 20 (underlining in original transcript).

91. Koop, "Address Presented to the National Religious Broadcasters, Washington, D.C.," 29.

92. Koop, "Address Presented to the National Religious Broadcasters, Washington, D.C.," 29–30. On the limitations of such tolerance, see Pellegrini and Jakobsen, *Love the Sin.*

93. Koop, "Address to Christian Life Commission," Charlotte, NC, March 23, 1987, Box 105, Folder 84, Koop Papers, National Library of Medicine.
94. Koop, "Address to Christian Life Commission."
95. Koop cites information from Gay Men's Health Crisis, a nonprofit AIDS organization founded in New York City in January 1982, but I have not yet found any record of a meeting with representatives from this group or similar organizations. As Brier, *Infectious Ideas*, 11–44, has argued, the contributions of these earlier organizations are often eclipsed by the more radical group ACT UP in histories of AIDS relief work and activism.
96. Koop, "Address to the 59th General Assembly of the Union of the American Hebrew Congregations," Chicago, Illinois, November 2, 1987, Box 106, Folder 39, Koop Papers, National Library of Medicine (underlining in original). The Union of the American Hebrew Congregations is now called the Union for Reform Judaism.
97. Koop, "Address to the 59th General Assembly of the Union of the American Hebrew Congregations," 15, underlining in original.
98. Koop, "Address to the 59th General Assembly of the Union of the American Hebrew Congregations," 15.
99. Koop, "Address to the 59th General Assembly of the Union of the American Hebrew Congregations," 15.
100. It may see odd that Koop delivered his most explicitly religious lecture, by which I mean one during which he cited several biblical passages and commented on shared religious traditions, to an audience of Reform Jews. This was no doubt an attempt to find common ground. But Koop's use of such religious arguments to support his conservative stance regarding sexuality and AIDS may also have been misplaced. By the late 1980s, Reform Jews had joined most liberal Protestant denominations in decrying the blame placed on homosexuals and drug users and focused their efforts instead on calling for care and compassion and supporting the civil rights of those populations most affected. See, for instance, Union of American Hebrew Congregations, "Statement on AIDS (1985)" and "Confronting the AIDS Crisis (1987)," reprinted in Melton, *Churches Speak on: AIDS*, 169–171; also see Freudenthal, *AIDS in Jewish Thought and Law*, especially 139–158.
101. The rhetoric of "Judeo-Christian" in the 1950s was itself a testament to this process. See, for instance, Will Herberg, *Protestant, Catholic, Jew: An Essay in American Religious Sociology* (Chicago: University of Chicago Press, 1955) and Wuthnow, *Restructuring of American Religion*.
102. Koop, "Address to the 59th General Assembly," 32.
103. Health and Human Services, *Understanding AIDS*, 4. Also see note 85 and the discussion in text on pages 83–84.
104. Treichler, *How to Have Theory in an Epidemic*, 57, but also see 42–98.
105. Crimp, "How to Have Promiscuity in an Epidemic;" Patton, *Fatal Advice*; Brier, *Infectious Ideas*, 11–44; Warner, *The Trouble with Normal*.

106. The pamphlet was first published in 1983 and is reprinted in Richard Berkowitz, *Stayin' Alive: The Invention of Safe Sex* (New York: Basic Books, 2003), 187–218; quotation on 200.

107. For reflections on safe sex practices among women, also see ACT UP NY/ Women's AIDS Book Group, *Women, AIDS, and Activism* (Boston: South End Press, 1990).

108. Crimp attributes one such narrative to Andrew Sullivan. Crimp, "Melancholia and Moralism: An Introduction," *Melancholia and Moralism: Essays on AIDS and Queer Politics* (Cambridge: MIT Press, 2002), 3–6.

109. Crimp, "Melancholia and Moralism," 16.

110. Irvine, *Talk about Sex*, and Gardner, *Making Chastity Sexy*, trenchantly examine the history of Christian abstinence campaigns, and Gardner carries this analysis into the 21st century. Also see Herzog, *Sex in Crisis*, 93–161.

111. Carlson, "A Doctor Prescribes Hard Truth," 82.

CHAPTER 3

1. Steinem named comedian Lily Tomlin and the volunteer group Meals on Wheels as the best things about New York. Gloria Steinem, "'Best and Worst' Feature," *New York Magazine*, December 23–30, 1985, 44; also cited in Nat Hentoff, *John Cardinal O'Connor: At the Storm Center of a Changing American Catholic Church* (New York: Scribner, 1988), 99.

2. On the Catholic Church and abortion in this period, see Timothy A. Byrnes and Mary C. Segers, eds., *The Catholic Church and the Politics of Abortion: A View from the States* (Boulder, CO: Westview Press, 1992), and Patricia Miller, *Good Catholics: The Battle over Abortion in the Catholic Church* (Berkeley: University of California Press, 2014). Tentler, *Catholics and Contraception*, examines the broader history of Catholic teaching on marriage, abortion, and sexual conduct over the twentieth century; and John T. McGreevy, *Catholicism and American Freedom: A History* (New York: W. W. Norton & Company, 2003), 216–281, places the history of Catholic debates about abortion and sexuality within longer struggles to become fully American.

3. José Casanova, "Catholicism in the United States," in *Public Religions in the Modern World* (Chicago: University of Chicago Press, 1994): 167–210; Herberg, *Protestant, Catholic, Jew*; Camilla J. Kari, *Public Witness: The Pastoral Letters of the American Catholic Bishops* (Collegeville, MN: Liturgical Press, 2004).

4. Casanova, *Public Religions*, 184. See Timothy A. Byrnes, *Catholic Bishops in American Politics* (Princeton, NJ: Princeton University Press, 1991), chapter three. The pastoral letter on *The Challenge of Peace: God's Promise and Our Response* was published in 1983 and the letter on *Economic Justice for All: Catholic Social Teaching and the U.S. Economy* in 1986.

5. For an excellent example, see Smith, *AIDS, Gays, and the American Catholic Church*, 87–116. As scholars of lived religion have argued, such personal negotiations should not be underemphasized. But we must avoid exaggerating the potential agency of such negotiations or understating the very real forms of institutional power against which they are often wrought. To wit, negotiations of power work differently in various religious traditions that have unique histories and constellations of institutional organization, knowledge, and participation. See David D. Hall, *Lived Religion in America: Toward A History of Practice* (Princeton, NJ: Princeton University Press, 1997); Orsi, *Between Heaven and Earth*; and Griffith, *God's Daughters*.

6. O'Connor also completed a doctoral degree in political science. See John J. O'Connor, "Cross-Cultural Interaction: An Evaluation of Some Conceptual Approaches," (Ph.D. dissertation, Georgetown University, 1970).

7. Hentoff, *John Cardinal O'Connor*, 117; Michael Norman, "Scranton Bishop Gets Cooke Post; Magnitude of Task Impresses Him," *New York Times*, February 1, 1984, A1, and Ari L. Goldman, "New York's Controversial Archbishop," *New York Times*, October 14, 1984, A38.

8. Cited in Michael Norman, "Scranton Bishop Gets Cooke Post; Magnitude of Task Impresses Him," *New York Times*, February 1, 1984, A1.

9. Norman, "Scranton Bishop," A1. O'Connor was elevated to the College of Cardinals in April of 1985.

10. The New York archdiocese included three boroughs (Manhattan, the Bronx, and Staten Island) along with several counties, including Westchester, Putnam, Dutchess, Rockland, Orange, Sullivan, and Ulster.

11. These statistics are compiled from "The Archdiocese; History," *New York Times*, February 1, 1984, B5, and Norman, "Scranton Bishop," A1; also see Florence D. Cohalan, *A Popular History of the Archdiocese of New York* (Yonkers, NY: United States Catholic Historical Society, 1999 [1983]); Christopher J. Kauffman, *Meaning and Ministry: A Religious History of Catholic Healthcare in the United States* (New York: Crossroad, 1995).

12. Quoted in Norman, "Scranton Bishops," A1.

13. Quoted in "Cuomo Opposed Cardinal on Abortion," *New York Times*, February 17, 1986. An article in the *Village Voice* quoted a similar statement from O'Connor as his "famous no-vote-for-abort fiat": "I do not see how a Catholic in good conscience can vote for an individual expressing himself or herself as favoring abortion." Cited in Wayne Barrett, "Holier Than Thou," *Village Voice*, December 25, 1984, 12.

14. "Cuomo Opposed Cardinal on Abortion," *New York Times*, February 17, 1986.

15. U.S. Catholic Conference, "Statement on Politics and Religion: Religion and the '84 Campaign," *Origins*, 14: 11, August 23, 1984. Unless otherwise noted, articles cited to *Origins* come from originsonline.com, which does not provide page numbers. On the "swirl of debate," see Kenneth A. Briggs,

"Politics and Morality: Dissent in Catholic Church," *New York Times*, August 11, 1984, 1, 7.

16. "O'Connor Critical of Ferraro Views," *New York Times*, September 9, 1984, A1, and Barrett, "Holier Than Thou," 12.

17. Mario Cuomo, "Religious Belief and Public Morality: A Catholic Governor's Perspective," reprinted in Patricia Beattie Jung and Thomas A. Shannon, editors, *Abortion and Catholicism: The American Debate* (New York: Crossroad, 1988), 202–216; Kenneth A. Briggs, "Cuomo vs. Bishops," *New York Times*, September 14, 1984, A22. Though probably overstating the point, Casanova described the speech as a turning point in the debate on abortion, after which conservative bishops could no longer question the logic by which Catholic politicians supported abortion rights. Casanova, *Public Religions*, 197–198.

18. Cuomo, "Religious Belief," 216; Jay Dolan, *The American Catholic Experience: A History from Colonial Times to the Present* (Notre Dame, IN: University of Notre Dame Press, 1992), 127–348.

19. Cuomo, "Religious Belief," 208–210.

20. Cuomo, "Religious Belief," 208–209.

21. Cuomo, "Religious Belief," 209.

22. Joseph Cardinal Bernardin, *Consistent Ethic of Life* (Kansas City, MO: Sheed & Ward, 1988).

23. Ari L. Goldman, "O'Connor Challenges Cuomo on Abortion but Lauds Stand," *New York Times*, September 24, 1984.

24. Cardinal John J. O'Connor, "Consistent Ethic of Death," *Catholic New York*, January 22, 1987, 5, and "From Theory to Practice in the Public-Policy Realm," in *Abortion and Catholicism*.

25. Ari L. Goldman, "New York's Controversial Archbishop," *New York Times*, October 14, 1984, A38. Bernardin headed the five-person committee that authored the letter, which was critical of the Reagan White House's nuclear policy. But O'Connor, who also served on the committee and signed the final letter, developed a reputation for defending the Reagan administration and pushed for language to moderate the letter's tone. On the pastoral letter, see Jim Castelli, *The Bishops and the Bomb: Waging Peace in a Nuclear Age* (Garden City, NY: Image Books, 1983).

26. While Vatican Two signaled a modernizing church in regard to many issues, it reaffirmed traditional positions on sexuality and marriage, including opposition to contraception. See Byrnes, *Catholic Bishops*, chapter three.

27. Casanova, *Public Religions*, 167–210; Kari, *Public Witness*.

28. Casanova, *Public Religions*, 193.

29. Casanova, *Public Religions*, 193.

30. Casanova, *Public Religions*, 193.

31. Casanova, *Public Religions*, 196.

32. Casanova, *Public Religions*, 200–201.

33. Casanova, *Public Religions*, 204; Byrnes, *Catholic Bishops*, 3–4.

34. Goldman, "New York's Controversial Archbishop," A38.

35. Eric Marcus, *Making Gay History: The Half-Century Fight for Lesbian and Gay Equal Rights* (New York: Harper Paperbacks, 2002), 185–242; John D'Emilio, *Sexual Politics, Sexual Communities* (Chicago: University of Chicago Press, 1998); Koch, "The Mayor: Gay Rights," in *His Eminence and Hizzoner: A Candid Exchange*, co-authored with O'Connor (San Francisco: HarperCollins Publishers, 1989), 293–299.

36. See Koch and O'Connor, *His Eminence and Hizzoner*, 93–132, and Goldman, "New York's Controversial Archbishop," A38.

37. O'Connor describes Executive Order 50 and his response in "The Cardinal: Executive Order 50 and Child Care," in *His Eminence and Hizzoner*, 113–132; 114. O'Connor's decision to challenge the executive order stood out in New York politics, even more since the Bishop of Brooklyn, Francis Mugavero, fully complied with the city's anti-discrimination requirement.

38. O'Connor, "The Cardinal: Executive Order 50 and Child Care," 120; see also Koch, "Executive Order 50," 96–98; Hentoff, *John Cardinal O'Connor*, 88–99.

39. Koch, "Executive Order 50," 98–99; Mary Ann Poust, "'Detrimental to Society,'" *Catholic New York*, March 27, 1986, 18, 32.

40. Cited in Larry Rohter, "Homosexual-Rights Bill Will Pass, Backers Say," *New York Times*, Jan 13, 1986, B2.

41. Mary Ann Poust, "Mayor Offers Another Homosexual Rights Bill," *Catholic New York*, Jan. 30, 1986, 19.

42. Quoted in Larry Rohter, "O'Connor Sees Council Bill Shielding Homosexual 'Sin,'" *New York Times*, May 17, 1986, www.nytimes.com/1986/03/17/nyregion/o-connor-sees-council-bill-shielding-homosexual-sin.html.

43. "Homosexuals' Rights Need Protection," *New York Times*, January 24, 1986, A26.

44. "Homosexuals' Rights Need Protection," *New York Times*, A26.

45. Cardinal John J. O'Connor, "What Kind of Mischief Is This?" *Catholic New York*, New York, Feb. 6, 1986, 5.

46. O'Connor, "What Kind of Mischief Is This?," 5.

47. "Homosexuals' Rights Need Protection," *New York Times*, A26.

48. Poust, "Mayor Offers Another Homosexual Rights Bill," 19.

49. "Homosexuals' Rights Need Protection," *New York Times*, A26.

50. "A United Voice: Cardinal O'Connor, Bishop Mugavero Oppose Homosexual Rights Bill," *Catholic New York*, Feb. 13, 1986, 3, 22 [The statement was reprinted here in full.]

51. "A United Voice: Cardinal O'Connor, Bishop Mugavero Oppose Homosexual Rights Bill," 3, 22.

52. "A United Voice: Cardinal O'Connor, Bishop Mugavero Oppose Homosexual Rights Bill," 3, 22.

53. Editorial, "A Clear Statement," *Catholic New York*, Feb. 13, 1986, 14. The statement was also provided in Spanish as "Posición Clara," *Catholic New York*, February 13, 1986, 14.

54. "An Unneeded Law," *Catholic New York*, March 13, 1986, 14, and "Le Innecesaria," *Catholic New York*, March 13, 1986, 14.

55. "An Unneeded Law," *Catholic New York*, 14.

56. Kevin T. O'Reilly, "Abomination," *Catholic New York*, March 13, 1986, 16.

57. Mary Ann Poust, "Behind the Bill," *Catholic New York*, March 13, 1986, 3.

58. Mary Ann Poust, "An Affront to Morality," *Catholic New York*, March 20, 1986, 3, 20, and Rohter, "O'Connor Sees Council Bill Shielding Homosexual 'Sin.'"

59. Poust, "An Affront to Morality," 3, 20.

60. Poust, "An Affront to Morality," 3, 20, and Rohter, "O'Connor Sees Council Bill Shielding Homosexual 'Sin.'"

61. "Homosexual Rights," *Catholic New York*, March 27, 1986, 14, and "Derechos Para Homosexuals," *Catholic New York*, March 27, 1986, 14. See also Mary Ann Poust, "Detrimental to Society," *Catholic New York*, March 27, 1986, 18, 32, and "Opposition Reaffirmed," *Catholic New York*, April 10, 1986, 27.

62. Thomas R. Riley, "AIDS and the Church," *Catholic New York*, November 28, 1985, 22. The conference proceedings, including Cooke's invocation and an introduction by Mayor Ed Koch, were subsequently published in Kevin M. Cahill, *The AIDS Epidemic* (New York: St. Martin's Press, 1983).

63. Cited in Greg Clarkin, "Health Care: Cardinal Discusses AIDS, Worker's Rights," *Catholic New York*, October 17, 1985, 16.

64. "Archdiocese Is Considering a Shelter for AIDS Patients," *New York Times*, August 19, 1985; "Mother Teresa Offer Helps to AIDS Patients," *Catholic New York*, October 31, 1985, 16; "AIDS Hospice," *Catholic New York*, November 7, 1985, 20; Mary Ann Poust, "Room in the Inn," *Catholic New York*, January 2, 1986, 9; Mary Ann Poust, "Efforts on AIDS," *Catholic New York*, January 9, 1986.

65. The hospital was managed through a joint effort by the archdiocese and the State of New York. In 1987, a state and federal plan proposed dedicating St. Clare's exclusively to the treatment of people with AIDS to meet the city's rising needs. O'Connor and the archdiocese "adamantly opposed" the plan, citing the range of services the hospital supplied to the local neighborhood and their desire for such services to continue. "AIDS Hospice," *Catholic New York*, November 7, 1985, 20; Mary Ann Poust, "Special Commitment: AIDS Patients Being Treated in Special Unit at St. Clare's Hospital," *Catholic New York*, December 19, 1985, 30; Poust, "'We'd Go to Court': Archdiocese Vows to Fight All-AIDS Proposal for St. Clare's Hospital," *Catholic New York*, June 4, 1987, 3; "AIDS: A Plan of Actions," editorial, *Catholic New York*, June 11, 1987, 16.

66. Brier, *Infectious Ideas*, 93–97.

67. Ari L. Goldman, "300 Fault O'Connor Role on AIDS Commission," *New York Times*, July 27, 1987, B3.

68. See "O'Connor Defends AIDS Panel Role," *New York Times*, July 31, 1987, A12; Sandra G. Boodman, "Cardinal O'Connor Says He May Quit AIDS Panel," *New York Times*, October 17, 1987, A3; Mary Ann Poust, "'Responsibility to Help': Cardinal O'Connor Says He'll Remain on Presidential AIDS Commission," *Catholic New York*, October 22, 1987, 19.

69. See *The Presidential Commission on the Human Immunodeficiency Virus Epidemic Report*, June 24, 1988, http://www.eric.ed.gov/ERICWebPortal/contentdelivery/servlet/ERICServlet?accno=ED299531. Also see Brier, *Infectious Ideas*, especially 97–98.

70. Two schools distributed contraceptives, including condoms, diaphragms, and birth control pills, directly to students, while the seven others provided prescriptions for students to receive them elsewhere. Jane Perlez, "In New York, Storm Over Contraceptives in Schools," *New York Times*, October 12, 1986, A6; "Sex Education Plan Draws Objections," *Catholic New York*, September 25, 1986, 22; Jane Perlez, "Quiñones Announces Review of Sex-Education Materials," *New York Times*, December 4, 1986, B14; Jane Perlez, "2 Groups Differ on Sex Education," *New York Times*, December 5, 1986, B4.

71. One clergy group supported the education program, calling the curriculum "sensitive and well-planned." See Mary Ann Poust, "'Valueless': Sex Education Program Target of Clerymen," *Catholic New York*, December 11, 1986, 17, 24; also see Poust, "Sex Curriculum," *Catholic New York*, December 18, 1986, 24.

72. Anne Buckley, "A 'Specific Morality': Priests Called to Get Sex Education with Values into School," *Catholic New York*, January 22, 1987, 11; Associated Press, "Vicar Assails Sex Education Plan," *New York Times*, March 19, 1987, B7

73. Buckley, "'Specific Morality,'" 11.

74. AP, "Vicar Assails," B7.

75. "The Condom Campaign," editorial, *Catholic New York*, May 21, 1987, 12. See also Sister Mary Ann Walsh, "'A False Solution,'" *Catholic New York*, February 19, 1987, 9; Mary Ann Poust, "Anti-AIDS Commercials Draw Church Criticism," *Catholic New York*, May 14, 1987.

76. O'Connor and Koch, *His Eminence and Hizzoner*, 240.

77. Mary DeTurris, "Reversal: Abstinence to Be Theme of AIDS Prevention Ads," *Catholic New York*, June 11, 1987, 1.

78. "AIDS Campaign: New City Ads Stress Sexual Abstinence," *Catholic New York*, November 2, 1987, 2.

79. See Aline H. Kalbian, *Sexing the Church: Gender, Power, and Ethics in Contemporary Catholicism* (Bloomington: Indiana University Press, 2005); Leslie Griffin, "American Catholic Sexual Ethics, 1789–1989," in Charles Curran and Richard McCormack, eds., *Dialogue about Catholic Sexual Teaching (Readings in Moral Theology*, vol 8) (New York: Paulist Press, 1993), 453–484; Charles Curran, *Catholic Moral Theology in the United States: A History* (Washington, D.C.: Georgetown University Press, 2008), 191–218; Jeannine Gramick and Pat

Furey, *The Vatican and Homosexuality: Reactions to the "Letter to the Bishops of the Catholic Church on the Pastoral Care of Homosexual Persons"* (New York: Crossroad Publishing Company, 1988); and Lisa Sowle Cahill, John Garvey, and T. Frank Kennedy, S.J, *Sexuality and the U.S. Catholic Church: Crisis and Renewal* (New York: Crossroad Publishing Company, 2006).

80. Alert to the politics of homosexuality and to the church's strong stand against it, *Catholic New York* covered the release of Ratzinger's letter, which it printed in full in response to criticism of the church's position on homosexuality in mainstream press. John Thavis, "'Objective Disorder,'" *Catholic New York*, November 5, 1986, 7, and "The Issue of Homosexuality," *Catholic New York*, November 27, 1986, 23, 26–27.

81. Congregation for the Doctrine of the Faith, "Letter to the Bishops of the Catholic Church on the Pastoral Care of Homosexual Persons," reprinted in Gramick and Furey, eds., *Vatican and Homosexuality*, 1–12.

82. Congregation for the Doctrine of the Faith, "Declaration on Certain Questions Concerning Sexual Ethics," especially Section Eight, in *Persona Humana*, at http://www.vatican.va/roman_curia/congregations/cfaith/documents/rc_con_cfaith_doc_19751229_persona-humana_en.html

83. Of course, the Vatican was not the only Catholic body to confront homosexuality in this period. Theological, pastoral, and activist considerations of homosexuality within the Catholic tradition advanced through the 1970s and 1980s. See Gramick and Furey, *Vatican and Homosexuality*, xiii–xxi; on Dignity, see White, "Homosexuality, Gay Communities, and American Churches," 139–144; also see John J. McNeill, *The Church and the Homosexual*, 4th ed. (Boston: Beacon Press, 1993 [1976]); Philip S. Keane, *Sexual Morality: A Catholic Perspective* (New York: Paulist Press, 1977); Jeannine Gramick, *Homosexuality and the Catholic Church* (Chicago: Thomas More Press, 1983); Robert Nugent, *A Challenge to Love: Gay and Lesbian Catholics in the Church* (New York: Crossroad Publishing Company, 1983); and Joseph Hughes, *Homosexuality: A Positive Catholic Perspective* (Baltimore: Archdiocesan Gay/Lesbian Outreach, 1985); on the longer history of the Catholic Church and homosexuality, see John Boswell's groundbreaking *Christianity, Social Tolerance, and Homosexuality: Gay People in Western Europe from the Beginning of the Christian Era to the Fourteenth Century*, 8th ed. (Chicago: University of Chicago Press, 2005 [1980]).

84. Ratzinger, "Letter," 5.

85. Ratzinger, "Letter," 2.

86. Ratzinger, "Letter," 2.

87. Ratzinger, "Letter," 5.

88. Ratzinger, "Letter," 7.

89. Ratzinger, "Letter," 9.

90. Ratzinger, "Letter," 5.

91. See my discussion of evangelical constructions in chapters one and two.

92. Michael G. Meyer, "The Catholic Church and AIDS," *America* 154, no. 24, June 21, 1986, 512–514.

93. The NCCB and the USCC were established in 1966 on the heels of the Second Vatican Council. The NCCB included only bishops and was charged with fulfilling the Vatican's mandate for the pastoral functions of the American Church. The USCC addressed the concerns of the church in the context of American society more generally, and its committees included bishops, lay people, clergy, and religious who collaborated to confront social issues. The two bodies were combined in 2001 to form the United States Conference of Catholic Bishops (USCCB). The statements on HIV/AIDS include USCC Administrative Board, "The Many Faces of AIDS: A Gospel Response," *Origins* 17, no. 28, December 24, 1987, 481–489, and National Conference of Catholic Bishops, "Called to Compassion and Responsibility: A Response to the HIV/ AIDS Crisis," *Origins* 19, no. 26, November 30, 1989, 421–436.

94. On this point, as well as for a broader discussion of the metaphors employed to describe AIDS in these two statements, see Smith, *AIDS, Gays, and the American Catholic Church*, 58–86; also see James F. Keenan, Jon D. Fuller, and Lisa Sowle Cahill, eds., *Catholic Ethicists on HIV/AIDS Prevention* (New York: Continuum, 2001), especially Fuller and Keenan, "Introduction: At the End of the First Generation of HIV Prevention," 21–40.

95. Moreover, while these stances are neither univocal nor necessarily theologically consistent, they have directed the Catholic Church's teaching on these topics for over two decades since their release.

96. Michael D. Place, "The Many Faces of AIDS: Some Clarifications of the Recent Debate (Cover story)," *America* 158, no. 6, February 13, 1988, 135–137.

97. See also, Place, "Many Faces," 136–137.

98. USCC, "Many Faces," 481, 483.

99. USCC, "Many Faces," 483.

100. USCC, "Many Faces," 483.

101. USCC, "Many Faces," 483.

102. USCC, "Many Faces," 484.

103. USCC, "Many Faces," 486.

104. USCC, "Many Faces," 486.

105. USCC, "Many Faces," 486.

106. USCC, "Many Faces," 486.

107. USCC, "Many Faces," 486.

108. USCC, "Many Faces," 486.

109. USCC, "Many Faces," 486.

110. USCC, "Many Faces," 486.

111. USCC, "Many Faces," 488–489.

112. The bishops explain their reasoning, and supply the appropriate citations, in footnote seven of the statement. USCC, "Many Faces," 489.

113. Ari L. Goldman, "U.S. Bishops Back Condom Education as a Move on AIDS," *New York Times*, December 11, 1987, A1. The *Times* also carried excerpts drawn directly from the statement: "Excerpts from Statement on AIDS and Condoms by Catholic Conference," *New York Times*, December 11, 1987, D17.

114. See, for instance, "Reaction to AIDS Statement," *Origins*, 1987, 489–493; and "Continued Reaction to AIDS Statement," *Origins*, 1988, 516–522.

115. Cardinal O'Connor, "Reaction to AIDS Statement," *Origins* 17, no. 28, December 24, 1987, 489, emphasis mine. See also Rick Hampson, "Bishops Quarrel Over AIDS Policy; Conservatives Oppose Discussing Condoms in Education Programs," *Washington Post*, December 15, 1987, A03.

116. Mary Ann Poust, "Silence on Condoms," *Catholic New York*, December 17, 1989, 21; 49.

117. Statement of Seventeen Bishops, "Reaction to AIDS Statement," *Origins* 17, no. 28, December 24, 1987, 490.

118. Cited in Military Services Archdiocese, "Continued Reaction to AIDS Statement," *Origins* 17, no. 30, January 7, 1988, 516. See also "Religion: Catholics, AIDS and Condoms," *Time*, Dec 21, 1987, http://www.time.com/time/ magazine/article/0,9171,966287,00.html. In my reading, the article did not misrepresent the argument in "Many Faces;" it presented the statement's position on condoms quite clearly. It is possible, of course, that the bishops of the Military Services Archdiocese, as well as some others, focused on criticizing media accounts as a way to deflect their criticism from the administrative board's statement itself.

119. Military Services Archdiocese, "Continued Reaction," 516.

120. The bishops who signed onto the statement included Archbishop James Hickey of Washington, Bishop John Keating of Arlington, and Auxiliary Bishops Thomas Lyons, Eugene Marino, and Alvaro Corrada of Washington. Bishop Timothy Harrington of Worcester, Massachusetts also criticized the statement and its coverage by the mainstream press. Bishops of Metropolitan Washington, "Reaction to AIDS Statement," *Origins* 17, no. 28, December 24, 1987, 490; Harrington, "Continued Reaction to AIDS Statement," *Origins* 17, no. 30, January 7, 1988, 516–517. Archbishop Roger Mahoney of Los Angeles released a statement addressed to the members of his archdiocese praising "Many Faces," which he adopted for use in Los Angeles, with some minor alterations. Noting the confusion concerning condoms to which some unclear phrasing in the statement had led, he reaffirmed the church's opposition both to safe sex education and to the use of condoms. Mahoney, "Reaction to AIDS Statement," *Origins* 17, no. 28, December 24, 1987, 491–492.

121. Cardinal John Krol and Archbishop Anthony Bevilacqua, "Reaction to AIDS Statement," *Origins* 17, no. 28, December 24, 1987, 493. See also U.S. Bishops, "Statement on School-Based Clinics," *Origins* 17, no. 25, December 3, 1987, 433.

122. Archbishop J. Francis Stafford, "Continued Reaction to AIDS Statement," *Origins* 17, no. 30, January 7, 1988, 519–520.

123. Bishop William Hughes, "Reaction to AIDS Statement," *Origins* 17, no. 28, December 24, 1987, 490.

124. Archbishop Daniel Pilarczyk, "Reaction to AIDS Statement," *Origins* 17, no. 28, Dec. 24, 1987, 491.

125. Archbishop John May, "Reaction to AIDS Statement," *Origins* 17, no. 28, Dec. 24, 1987, 489–490. Bishop Howard Hubbard of Albany and Archbishop John Roach of St. Paul and Minneapolis also raised this point and underscored the need for the church to present information on condoms, not in order to promote their use, but to use the opportunity to place condoms within the context of Catholic moral thought. Hubbard and Roach, separate entries, in "Continued Reaction to AIDS Statement," *Origins* 17, no. 30, Jan. 7, 1988, 516–517 and 522.

126. Cardinal Joseph Bernardin, "Continued Reaction to AIDS Statement," *Origins* 17, no. 30, January 7, 1988, 517–518.

127. Bernardin, "Continued Reaction to AIDS Statement," 517–518.

128. Cited in Robert Suro, "Vatican and the AIDS Fight," *New York Times*, January 29, 1988, A1.

129. Cardinal Joseph Ratzinger, "Cardinal Ratzinger's Letter on AIDS Document," *Origins* 18, no. 8, July 7, 1988, 117–118.

130. Cited in Ratzinger, "Letter on AIDS Document," 117. *L'Osservatore Romano* is the Vatican newspaper, which carries important communications and statements from church authorities.

131. Ratzinger, "Letter on AIDS Document," 117.

132. Cardinal Joseph Bernardin, "AIDS Statement: Proposal of Cardinal Bernardin Accepted," *Origins* 18, no. 8, July 7, 1988, 119.

133. Bernardin, "AIDS Statement," 118–120.

134. NCCB, "Called to Compassion," 421–436. The ad hoc committee that drafted this statement included its chair, Archbishop Roger Mahoney of Los Angeles, as well as Cardinal Bernardin, Cardinal Law, Archbishop William Keeler of Baltimore, and Bishop Raymond Lessard of Savannah, Georgia.

135. NCCB, "Called to Compassion," 423; Pope John Paul VI, "The Pastoral Constitution of the Church in the Modern World," *Gaudium et Spes*, Dec. 7, 1965, http://www.vatican.va/archive.

136. NCCB, "Called to Compassion," 425.

137. NCCB, "Called to Compassion," 425.

138. The key fault-lines in such debates over politics and medicine in public health find useful discussion in Bayer, *Private Acts, Social Consequences*, and Epstein, *Impure Science*, especially 1–44.

139. NCCB, "Called to Compassion," 427–429.

140. NCCB, "Called to Compassion," 425.

141. NCCB, "Called to Compassion," 424.

142. NCCB, "Called to Compassion," 424–425.

143. Of course, even as HIV spread among minority communities, and through the sharing of needles, sexual transmission (through same- and opposite-sex encounters) remained prevalent.

144. It is footnote number 30, which follows "lives" in the sentence previously quoted. Though it goes undefined, one could assume the practices described by the study included unprotected anal (and possibly oral) sex.

145. NCCB, "Called to Compassion," 426–427. On complementarianism, see Kalbian, *Sexing the Church*, 21–54.

146. NCCB, "Called to Compassion," 427.

147. NCCB, "Called to Compassion," 427.

148. Much of the Catholic Church's discourse (and that of many social and political conservatives) about condoms emphasized the medical fact that condoms are not 100% effective, and they often cited a "failure rate" ranging from 10% to 50%. These arguments, unlike those of Surgeon General Koop, for instance, made little of the fact that some protection is better than no protection, and that when used properly, condoms had been proven to reduce the spread of HIV. They also imagined heterosexual marriage to be monogamous, and free from infidelity, and thus safer than condom use. See NCCB, "Called to Compassion," 429, 433.

149. NCCB, "Called to Compassion," 429.

150. David Hollenbach, "AIDS Education: The Moral Substance," *America*, December 26, 1987, 493–494; Michael D. Place, "The Many Faces of AIDS: Some Clarifications of the Recent Debate," *America*, February 13, 1988, 135–171; Bela Somfai, "AIDS, Condoms, and the Church," *Compass*, November 1987, 25–26, 43–44. On the opposite side, see attorney for the Archdiocese of New York, John P. Hale's "The Bishops' Blunder," *America*, February 13, 1988, 156–158, 171.

151. Cited in AP, "Vatican AIDS Meeting Hears O'Connor Assail Condom Use," *New York Times*, November 14, 1989, A10.

152. AP, "Vatican AIDS Meeting," A10.

CHAPTER 4

1. Cardinal John J. O'Connor, "A Sacrilege Recalled," *Catholic New York*, December 17, 1992, 5; first found in Reel 13, Box 18, Folder 14, ACT UP/NY Collection, New York Public Library (NYPL).

2. O'Connor, "Sacrilege Recalled," 5.

3. Robert Hilferty, *Stop the Church* [video recording] (New York: PDR Productions, 1990).

4. On the PBS debates, see B.J. Bullert, "Stop the Church," in *Public Television: Politics and the Battle over Documentary Film* (New Brunswick, NJ: Rutgers University

Press, 1997). Media coverage included Eleanor Blau, "PBS Cancels Act-Up Film," *New York Times*, August 13, 1991, C16; "An Attack That Exceeded Ridicule," *Washington Post*, August 25, 1991, C6; Walter Goodman, "Prime Time vs. the Art of Ridicule," *New York Times*, September 1, 1991, A21; "L.A. Cardinal Rips AIDS Film," *San Diego Tribune*, September 6, 1991, A10; Howard Rosenberg, "'Stop the Church': All Parties Do Their Part," *Los Angeles Times*, September 9, 1991, 1; Gunther Freehill and Eliseo Acevedo Martinez, "Blasphemy, Lies, Videotape: The Encounter Over AIDS Public TV," *Los Angeles Times*, September 13, 1991, 7; Peter Steinfels, "Beliefs," *New York Times*, September 14, 1991, http://www.nytimes.com/1991/09/14/us/beliefs-038191.html; Howard Rosenberg, "Stop the Charges: No Double Standard in 'Church' Stance," *Los Angeles Times*, September 16, 1991, http://articles.latimes.com/1991-09-16/entertainment/ca-1813_1_double-standard; George Weigel, "KCET's Action," *Los Angeles Times*, September 17, 1991, 7. Also see Robert Hilferty's take in "Why 'Stop the Church' Was Televised," *New York Times*, October 4, 1991, A30.

5. ACT UP hosted a press conference on December 12, 1999 to commemorate the tenth anniversary of the original protest. During this event, members handed out condoms and safe-sex brochures outside of St. Patrick's because, as they stated, "so little has changed in ten years." See http://www.actupny.org/YELL/stopchurch99.html.

6. O'Connor, "Sacrilege Recalled," 5.

7. O'Connor, "Sacrilege Recalled," 5.

8. Robert Orsi, "Abundant History: Marian Apparitions as Alternative Modernity," *Historically Speaking* (September/October 2008), 12–16.

9. Ray Kerrison, "Opinion Column," *New York Post*, December 11, 1989, Real 10, Box 15, Folder 1, ACT UP/NY Collection, NYPL.

10. Given my focus on the politics of AIDS activism, this chapter emphasizes ACT UP's participation in the protest. For more on WHAM!, see Tracy Morgan, "From WHAM! to ACT UP," in Benjamin Shepard and Ronald Hayduk, eds., *From ACT UP to the WTO: Urban Protest and Community Building in the Era of Globalization* (London and New York: Verso, 2002), 141–149.

11. For an excellent counterargument to the all-too-common historiographical assumptions which pit ostensibly secular gays and lesbians against supposed conservative religion, see White, "Homosexuality, Gay Communities, and American Churches."

12. This chapter focuses on ACT UP/New York, the first and largest branch of the AIDS organization. Deborah B. Gould, *Moving Politics: Emotion and ACT UP's Fight against AIDS* (Chicago: University of Chicago Press, 2009), offers an in-depth sociological and historical discussion of ACT UP, especially focused on the New York and Chicago chapters; on ACT UP/NY, see Jennifer Brier's excellent chapter, "Drugs into Bodies, Bodies into Healthcare: The AIDS Coalition to Unleash Power and the Struggle over How Best to Fight AIDS," *Infectious*

Ideas, 156–189; Gilbert Elbaz, "The Sociology of AIDS Activism: The Case of ACT UP/New York, 1987–1992, Volumes I and II," (United States—New York: City University of New York, 1992); Douglas Crimp with Adam Rolston, *AIDS Demo Graphics* (Seattle: Bay Press, 1990); Douglas Crimp, *Melancholia and Moralism: Essays on AIDS and Queer Politics* (Cambridge, MA: MIT Press, 2004); and Peter F. Cohen, *Love and Anger: Essays on AIDS, Activism, and Politics* (New York: Haworth Press, 1998).

13. For an account of this early history, see Larry Kramer, "The First Defense," reprinted in *Reports from the Holocaust: The Story of an AIDS Activist* (New York: St. Martin's Press, 1994), 10–23, especially 13. This piece was first printed in the *New York Native*, Issue 27, December 21, 1981–January 3, 1982. For the activities of GMHC in its first year, see the *GMHC Newsletter*, "Where Are We Now?" also reprinted in *Reports from the Holocaust*, 24–32.

14. Centers for Disease Control and Prevention, "HIV Surveillance—United States, 1981–2008," *Morbidity and Mortality Weekly Report*, 60:21, June 3, 2003: 689–693.

15. Elbaz, "Sociology of AIDS Activism," 56–58; *Bowers v. Hardwick*, 478 U.S. 186 (1986) (Berger, C.J., concurring).

16. Larry Kramer, "An Open Letter to Richard Dunne and Gay Men's Health Crisis," in *Reports from the Holocaust*, 100–116. It was first published in the *New York Native*, Issue 197, January 26, 1987.

17. Kramer was a divisive figure in the gay community even before the AIDS crisis emerged. He gained notoriety in the years preceding the epidemic when he authored *Faggots* (New York: Random House, 1978), a novel critical of the sexual promiscuity celebrated among many urban gay men. His reputation as a sexual naysayer also contributed to his falling out with GMHC, since many gay men saw Kramer as simply sex-negative and his AIDS work as another way in effect of saying "I told you so." By the mid-1980s Kramer had re-established his political voice and captured the developing radical spirit of gay activism. For useful assessments of Kramer's role as a gay writer and activist, see Lawrence D. Mass, ed., *We Must Love One Another Or Die: The Life and Legacies of Larry Kramer* (New York: St. Martin's, 1997).

18. Kramer's speech reprised an earlier AIDS screed, "1,112 and Counting," which fell on deaf ears when it was first published in 1983. At that time, the gay community found itself largely on the defensive, with little information about the new epidemic. In order to present the best face of the gay community, many favored the approach taken by GMHC. Deborah Gould, in *Moving Politics*, 163, describes the affective shift that occurred in the mid-1980s, especially following *Bowers*, which pushed gay political responses from "respectable" to more angry and militant approaches. See Kramer's 1983 article from the *New York Native* and his 1987 speech: "1,112 and Counting" and "The Beginning of ACTing UP," in *Reports from the Holocaust*, 33–51; 127–130.

19. Kramer, "Beginning of ACTing UP," 127–139.
20. "ACT UP Working Document" (last updated in 2003), http://www.actupny.org/documents/workdoc.html.
21. "ACT UP Working Document."
22. See, for instance, the ACT UP/New York Women and AIDS Book Group, *Women, AIDS, and Activism* (Boston: South End Press, 1990).
23. Elbaz, "Sociology of AIDS Activism," 86.
24. On the specific structure and governance of ACT UP/NY, see Elbaz, "Sociology of AIDS Activism," 84–90.
25. See, for instance, ACT UP members Jim Eigo, Mark Harrington, Margaret McCarthy, Stephen Spinella, and Rick Sugden, "FDA Action Handbook," September 12, 1988, available in the ACT UP Archive and at http://www.actupny.org/documents/FDAhandbook1.html.
26. See http://www.actupny.org/documents/1stFlyer.html.
27. ACT UP, "Civil Disobedience Training," http://www.actupny.org/documents/CDdocuments/ACTUP_CivilDisobedience.pdf.
28. See especially Epstein, *Impure Science*, and Patton, *Inventing AIDS*; also see Brier, "Drugs into Bodies, Bodies into Healthcare," *Infectious Ideas*, 156–189, and Gould, *Moving Politics*.
29. See, for instance, Scott Long and Julie Dorf, "ACT UP," in George E. Haggerty, ed., *Gay Histories and Cultures: An Encyclopedia* (New York and London: Taylor & Francis, 2000), 5; and Brett C. Stockdill, "ACT UP," in Roger S. Powers et al., eds., *Protest, Power, and Change: An Encyclopedia of Nonviolent Action from ACT-UP to Women's Suffrage* (New York and London: Taylor & Francis, 1997), 9.
30. Gould, *Moving Politics*, 362–363.
31. Elbaz conducted this research for his doctoral dissertation in sociology at CUNY. He distributed 450 surveys in total and received back 413. See "Who's Who in ACT UP," in Elbaz, "Sociology of AIDS Activism," 65–83. This survey was particularly well timed for gaining a demographic portrait of ACT UP in the months leading up to the Stop the Church demonstration. After 1989, and especially once the organization began to lose cohesion, the demographics changed.
32. The options on the survey for gender were male or female. The survey asked the respondent to fill in race or ethnic background. Elbaz does not list "Asian" or "Pacific Islander" in his description of the data. He does note, however, that the demographic composition of the organization was in flux and changed after 1989. The survey is included in the appendix of Elbaz, "Sociology of AIDS Activism," 545–567.
33. The first question read: "In what religion were you raised? Please specify the denomination, for example: Protestant: Baptist, Jewish: Reform." The options included, in the order listed: Catholic, Hindu, Jewish, Moslem, Protestant,

None, Other (please specify). The second question read: "What is your religious preference? (Please specify)" and included the same options as above. Elbaz, "Sociology of AIDS Activism," 552.

34. This number certainly falls well behind the average for the general American population at the time, which saw far more people identifying as religious. My point here is merely to note that any characterization of ACT UP's overall membership as nonreligious would be inaccurate, since a substantial percentage did identify as such and many more were raised in religious traditions. But I also do not want to overemphasize the importance of religious identity and demographics, as though one must identity as belonging to a particular religious tradition in order to participate in religious work or rhetoric. This would be a quite reductive understanding of what "religion" or "religious" have meant historically.

35. For sociological accounts of this shift, see Robert Wuthnow, *After Heaven: Spirituality in America since the 1950s* (Berkeley: University of California Press, 1998) and *Restructuring of American Religion*; Robert N. Bellah et al., *Habits of the Heart: Individualism and Commitment in American Life* (Berkeley: University of California Press, 1996 [1985]), and for an ethnographic assessment of contemporary New Age spirituality and New Agers' (often-unrecognized) dependence upon institutional forms, see Bender, *New Metaphysicals*. On the history of American spirituality, see Schmidt, *Restless Souls*. For a more capacious, critical analysis of modern American forms of "religion," see Lofton, *Oprah*.

36. Thomas was also one of the founding members of the Majority Action Committee. Maria Maggenti, Interview for ACT UP Oral History Project, January 20, 2003, 10–12; Kendall Thomas, Interview for ACT UP Oral History Project, May 3, 2003, 12–13. The ACT UP Oral History Project is coordinated by filmmaker Jim Hubbard and writer and activist Sarah Schulman, who also conducted the interviews. It is available at http://www.actuporalhistory.org/. See also Elbaz, "Sociology of AIDS Activism," 266–269, and Brier, *Infectious Ideas*, 170–171.

37. See Kendall Thomas, Interview for ACT UP Oral History Project, May 3, 2003, 19–20.

38. Kendall Thomas, Interview for ACT UP Oral History Project, 20. Gran Fury was a collective of activists and artists that formed following ACT UP's participation in the "Let the Record Show . . ." installation at The New Museum for Contemporary Art in December of 1987. Its membership overlapped with ACT UP's.

39. Larry Kramer, "Before the President's Commission," *Reports from the Holocaust*, 182.

40. Kramer, "Before the President's Commission," 183. As I noted in the previous chapter, the commission's report largely sidestepped the question of sexuality, though it did praise the gay community for the excellent work it had done to fight AIDS.

41. Kramer, "Before the President's Commission," 184.

42. Kramer, "Before the President's Commission," 185.

43. The scene is captured in Hilferty, *Stop the Church*. My narrative in the following three paragraphs is culled partly from this film as well as from the subsequently cited newspaper articles and documents from the ACT UP archives. For a brief essay on the protest, and a description of the activist who crumbled the host as a former altar boy, see the final chapter of Crimp, *AIDS Demo Graphics*, 131–142; for a reading of the protest as an appropriation of religious ritual, see Jordan, *Recruiting Young Love*, 185–190.

44. See Ray Kerrison, "Opinion Column," *New York Post*, December 11, 1989, and "Sacrilege in St. Pat's [Editorial]," *New York Post*, December 12, 1989, Real 10, Box 15, Folder 1, ACT UP/NY Collection, NYPL.

45. Quoted in Hilferty, *Stop the Church*.

46. On the Lavender Hill Mob and their actions as a precursor to ACT UP's work, see Gilbert Elbaz, "The Sociology of AIDS Activism," 56–57. On O'Connor's support for Vatican actions taken against Hunthausen and Curran, see Hentoff, *John Cardinal O'Connor*, 73, and Jane Gross, "O'Connor Backs a Curb on Dissenting Speakers," *New York Times*, September 8, 1986, B3. I describe Cardinal Ratzinger's letter in chapter three.

47. Mary Ann Poust, "Occasion of Disunity," *Catholic New York*, March 12, 1987, 21.

48. Andrew Miller and Rex Wockner, "AIDS/Abortion Rights Demo Halts High Mass at St. Pat's," *OutWeek*, December 24, 1989, Real 10, Box 14, Folder 2, ACT UP/NY Collection, NYPL.

49. Associated Press, "Vatican AIDS Meeting Hears O'Connor Assail Condom Use," *New York Times*, November 14, 1989, A10.

50. I discuss this history, including these two statements, in greater depth in chapter three.

51. Michael Hirsely, "Catholic Bishops Renew Abortion Fight," *Chicago Tribune*, November 8, 1989, 7.

52. Hirsely, "Catholic Bishops Renew Abortion Fight," 7.

53. Ari L. Goldman, "O'Connor Challenges Cuomo on Abortion But Lauds Stand," *New York Times*, September 24, 1984, B3.

54. Tyree Johnson, "Cardinal O'Connor Hails Jailed Bishop," *Philadelphia Daily News*, November 29, 1988, 13.

55. "Cardinal Hails Protesters in Operation Rescue," *The Buffalo News*, October 12, 1989, A18; Associated Press, "Cardinal O'Connor Won't Join an Operation Rescue," *Philadelphia Daily News*, October 9, 1989, 12.

56. Vincent Gagliostro, Interview for ACT UP Oral History Project, July 8, 2005, 49. This story is also recounted in Morgan, "From WHAM! to ACT UP," 141–149.

57. Gagliostro, Interview, 49–50.

58. Gagliostro, Interview, 51.

59. Gagliostro, Interview, 51.

60. This scene is captured in Hilferty, *Stop the Church.* I have attempted to verify the historical claims, but have not yet been successful in doing so. At the very least, this narrative illustrates the historical trajectory in which members placed their protest. Notably, it was not a context that opposed religion but rather a history about the fight for religious inclusion.

61. Gagliostro, Interview, 52.

62. Gagliostro, Interview, 53.

63. ACT UP and WHAM!, "Stop the Church Action Update," in Mark Blasius and Shane Phelan, eds., *We Are Everywhere: A Historical Sourcebook of Gay and Lesbian Politics* (New York: Routledge, 1997), 623–624, capitalization in original.

64. Elbaz, "The Sociology of AIDS Activism," 86, notes that affinity groups were commonly formed to provide a way for activists to engage in demonstrations that could not be approved of by the floor. Hence, their actions were not formally supported by ACT UP, but neither can they be fully disentangled from the larger body.

65. The various activities planned to advertise the demonstration are clearly seen in notes taken at ACT UP meetings. See, for instance, "Things to do," unpublished notes, Reel 10, Box 15, Folder 2, ACT UP/NY Collection, NYPL.

66. Jay Blotcher, Interview for ACT UP Oral History Project, April 24, 2004, 39–42.

67. ACT UP, "Letter to the Press," December 6, 1989, Reel 10, Box 15, Folder 1. ACT UP/NY Collection, NYPL.

68. ACT UP, "Media Advisory Update," December 6, 1989, Reel 10, Box 15, Folder 1, ACT UP/NY Collection, NYPL.

69. ACT UP and WHAM!, "Letter to the Parishioners of Saint Patrick's Cathedral," in Blasius and Phelan, eds., *We Are Everywhere,* 624–625.

70. ACT UP and WHAM!, "Letter to the Parishioners of Saint Patrick's Cathedral." 624–625.

71. Gay Men's Health Crisis, "Gay Men's Health Crisis Statement on Action at St. Patrick's Cathedral," News from GMHC, December 13, 1989, Reel 10, Box 15, Folder 1, ACT UP/NY Collection, NYPL.

72. The statement by ACT UP was released in English and Spanish. See "Position Statement," December 13, 1989 and "Posición," December 14, 1989, in Reel 10, Box 15, Folder 1, ACT UP/NY Collection, NYPL.

73. ACT UP, "Position Statement."

74. ACT UP, "Position Statement," 57.

75. ACT UP, "Stop the Church Media Update," unpublished notes, Reel 153, Box 194, Folder 37, ACT UP/NY Collection, NYPL. See also ACT UP Media Report, "Stop the Church," in Blasius and Phelan, eds., *We Are Everywhere,* 626–627.

76. "Unjoyful Noise: Worshippers Rights Violated [Editorial]," *New York Newsday,* December 12, 1989, Real 10, Box 15, Folder 1, ACT UP/NY Collection, NYPL; "Sacrilege in St. Pat's [Editorial]," *New York Post,* December 12, 1989; "The

Storming of St. Pat's [Editorial]," *New York Times*, December 12, 1989, A24; Ray Kerrison, "Opinion Column," *New York Post*, December 11, 1989.

77. "Unjoyful Noise [Editorial]."

78. "The Storming of St. Pat's," A24.

79. "Church Service Disrupted at St. Patrick's in N.Y.," *San Francisco Chronicle*, December 11, 1989, A3, and "Sacrilege in St. Pat's," *New York Post*, in Real 10, Box 15, Folder 1, ACT UP/NY Collection, NYPL.

80. "Attacks on Catholic Churches [Editorial]," *San Francisco Chronicle*, December 12, 1989, A24.

81. Randy Shilts, "AIDS Protests at Churches," *San Francisco Chronicle*, December 18, 1989, A4. The simultaneous protests on the West Coast garnered less media attention, largely because they were less controversial, since the demonstrations remained outside the churches. Their relative lack of coverage also illustrated in part the bind in which AIDS activists found themselves—in order to gain substantial mainstream coverage concerning AIDS, they had to cross certain lines of decorum. But in doing so, they risked losing the sympathy of the media and its readership.

82. Randy Shilts, "AIDS Protests at Churches," A4. Though Shilts authored a highly influential, critical study of the early history of the AIDS crisis, *And the Band Played On*, AIDS activists, including those aligned with ACT UP, often found in his work a moralistic critique of gay sexual culture and an uncritical dependence on science. Shilts represented a more established and "respectable" side of gay politics, in contrast to the grassroots, direct-action protests organized by ACT UP.

83. Gerald M. Costello, "Editor's Report: Faces of Hate," *Catholic New York*, December 14, 1989, 2. It is not clear exactly how many demonstrators repeated the action of crumbling the host, since the reports are conflicting, including those offered by people who were inside the cathedral. Most accounts report only one instance, which I describe in more detail later in this chapter, but more were certainly possible.

84. Mary Ann Poust and Gerald M. Costello, "Unfair, Unjustified and Offensive," *Catholic New York*, December 14, 1989, 3, 17.

85. Poust and Costello, "Unfair, Unjustified and Offensive," 3, 17.

86. Poust and Costello, "Unfair, Unjustified and Offensive," 3, 17. The list of organizations, some of which also issued separate statements, included the American Jewish Congress, Metropolitan Region; the American Jewish Committee, New York Chapter; B'nai B'rith, District One; the Jewish Community Relations Council of New York; the New York Board of Rabbis; and the Synagogue Council of America.

87. Poust and Costello, "Unfair, Unjustified and Offensive," 3, 17. Those signed onto the statement included Reverend Carl Flemister of the American Baptist Churches, Archbishop Iakovos of the Greek Orthodox Archdiocese of North

and South America, Bishop William H. Lazarus of the Metropolitan New York Synod of the Evangelical Lutheran Church of America, Bishop Torkom Manoogian of the Armenian Orthodox Church, and Bishop C. Dale White of the United Methodist Church.

88. Poust and Costello, "Unfair, Unjustified and Offensive," 3, 17.

89. Mary Ann Poust, "Cathedral Disturbance: Fallout Continues as Cardinal Praises Congregation for Restraint," *Catholic New York*, December 21, 1989, 15.

90. Poust, "Cathedral Disturbance: Fallout Continues as Cardinal Praises Congregation for Restraint," 15.

91. I discuss their positions more fully in a later section.

92. The sensitivity toward anti-Catholicism at least historically was well founded, as American Catholics often found themselves the object of Protestant ridicule and oppression throughout much of the nineteenth and early twentieth centuries. After World War II, however, Catholics, along with Jews, were largely brought into the fold of the American religious mainstream, though this has not been a complete or smooth transition. Claims of anti-Catholicism reemerged after the cultural upheavals of the 1960s and 1970s, and throughout the culture wars of the 1980s, as conservative Catholics argued that protests against the Catholic Church organized by feminist and gay activists represented a new form of anti-Catholic oppression and Catholics became one of the last groups that one could openly bash in public. See, for instance, Mark S. Massa, *Anti-Catholicism in America: The Last Acceptable Prejudice*, 2nd ed. (New York: Crossroad Publishing Company, 2005) and Philip Jenkins, *The New Anti-Catholicism: The Last Acceptable Prejudice* (New York: Oxford University Press, 2004).

93. On the demographics of the *Catholic New York* readership, see Gerard J. Hekker, "CNY Poll," *Catholic New York*, November 12, 1987, 16, which details the findings of a Gallup poll taken that year. Most readers considered the newspaper their best source for information about Catholicism and Catholic culture and reported reading the paper regularly. In addition, the majority of readers claimed Irish descent and were over 50. As a whole, the readers considered themselves and the paper to be conservative on both political and theological issues, and most thought themselves more conservative than the paper. Most subscribers to the paper were married women who owned homes, while the largest number picking up copies of the paper in church were single men who rented apartments in the city.

94. Mariann Beals, "Letters: Make Reparation," *Catholic New York*, January 4, 1990, 16.

95. Barbara Braum, "Letters: Sorrow at Sacrilege," *Catholic New York*, January 4, 1990, 16.

96. Richard D McKeon, "Letters: Circle the Wagon," *Catholic New York*, January 4, 1990, 16.

97. Edward Scully, "Letters: Fighting Back," *Catholic New York*, January 4, 1990, 16. Also see Rafael Ocasio, "Letters: Support the Cardinal," *Catholic New York*, January 4, 1990, 16.

98. Benedict J. Groeschel, "Two Demonstrations," *Catholic New York*, January 4, 1990, 15.

99. Groeschel, "Two Demonstrations," 15.

100. Groeschel, "Two Demonstrations," 15.

101. Now called *Culture Wars*, *Fidelity* was founded in 1981 by E. Michael Jones as an orthodox Catholic magazine following his departure from St. Mary's College in Notre Dame, Indiana, where he was let go for his extremist religious positions. J. Joseph Garvey, "The Homofascist Invasion of St. Patrick's Cathedral: The Curtain Goes Up on the Gay '90s," *Fidelity*, February 1990, 24–30.

102. Garvey, "Homofascist Invasion," 24. A number of pro-lifers accused Koop of turning his back on the movement when the surgeon general reported his findings to President Reagan concerning the potential health effects of abortions on women. Koop told the president that, based on his research, no substantial health effects could be noted. See Philip D. Yancey, "The Embattled Career of Dr. Koop," *Christianity Today*, October 20, 1989, 20–21.

103. Garvey, "Homofascist Invasion," 24.

104. Garvey, "Homofascist Invasion," 24.

105. Garvey, "Homofascist Invasion," 25.

106. Garvey, "Homofascist Invasion," 26.

107. Garvey, "Homofascist Invasion," 26.

108. David Hume, "Of Superstition and Enthusiasm," in Eugene F. Miller, ed., *Essays, Moral, Political, and Literary* (Indianapolis: Liberty Fund, Inc., 1987); Talal Asad, *Genealogies of Religion: Discipline and Reasons of Power in Christianity and Islam* (Baltimore: Johns Hopkins University Press, 1993), especially 1–82, and *Formations of the Secular*; Mahmood, *Politics of Piety*, and "Secularism, Hermeneutics, and Empire: The Politics of Islamic Reformation," *Public Culture* 18:2 (2006): 323–347. Within American religion, see Winnifred Fallers Sullivan, *The Impossibility of Religious Freedom* (Princeton, NJ: Princeton University Press, 2005); Tisa Wenger, *We Have a Religion: The 1920s Pueblo Indian Dance Controversy and American Religious Freedom* (Chapel Hill: University of North Carolina Press, 2009); Susan Harding, "Representing Fundamentalism: The Problem of the Repugnant Culture Other," *Social Research* 58:2 (Summer 1991): 373–393; and Tracy Fessenden, "Religious Liberalism and the Liberal Geopolitics of Religion," in Leigh E. Schmidt and Sally M. Promey, eds., *American Religious Liberalism* (Bloomington: Indiana University Press, 2012), 359–373.

109. Garvey, "Homofascist Invasion," 27.

110. Garvey, "Homofascist Invasion," 27.

111. Jenkins, *New Anti-Catholicism*, 3; 22. The other example Jenkins cites was of a feminist protest in the Catholic cathedral of Marie, Reine du Monde in Montreal in 2000.

112. Jenkins, *New Anti-Catholicism*, 93; 102.

113. *OutWeek* was published in New York from June 1989 to July 1991. Founded by ACT UP members Gabriel Rotello and Kendall Morrison, the magazine had a circulation estimated at thirty to forty thousand. *OutWeek* has been archived online at http://www.outweek.net/archive.html. Deirdre Carmody, "Outweek, Gay and Lesbian Magazine, Ceases Publication," *New York Times*, June 28, 1991, D9; "Open Closets, Closed Doors," *Time*, 138, issue 1, July 8, 1991, 47.

114. "Outspoken: Gays and the Church" [Editorial] *OutWeek*, December 3, 1989, 4.

115. "Outspoken: Gays and the Church," 4.

116. Andy Humm, "Letters: Humm Bug," *OutWeek*, December 24, 1989, 6. Humm's remarks in *OutWeek* followed an editorial he authored for the *New York Post*.

117. Humm, "Letters: Humm Bug," 6.

118. Michael Flynn, "Letters: Stop ACT UP," *OutWeek*, January 7, 1990, 8–9.

119. Bob Johnston, "Letters: Ban ACT UP," *OutWeek*, January 7, 1990, 9.

120. Ronald Najman, "Letters: Religious Right," *OutWeek*, December 17, 1989, 6.

121. Najman, "Letters: Religious Right," 6.

122. James E. Keenan, "ACT DOWN," *OutWeek*, January 7, 1990, 11.

123. Keenan, "ACT DOWN," 11.

124. Terry McGovern, "Letters: Ho Humm," *OutWeek*, December 24, 1989, 6–7. She attributed this hypocrisy in part to the gendered bifurcation of authority in the church: "There are, of course, exceptional people working within the church, but these are not the powerful. Often they are women."

125. McGovern, "Letters: Ho Humm," 6–7.

126. Dan Hunter and Servalan Erik, "Letters: If You Can't Take the Heat . . ." *OutWeek*, December 24, 1989, 7–8.

127. Hunter and Erik, "Letters: If You Can't Take the Heat . . .," 7–8.

128. Victor Mendolia, "Letters: Mission Accomplished," *OutWeek*, January 7, 1990, 5–6.

129. Mendolia, "Letters: Mission Accomplished," 5–6.

130. Michelangelo Signorile, "Liturgical Loophole?" *OutWeek*, December 24, 1989, 18.

131. Cited in Signorile, "Liturgical Loophole?" 18.

132. John N. Calve, "Letters: Cardinal Hypocrisy," *OutWeek*, December 24, 1989, 8–9.

133. Calve, "Letters: Cardinal Hypocrisy," 8–9, capitalization in original.

134. Paul Guzzardo, "Letter to the Editor," *OutWeek*, January 14, 1990, 6–7.

135. Tom Shultz, "Letters: Freedom from Religion," *OutWeek*, January 7, 1990, 6–8.

136. Shultz, "Letters: Freedom from Religion," 7.

137. Shultz, "Letters: Freedom from Religion," 7–8.

138. Shultz, "Letters: Freedom from Religion," 7–8.

139. Asad, *Formations of the Secular*, 1–20, and *Genealogies of Religion*, 55–82. Following Asad and scholars of lived religion and material culture, this approach would also emphasize the role of practice, including bodily interaction with visual and material objects, over belief or identity. That is, it takes the emphasis off of the question of whether the demonstrator who desecrated the host was himself religious or even Catholic to underscore instead the instrumental effects of his actions (along with the actions of the broader protest, including the visual imagery reproduced in this chapter). On the study of visual and material religious culture, see David Morgan, *The Sacred Gaze: Religious Visual Culture in Theory and Practice* (Berkeley: University of California, 2005), 48–74, and Sally M. Promey, *Sensational Religion: Sensory Cultures in Material Practice* (New Haven, CT: Yale University Press, 2014).

140. At least by the medieval period, the term referred more broadly to any form of violation or outrage committed against a sacred object. "Sacrilege, n.1," OED Online, June 2014, Oxford University Press, http://www.oed.com/view/Entry/169585. O'Connor's reference to the "demonic" also suggests an alternative reading. As the Christian movement was forming in the first couple centuries of the Common Era, it turned the variety of divine beings or spirits, called *daimones* in Greek, into evil forces eventually subdued to the one, powerful God—today we call these evil forces *demons*. To call the protestor demonic, then, could suggest not a secular madness but a supernatural one. Joseph H. Lynch, *Early Christianity: A Brief History* (New York: Oxford University Press, 2010), 28, 32–33.

141. The demonstrator's name appears in the ACT UP archive, but I have withheld it here, as I have not yet been able to reach him. The archive suggests he was Catholic, or raised Catholic, which would not be unusual given ACT UP's demographics. But as I mention in the notes here, we might also emphasize his action rather than his beliefs or intention, by reading the crumbling of the wafer as another kind of ritual. Groeschel, "Two Demonstrations," *Catholic New York*, 15. Former Jesuit priest Robert Goss offers a very different, activist reading in *Jesus Acted Up*, though he also contends that the act of crumbling was "counterproductive" to the goals of the AIDS activists (147). As a historian, I am less interested in debating whether or not the act went too far than I am in the history of its interpretation and its effects. By most accounts (from Catholics in New York and mainstream journalists to several gays and lesbians and AIDS activists), the act crossed a line of some sort. I want to suggest other possible interpretations less to displace these readings than to suggest other ways it *could* have been interpreted—and then to ask why, given other possibilities, dominant narratives depicted it more narrowly as an attack upon religion or religious freedom, if not Jesus himself.

142. Aside from obvious examples of religious protestors, such as Jesus or Martin Luther, for instance, Caroline Walker Bynum offers another instructive historical precedent. She describes how medieval women who fasted, and thus could not take regular bread, exerted religious authority by refusing to take the host or by spitting it out—a sign that the priest had corrupted the Communion wafer in some way. Faithful onlookers, Bynum writes, "might see the pious woman's rejection of the host as a reason for questioning the priest's act of consecration. However theologically unsound the conclusion might be, they tended to deduce in some unspecified way he was disqualified by immorality (usually sexual immorality)." Bynum, *Holy Feast and Holy Fast: The Religious Significance of Food to Medieval Women* (Berkeley and Los Angeles: University of California Press, 1988), 228.

AFTERWORD I

1. Paul Monette, *Last Watch of the Night: Essays Too Personal and Otherwise* (New York: Harcourt Brace, 1994), 81, 120, 303. Monette expressed similar sentiments in his account of his partner's battle with AIDS in *Borrowed Time: An AIDS Memoir* (San Diego: Harcourt Brace, 1988) and in his autobiographical work *Becoming a Man: Half a Life Story* (New York: Harcourt Brace, 1992).
2. Rafael Campo, "AIDS and the Poetry of Healing," in Marie Howe and Michael Klein, eds., *In the Company of My Solitude: American Writing from the AIDS Pandemic* (New York: Persea Books, 1995), 24.
3. Susan Harding describes Falwell's claim that AIDS is a national punishment in *Book of Jerry Falwell*, 160.
4. Statistics had been gathered since 1973. See American Enterprise Institute for Public Policy Research, "Attitudes about Homosexuality and Gay Marriage" (updated June 3, 2008), compiled by Karlyn Bowman and Adam Foster, 2, http://www.aei.org/paper/14882). Cited in George Chauncey, *Why Marriage?* (New York: Basic Books, 2004), 43.
5. I do not want to suggest a rigid distinction here between mainline or progressive Christians on the one hand and evangelicals and Catholics on the other. First, because the official statements of denominations and Christian elites often did not represent the feelings of American Christians more broadly, who tended to be less progressive than mainline Protestant elites and less conservative on sexual issues than leaders within the Catholic Church and the Christian Right. I am not pointing out a distinction between two opposing sides but rather suggesting two points on a continuum of Christian reactions to the AIDS crisis. Second, the moral discourse about AIDS that I describe among evangelicals and the Catholic bishops was not limited to specific religious groups; it pervaded mainstream, secular coverage of the epidemic in the media and was even translated into the secular terms of public health. In other words,

we can see this moral religious discourse *as moral* and *as steeped in religious history* most clearly in work of the evangelicals and Catholic leaders I describe here, but it was in no way limited to them.

6. Michael Warner, "Introduction," *Fear of a Queer Planet: Queer Politics and Social Theory* (Minneapolis: University of Minnesota Press, 1993), xviii–xix.

7. The church hierarchy has more recently signaled the potential for some movement on its opposition to condom use as a tool to prevent HIV infection. In 2010, Pope Benedict XVI (formerly Cardinal Ratzinger) made headlines for suggesting condoms could sometimes be used for prevention, such as by male sex workers—though the Vatican clarified that they should not be used to prevent pregnancy. Rachel Donadio, "Vatican Adds Nuance to Pope's Condom Remarks," *New York Times*, December 21, 2010, http://www.nytimes. com/2010/12/22/world/europe/22pope.html. The clarification can be found in Congregation for the Doctrine of the Faith, "Note on the Banalization of Sexuality regarding Certain Interpretations of 'Light of the World,'" December 21, 2010, http://www.vatican.va/roman_curia/congregations/cfaith/documents/rc_con_cfaith_doc_20101221_luce-del-mondo_en.html. Pope Francis' emphasis on social justice has led many to wonder if he would take this position further, though there has not been much change to date. In 2014, Pope Francis praised members of the church working in health-related positions in Africa for educating people in "sexual responsibility and chastity" to curb the spread of HIV. Cited in Associated Press, "Pope Francis Praises Chastity as a Strategy to Prevent the Spread of HIV in Africa," *Huffington Post*, April 7, 2014, http://www.huffingtonpost.com/2014/04/07/pope-francis-chastity_n_5105240.html.

8. Fears about protecting the national body, assumed to be HIV negative, were played out in a 1987 law banning entry to the United States for noncitizens who tested positive, a law not lifted in until 2013. As Jennifer Brier sharply demonstrates, requirements for HIV tests for immigrants and federal prisoners— supported by both Reagan and Surgeon General Koop—were rooted in a number of fears, especially of racial otherness. They tapped into a longer history of white Americans' fears about polluting the population as well as more particular fears in the 1980s, as AIDS was coded as Haitian and African. According to a 1987 Gallup poll, 90% of Americans supported testing for potential immigrants and 66% supported testing for foreign visitors. Brier, *Infectious Ideas*, 107, but see 78–121.

9. Harding, *Book of Jerry Falwell*, 167, discusses the negative sexual politics of "moral majority jeremiads."

10. I do not mean to suggest that moral prescriptions for sex were new. The early twentieth century witnessed a proliferation of morally inflected sex education, but this was often produced by progressives within the medical establishment. The more recent, positive discourse I am referring to developed as a reaction

to what many evangelicals and other Christians took as the sexual license, or moral declension, wrought by the sexual revolution of the two decades preceding AIDS. On the earlier period, see Moran, *Teaching Sex*. By "positive," I do not mean to imply that their stances mirrored the "sex-positive" approaches articulated by a number of gay and AIDS activists described elsewhere in this book. A good bit of sex-negativity still reigned. But the impulse to malign homosexuality and other forms of perceived sexual immorality was suppressed in order to articulate a specific program in which people could (and even should) have sex.

11. In the Foucaultian sense, that is; see *History of Sexuality*, 15–50.

12. Chauncey uses this phrasing to describe the shift in gay politics in *Why Marriage?*, 121; see also 87–136.

13. Chauncey, *Why Marriage?*, 87–136.

14. Chauncey, *Why Marriage?*, 120–123; for conservative gay voices, see Andrew Sullivan, *Virtually Normal: An Argument about Homosexuality* (New York: Knopf, 1989), and Jonathan Rauch, *Gay Marriage: Why It Is Good for Gays, Good for Straights, and Good for America* (New York: Holt, 2004). For a historical analysis of the rise of gay conservatives, see Paul Robinson, *Queer Wars: The New Gay Right and Its Critics* (Chicago: University of Chicago Press, 2006); for different but trenchant critiques of this conservative narrative, see Crimp, "Melancholia and Moralism," 1–26, and Lisa Duggan, "The New Homonormativity: The Sexual Politics of Neoliberalism," in Russ Castronovo and Dana D. Nelson, eds., *Materializing Democracy: Toward a Revitalized Cultural Politics* (Durham, NC: Duke University Press, 2002), 175–194.

15. For an early account of gay sexual politics and battles with political and religious conservatism, see Gayle Rubin, "Thinking Sex: Notes for a Radical Theory of the Politics of Sexuality," in Carol S. Vance, ed., *Pleasure and Danger: Exploring Female Sexuality* (Boston: Routledge and K. Paul, 1984), 267–319. Republished numerous times, Rubin's essay has become a classic text in feminist and queer politics. Released in 1984, as the AIDS epidemic was still emerging in public consciousness and gay marriage was barely a dream for most activists, this essay remains one of the most developed articulations of queer sexual ethics.

16. Saundra Young, "Imprisoned Over HIV: One Man's Story," *CNN*, November 9, 2012, http://www.cnn.com/2012/08/02/health/criminalizing-hiv/index.html; Sean Strub, "Criminalization 101," *POZ*, November 2, 2010, http://blogs.poz.com/sean/archives/2010/11/criminalization_101.html. Also see the suite of articles available on the *POZ* website, http://www.poz.com/criminalization.shtml. The Center for HIV Law and Policy (http://www.hivlawandpolicy.org/) monitors the criminalization of HIV and advocates against such laws, and there has been more success in the decriminalization of HIV in the United

States under the Obama administration. Other countries have not fared as well. The criminalization of HIV and homosexuality in Uganda, for instance, remains a central concern for public health workers and activists working to curb the epidemic. Much of the resistance to homosexuality and to public health policies against criminalization has been supported by conservative American evangelical leaders, such as Scott Lively. For a report on American evangelicals and the ongoing culture wars around sexuality in African churches, see Kapya Kaoma, *Globalizing the Culture Wars: U.S. Conservatives, African Churches, and Homophobia* (Somerville, MA: Political Research Associates, 2009).

17. Soumya Karlamangla, "Get Me to the Float on Time: Gay Grooms Exchange Rolling Vows," *Los Angeles Times*, January 1, 2014, http://www.latimes.com/local/lanow/la-me-ln-marriage-float-20131231-story.html; Jerry Portwood, "Danny Leclair and Aubrey Loots," *OUT*, January 2, 2014, http://www.out.com/out-exclusives/wedding-guide/vows/2014/01/02/rose-bowl-parade-wedding-danny-leclair-aubrey-loots. For a critique of the focus on gay marriage to the exclusion of HIV/AIDS, and a subsequent response, see Peter Staley, "Gay Marriage Is Great, But How about Some Love for the AIDS Fight," *Washington Post*, June 28, 2013, http://www.washingtonpost.com/opinions/gay-marriage-is-great-but-how-about-some-love-for-the-aids-fightlove-will-tear-us-apart/2013/06/28/5b18c50c-dddo-11e2-948c-d644453cf169_story.html, and Peter Halkitis, "How Gay Marriage Helps Fight AIDS," *New York Daily News*, July 11, 2013, http://www.nydailynews.com/opinion/gay-marriage-helps-fight-aids-article-1.1395315.

18. Of course, PrEP can also be used by women who sleep with women or with men, though most media coverage on the use of PrEP in the United States has focused on gay men and MSMs. United States Public Health Service, "Preexposure Prophylaxis for the Prevention of HIV Infection in the United States – 2014: A Clinical Guidline," May 14, 2014, http://www.cdc.gov/hiv/pdf/PrEP-guidelines2014.pdf; also see the Centers for Disease Control information page on PrEP, http://www.cdc.gov/hiv/prevention/research/prep/; Tim Murphy, "Sex without Fear," July 13, 2014, *New York Magazine*, http://nymag.com/news/features/truvada-hiv-2014-7/.

19. Paul Jeffrey, "AIDS Activists Praise Progress, Warn about Lingering Danger of HIV," *Catholic News Service*, July 30, 2014, http://www.catholicnews.com/data/stories/cns/1403163.htm. The article was carried in the *National Catholic Reporter* and *National Catholic Register*. The text of the "Melbourne Declaration" is available at www.aids2014.org/declaration.aspx.

20. Linda Harvey, "Condoms Out, Drugs In: America's New Message to Youth," *Barbwire*, May 21, 2014, http://barbwire.com/2014/05/21/condoms-drugs-americas-new-message-youth/.

21. Karlamangla, "Get Me to the Float on Time."

22. David Crary for AP, "Truvada, HIV Prevention Drug, Divides Gay Community," *Huffington Post*, April 7, 2014, http://www.huffingtonpost.com/2014/04/07/truvada-gay-men-hiv_n_5102515.html; Tony Merevick, "Head Of Largest U.S. HIV/AIDS Health Care Organization Still Insists Truvada Is A 'Party Drug,'" *Buzzfeed*, April 17, 2014, http://www.buzzfeed.com/tonymerevick/head-of-largest-us-hivaids-healthcare-organization-still-ins#x308eg.

23. Cited in Patrick Healy, "A Lion Still Roars, with Gratitude," *New York Times*, May 21, 2014, http://www.nytimes.com/2014/05/25/arts/television/larry-kramer-lives-to-see-his-normal-heart-filmed-for-tv.html.

24. Larry Kramer, *The Normal Heart and The Destiny of Me* (New York: Grove Press, 2000; *The Normal Heart* [1985]) 70; 78; 117. For a critique of Kramer's position, see Crimp, "How to Have Promiscuity," 237–271 (discussion of *Normal Heart* on 247) and Max Fox, "The Silences of Larry Kramer's 'Normal Heart,'" *Al-jazeera America*, May 31, 2014, http://america.aljazeera.com/opinions/2014/5/probing-larry-kramersnormalheart.html.

25. For many Americans, including most conservative Christians and some gay and AIDS activists alike, the idea that marriage would limit sexual partners and thus reduce risk of HIV infection appears to be common sense, or even natural. Yet, as public health researchers have shown, for many women across the world marriage is a major risk factor for contracting HIV. The normative ideal of marriage today, as an intimate monogamous union between equals, is neither the reality of most marriages (gay or straight), historically speaking, nor the best model for the prevention of HIV. Jennifer S. Hirsch, Sergio Meneses, Brenda Thompson, Mirka Negroni, Blanca Pelcastre, and Carlos del Rio, "The Inevitability of Infidelity: Sexual Reputation, Social Geographies, and Marital HIV Risk in Rural Mexico," *American Journal of Public Health* 97 (6) (June 2007), 986–996; Daniel Jordan Smith, "Modern Marriage, Men's Extramarital Sex, and HIV Risk in Southeastern Nigeria," *American Journal of Public Health* 97 (6) (June 2007), 997–1005; Lucy Mkandawire-Valhmu, Claire Wendland, Patricia E. Stevens, Peninnah M. Kako, Anne Dressel, and Jennifer Kibicho, "Marriage as a Risk Factor for HIV: Learning from the Experiences of HIV-infected Women in Malawi," *Global Public Health* 8 (2) (January 2013), 187–201. On the particular history of American monogamy, see Cott, *Public Vows*, and Davis, *More Perfect Unions*.

Selected Bibliography

PERIODICALS

The Advocate
AIDS Weekly
America
BLK
The Body
Body Politic
Catholic Almanac
Catholic New York
The Chicago Catholic
Chicago Tribune
The Christian Century
Christianity Today
Commonweal
Fidelity Magazine
Gay Community News
Liberty Report
LIFE
Los Angeles Times
Morbidity and Mortality Weekly
National Catholic Register
National Catholic Reporter
New York Magazine
New York Native
New York Newsday
New York Post
New York Times
Origins

OutWeek
San Diego Tribune
San Francisco Chronicle
Time
USA Today
The Village Voice
The Washington Post

MONOGRAPHS AND ESSAYS

ACT UP NY/Women AIDS Book. *Women, AIDS, and Activism.* Boston: South End Press, 1999.

Adam, Barry D. *The Rise of a Gay and Lesbian Movement.* Boston: Twayne Publishers, 1987.

Adams, Vincanne, and Stacy Leigh Pigg. *Sex in Development.* Durham, NC: Duke University Press, 2005.

Ahmed, Sara. "Affective Economies," *Social Text* 22.2 (2004): 117–139.

Alcorn, Randy. *Christians in the Wake of Sexual Revolution: Recovering Our Sexual Sanity.* Portland, OR: Multnomah Press, 1985.

Alison, James. *Catholics and AIDS: Questions and Answers.* London: Catholic Truth Society, 1987.

Allen, Jimmy. *Burden of a Secret.* New York: Random House, 1995.

Allen, Peter Lewis. *The Wages of Sin: Sex and Disease, Past and Present.* Chicago: University of Chicago Press, 2000.

Allitt, Patrick. *Catholic Intellectuals and Conservative Politics in America, 1950–1985.* Ithaca, NY: Cornell University Press, 1995.

Allyn, David. *Make Love, Not War: The Sexual Revolution: An Unfettered History.* New York: Routledge, 2001.

Altman, Dennis. *AIDS in the Mind of America.* Garden City, NY: Anchor/Doubleday Press, 1986.

———. *AIDS and the New Puritanism.* London: Pluto Press, 1986.

Amos, Jr., William E. *When AIDS Comes to Church.* Philadelphia: Westminster Press, 1988.

Anderson, Benedict. *Imagined Communities: Reflections on the Origin and Spread of Nationalism.* London and New York: Verso, 1991.

Andriote, John-Manuel. *Victory Deferred: How AIDS Changed Gay Life in America.* Chicago: University of Chicago Press, 1999.

Antonio, Gene. *The AIDS Cover-Up? The Real and Alarming Facts about AIDS.* San Francisco: Ignatius Press, 1986.

Appleby, R. Scott. "Review: Public Catholicism and Clerical Activities." *The Review of Politics* 59, no. 2 (Spring 1997): 377–381.

Armstrong, Elizabeth A. *Forging Gay Identities: Organizing Sexuality in San Francisco, 1950–1994.* Chicago: University of Chicago Press, 2002.

Asad, Talal. *Genealogies of Religion: Discipline and Reasons of Power in Christianity and Islam.* Baltimore: Johns Hopkins University Press, 1993.

———. *Formations of the Secular: Christianity, Islam, Modernity.* Stanford: Stanford University Press, 2003.

Badaracco, Claire. *Prescribing Faith: Medicine, Media, and Religion in American Culture.* Waco, TX: Baylor University Press, 2007.

Bailey, Beth. *Sex in the Heartland.* Cambridge, MA: Harvard University Press, 2002.

Balmer, Randall. *Thy Kingdom Come: How the Religious Right Distorts Faith and Threatens the Nation.* New York: Basic Books, 2006.

———. *Mine Eyes Have Seen the Glory: A Journey into the Evangelical Subculture in America,* 4th ed. New York: Oxford University Press, 2006.

———. *God in the White House: A History: How Faith Shaped the Presidency from John F. Kennedy to George W. Bush.* New York: HarperOne, 2008.

Bamforth, Nick. *AIDS and the Healer Within.* New York and London: Amethyst Books, 1987.

Barnes, Sandra L. *Live Long and Prosper: How Black Megachurches Address HIV/AIDS and Poverty in the Age of Prosperity Theology.* New York: Fordham University Press, 2013.

Barnes, Linda L., and Susan S. Sered. *Religion and Healing in America.* New York: Oxford University Press, 2004.

Bataille, Georges. "Attraction and Repulsion II: Social Structure," in Denis Hollier, ed., translated by B. Wing, *The College of Sociology (1937–1939).* Minneapolis: University of Minnesota Press, 1988, 113–136.

Bayer, Ronald. *Private Acts, Social Consequences: AIDS and the Politics of Public Health.* New Brunswick, NJ: Rutgers University Press, 1991.

Bean, Carl, with David Ritz. *I Was Born This Way: A Gay Preacher's Journey through Gospel Music, Disco Stardom, and a Ministry in Christ.* New York: Simon and Schuster, 2010.

Bebbington, David. *Evangelicalism in Modern Britain: A History from the 1730s to the 1980s.* London: Unwin Hyman, 1989.

Beckley, Robert E., and Jerome R. Koch. *The Continuing Challenge of AIDS: Clergy Responses to Patients, Friends, and Families.* Westport, CT: Auburn House, 2002.

Bellah, Robert N., Richard Madsen, William M. Sullivan, Ann Swidler, and Steven M. Tipton. *Habits of the Heart: Individualism and Commitment in American Life.* Berkeley: University of California Press, 1996.

Bender, Courtney. *Heaven's Kitchen: Living Religion at God's Love We Deliver.* Chicago: University of Chicago Press, 2003.

———. *The New Metaphysicals: Spirituality and the American Religious Imagination.* Chicago: University of Chicago Press, 2010.

Berkovitch, Sacvan. *The American Jeremiad.* Madison: University of Wisconsin Press, 1978.

Berkowitz, Richard. *Stayin' Alive: The Invention of Safe Sex*. New York: Basic Books, 2003.

Berlant, Lauren. *The Queen of America Goes to Washington City: Essays on Sex and Citizenship*. Durham, NC: Duke University Press, 1997.

———. "Citizenship," in Bruce Burgett and Glenn Hendler, eds., *Keywords in American Cultural Studies*. New York and London: NYU Press, 2007, 37–42.

———. *The Female Complaint: The Unfinished Business of Sentimentality in American Culture*. Durham, NC: Duke University Press, 2008.

Bernardin, Joseph Cardinal. *Consistent Ethic of Life*. Kansas City, MO: Sheed & Ward, 1988.

Berridge, Virginia and Philip Strong, eds., *AIDS and Contemporary History*. Cambridge: Cambridge University Press, 1993.

Bivins, Jason. *Religion of Fear: The Politics of Horror in American Evangelicalism*. New York: Oxford University Press, 2008.

Blasius, Mark, and Shane Phelan. *We Are Everywhere: A Historical Sourcebook of Gay and Lesbian Politics*. New York: Routledge, 1997.

Boswell, John. *Christianity, Social Tolerance, and Homosexuality: Gay People in Western Europe from the Beginning of the Christian Era to the Fourteenth Century*, 8th ed. Chicago: University of Chicago Press, 2005 [1981].

Bourke, Dale Hanson. *The Skeptic's Guide to the Global AIDS Crisis: Tough Questions, Direct Answers*. Waynesboro, GA: Authentic Media 2004.

Boyle, Philip, and Kevin D. O'Rourke. *Medical Ethics: Sources of Catholic Teachings*, 3rd ed. Washington, DC: Georgetown University Press, 1999.

Brandt, Allan M. *No Magic Bullet: A Social History of Venereal Disease in the United States Since 1880*. New York: Oxford University Press, 1987.

———. "AIDS in Historical Perspective: Four Lessons from the History of Sexually Transmitted Diseases," *American Journal of Public Health* 78, no. 4 (April 1988): 367–371.

———. "The Syphilis Epidemic and Its Relation to AIDS." *Science* 239, no. 4838 (January 22, 1988): 375–380.

Brandt, Allan M., and Martha Gardner. "Antagonism and Accommodation: Interpreting the Relationship between Public Health and Medicine in the United States during the 20th Century," *American Journal of Public Health* 90, no. 5 (May 2000): 707–715.

Brandt, Allan M., and Paul Rozin. *Morality and Health*. New York: Routledge, 1997.

Brenneman, Todd M. *Homespun Gospel: The Triumph of Sentimentality in Contemporary American Evangelicalism*. New York: Oxford University Press, 2013.

Brier, Jennifer. *Infectious Ideas: U.S. Political Responses to the AIDS Crisis*. Chapel Hill, NC: University of North Carolina Press, 2009.

Bronski, Michael. *Taking Liberties: Gay Men's Essays on Politics, Culture, and Sex*. New York: Masquerade Books, 1996.

———. *Culture Clash: The Making of Gay Sensibility*. Boston: South End Press, 1999.

————. *The Pleasure Principle: Sex, Backlash, and the Struggle for Gay Freedom.* New York: Stonewall Inn Edition, St. Martin's Press, 2000.

Brown, Ruth Murray. *For a "Christian America": A History of the Religious Right.* Amherst, NY: Prometheus Books, 2002.

Brown, Candy Gunther. *The Healing Gods: Complementary and Alternative Medicine in Christian America.* Oxford and New York: Oxford University Press, 2013.

Brown, Dorothy M., and Elizabeth McKeown. *The Poor Belong to Us: Catholic Charities and American Welfare.* Cambridge, MA: Harvard University Press, 2000.

Bullert, B.J. *Public Television: Politics and the Battle over Documentary Film.* New Brunswick, NJ: Rutgers University Press, 1997.

Burkett, Elinor. *The Gravest Show on Earth: America in the Age of AIDS.* New York: Picador, 1996.

Burns, Jeffrey M. "Beyond the Immigrant Church: Gays and Lesbians and the Catholic Church in San Francisco, 1977–1987," *U.S. Catholic Historian* 19, no. 1 (Winter 2001): 79–92.

Busch, Andrew E. *Reagan's Victory: The Presidential Election of 1980 and the Rise of the Right.* Lawrence: University of Kansas Press, 2005.

Butler, Judith. *Gender Trouble: Feminism and the Subversion of Identity.* New York: Routledge, 1999.

Bynum, Caroline Walker. *Holy Feast and Holy Fast: The Religious Significance of Food to Medieval Women.* Berkeley and Los Angeles: University of California Press, 1988.

Byrnes, Timothy. *Catholic Bishops in American Politics.* Princeton, NJ: Princeton University Press, 1991.

————. "The Cardinal and the Governor: The Politics of Abortion in New York State." In *The Catholic Church and the Politics of Abortion.* Boulder, CO: Westview Press, 1992.

————. "The Politics of Abortion: The Catholic Bishops." In *The Catholic Church and the Politics of Abortion.* Boulder, CO: Westview Press, 1992.

Byrnes, Timothy A., and Mary C. Segers. *The Catholic Church and the Politics of Abortion: A View from the States.* Boulder, CO: Westview Press, 1992.

Cabezón, José Ignacio. "Homosexuality and Buddhism," in Arlene Swidler, ed., *Homosexuality and World Religions.* Valley Forge, PA: Trinity Press International, 1993: 81–10.

Cadge, Wendy. "Lesbian, Gay, and Bisexual Buddhist Practitioners," in Scott Thumma and Edward R. Gray, eds., *Gay Religion.* Walnut Creek, CA: Altamira, 2004: 139–152.

Cahill, Kevin M. *The AIDS Epidemic.* New York: St. Martin's Press, 1983.

Cahill, Lisa Sowle, John Garvey, and T. Frank Kennedy, S.J. *Sexuality and the U.S. Catholic Church: Crisis and Renewal.* New York: Crossroad, 2006.

Callen, Michael. *Surviving AIDS.* New York: HarperPerennial, 1991.

Cameron, Paul. *Exposing the AIDS Scandal.* Lafayette, LA: Huntington House, 1988.

Campo, Rafael. "AIDS and the Poetry of Healing," in Marie Howe and Michael Klein, eds., *In the Company of My Solitude: American Writing from the AIDS Pandemic.* New York: Persea Books, 1995.

Canaday, Margot. *The Straight State: Sexuality and Citizenship in Twentieth-Century America.* Princeton, NJ: Princeton University Press, 2009.

Carter, Dan. *The Politics of Rage: George Wallace, the Origins of New Conservatism, and the Transformation of American Politics.* New York: Simon and Schuster, 1995.

Carter, David. *Stonewall: The Riots That Sparked the Gay Revolution.* New York: St. Martin's Griffin, 2010.

Carter, Erica and Simon Watney, eds., *Taking Liberties: AIDS and Cultural Politics.* London: Serpent's Tail, 1989.

Casanova, José. *Public Religions in the Modern World.* Chicago: University of Chicago Press, 1994.

Castelli, Jim. *The Bishops and the Bomb: Waging Peace in a Nuclear Age.* Garden City, NY: Image Books, 1983.

Chambré, Susan M. "The Changing Nature of 'Faith' in Faith-Based Organizations: Secularization and Ecumenicism in Four AIDS Organizations in New York City," *The Social Service Review* 75, no. 3 (September 2001): 435–455.

———. *Fighting For Our Lives: New York's AIDS Community and the Politics of Disease.* New Brunswick, NJ: Rutgers University Press, 2006.

Chauncey, George. *Gay New York: Gender, Urban Culture, and the Making of the Gay Male World, 1890–1940.* New York: Basic Books, 1994.

———. *Why Marriage? The History Shaping Today's Debate Over Gay Equality.* New York: Basic Books, 2004.

Chilton, David. *The Power in the Blood: A Christian Response to AIDS.* Brentwood, TN: Wolgemuth and Hyatt, 1987.

Clark, J. Michael. *Defying the Darkness: Gay Theology in the Shadows.* Cleveland, OH: Pilgrim Press, 1997.

Clendinen, Dudley, and Adam Nagourney. *Out For Good: The Struggle to Build a Gay Rights Movement in America.* New York: Simon & Schuster, 2001.

Cochran, Clarke E., and David Carroll Cochran. *Catholics, Politics, and Public Policy: Beyond Left and Right.* Maryknoll, NY: Orbis Books, 2003.

Cochrane, Michelle. *When AIDS Began: San Francisco and the Making of an Epidemic.* New York: Routledge, 2004.

Coffman, Elesha J. *The Christian Century and the Rise of the Protestant Mainline.* New York: Oxford University Press, 2013.

Cohalan, Florence D. *A Popular History of the Archdiocese of New York.* Yonkers, NY: United States Catholic Historical Society, 1999.

Cohen, Peter F. *Love and Anger: Essays on AIDS, Activism, and Politics.* New York: Haworth Press, 1998.

Cohen, Cathy. *The Boundaries of Blackness: AIDS and the Breakdown of Black Politics.* Chicago: University of Chicago Press, 1999.

Collins, Robert M. *Transforming America: Politics and Culture during the Reagan Years*. New York: Columbia University Press, 2009.

Cott, Nancy. *Public Vows: A History of Marriage and the Nation*. Cambridge, MA: Harvard University Press, 2000.

Courtenay, Bradley C., Sharan B. Merriam, and Patricia M. Reeves. "Faith Development in the Lives of HIV-Positive Adults," *Journal of Religion and Health* 38, no. 3 (Fall 1999): 203–218.

Crimp, Douglas. "How to Have Promiscuity in an Epidemic," *October* 43 (Winter 1987): 237–271.

———. *Melancholia and Moralism: Essays on AIDS and Queer Politics*. Cambridge, MA: MIT Press, 2004.

———. with Adam Rolston. *AIDS Demo Graphics*. Seattle: Bay Press, 1990.

Crimp, Douglas, ed. *AIDS: Cultural Analysis, Cultural Activism*. Cambridge, MA: MIT Press, 1988.

Cuneo, Michael W. *The Smoke of Satan: Conservative and Traditionalist Dissent in Contemporary American Catholicism*. Baltimore, MD: Johns Hopkins University Press, 1999.

Cuomo, Mario. "Religious Belief and Public Morality: A Catholic Governor's Perspective," in Patricia Beattie Jung and Thomas A. Shannon, eds., *Abortion and Catholicism: The American Debate*. New York: Crossroad, 1988: 202–216.

Curran, Charles E. *Catholic Moral Theology in the United States: A History*. Washington, DC: Georgetown University Press, 2008.

Curtis, Heather D. *Faith in the Great Physician: Suffering and Divine Healing in American Culture, 1860—1900*. Baltimore, MD: Johns Hopkins University Press, 2007.

D'Antonio, William V., James D. Davidson, Dean R. Hoge, and Mary L. Gautier. *American Catholics Today: New Realities of Their Faith and Their Church*. Lanham, MD: Rowman & Littlefield Publishers, Inc., 2007.

Davis, Rebecca L. *More Perfect Unions: The American Search for Marital Bliss*. Cambridge, MA: Harvard University Press, 2010.

D'Emilio, John. *Sexual Politics, Sexual Communities*. Chicago: University of Chicago Press, 1998.

D'Emilio, John, and Estelle B. Freedman. *Intimate Matters: A History of Sexuality in America*. Chicago: University of Chicago Press, 1988.

D'Emilio, John, William B. Turner, and Urvashi Vaid. *Creating Change: Sexuality, Public Policy, and Civil Rights*. New York: Stonewall Inn Editions, St. Martin's, 2002.

DeRogatis, Amy., "What Would Jesus Do? Sexuality and Salvation in Protestant Evangelical Sex Manuals, 1950s–Present," *Church History*, 74:1 (March 2005): 97–137.

Derthick, Martha. *Up in Smoke: From Legislation to Litigation in Tobacco Politics*. Washington, DC: CQ Press, 2004.

Diaz, Rafael M. *Latino Gay Men and HIV: Culture, Sexuality, and Risk Behavior*. New York: Routledge, 1997.

Dochuck, Darren. *From Bible Belt to Sunbelt: Plain-Folk Religion, Grassroots Politics, and the Rise of Evangelical Conservatism.* New York: W. W. Norton, 2010.

Dolan, Jay P. *The American Catholic Experience: A History from Colonial Times to the Present.* Notre Dame, IN: University of Notre Dame Press, 1992.

Dortzbach, Deborah and W. Meredith Long, *The AIDS Crisis: What We Can Do.* Downers Grove, IL: Intervarsity Press, 2006.

Doty, Mark. *Heaven's Coast: A Memoir.* New York: Harper Perennial, 1997.

Douglas, Ann. *The Feminization of American Culture.* New York: Knopf, 1977.

Dowland, Seth. "'Family Values' and the Formation of a Christian Right Agenda," *Church History* 78:3 (September 2009): 606–631.

Duffy, John. *The Sanitarians: A History of American Public Health.* Chicago: University of Illinois Press, 1992.

Duggan, Lisa. "The New Homonormativity: The Sexual Politics of Neoliberalism," in Russ Castronovo and Dana D. Nelson, eds., *Materializing Democracy: Toward a Revitalized Cultural Politics.* Durham, NC: Duke University Press, 2002, 175–194.

Dynes, Wayne R., and Stephen Donaldson. *Homosexuality and Medicine, Health, and Science.* New York: Garland, 1992.

Eaton, Jenny and Kate Etue, eds., *The aWAKE Project: Uniting Against the African AIDS Crisis.* Nashville, TN: W Publishing Group, 2002.

Ehrman, John. *The Rise of Neoconservatism: Intellectuals and Foreign Affairs, 1945–1994.* New Haven, CT: Yale University Press, 1996.

———. *The Eighties: America in the Age of Reagan.* New Haven, CT: Yale University Press, 2006.

Elbaz, Gilbert. "The Sociology of AIDS Activism, the Case of ACT UP/New York, 1987–1992. (Volumes I and II)." Ph.D. Dissertation. United States—New York: City University of New York, 1992.

Elisha, Omri. "Moral Ambitions of Grace: The Paradox of Compassion and Accountability in Evangelical Faith-Based Activism," *Cultural Anthropology* 23: 1 (2008): 173–174.

Engel, Jonathan. *The Epidemic: A Global History of AIDS.* New York: Smithsonian Books/Collins, 2006.

Epstein, Steven. *Impure Science: AIDS, Activism, and the Politics of Knowledge.* Berkeley: University of California Press, 1996.

Erzen, Tanya. *Straight to Jesus: Sexual and Christian Conversions in the Ex-Gay Movement.* Berkeley: University of California Press, 2006.

Esack, Farid, and Sarah Chiddy. *Islam and AIDS: Between Scorn, Pity and Justice.* Oxford: Oneworld Publications, 2009.

Farmer, Paul. *AIDS and Accusation: Haiti and the Geography of Blame.* Berkeley: University of California Press, 2006.

Fee, Elizabeth, and Daniel M. Fox, eds., *AIDS: The Burdens of History.* Berkeley: University of California Press, 1988.

———. eds. *AIDS: The Making of a Chronic Disease*. Berkeley: University of California Press, 1991.

Fernandez, Joseph A., and John Underwood. *Tales Out of School: Joseph Fernandez's Crusade to Rescue American Education*. Boston: Little Brown & Co, 1993.

Fessenden, Tracy. *Culture and Redemption: Religion, the Secular, and American Literature*. Princeton, NJ: Princeton University Press, 2006.

———. "Religious Liberalism and the Liberal Geopolitics of Religion," in Leigh E. Schmidt and Sally M. Promey, eds., *American Religious Liberalism*. Bloomington: Indiana University Press, 2012: 359–373.

Fessenden, Tracy, Magdalena J. Zaborowska, and Nicholas F. Radel, eds. *The Puritan Origins of American Sex: Religion, Sexuality, and National Identity in American Literature*. New York: Routledge, 2001.

Fetner, Tina. *How the Religious Right Shaped Lesbian and Gay Activism*. Minneapolis: University of Minnesota Press, 2008.

Finnis, John, Joseph Boyle, Jr., and Germain Grisez. *Nuclear Deterrence, Morality and Realism*. New York: Oxford University Press, 1988.

Fletcher, James. "Homosexuality: Kick and Kickback," *Southern Medical Journal* 77:2 (Feb. 1984): 149–150.

Flippen, J. Brooks. *Jimmy Carter, the Politics of the Family, and the Rise of the Religious Right*. Athens: University of Georgia Press, 2011.

Flynn, Eileen P. *AIDS: A Catholic Call for Compassion*. Kansas City, MO: Sheed & Ward, 1985.

Fogarty, Gerald P. "Public Patriotism and Private Politics: The Tradition of American Catholicism," *U.S. Catholic Historian* 4, no. 1 (1984): 1–48.

Fortunato, John E. *AIDS: The Spiritual Dilemma*. San Francisco: Harper and Row, 1987.

Foster, Pamela Payne. *Is there a Balm in Black America?: Perspectives on HIV/AIDS in the African American Community*. Montgomery, AL: AframSouth, Inc., 2007.

Foucault, Michel. *The History of Sexuality, Vol. 1: An Introduction*. Robert Hurley, trans. New York: Vintage, 1990.

———. *Ethics: Subjectivity and Truth*. Paul Rabinow, ed. New York: New Press, 1997.

———. *"Society Must Be Defended": Lectures at the College de France 1975–1976*. David Macy, trans. New York: Picador, 2003.

———. *Security, Territory, Population: Lectures at the College de France 1977–1978*. Graham Burchell, trans. New York: Picador, 2009.

Fox, Thomas C. *Sexuality and Catholicism*. New York: George Braziller, 2000.

Franchot, Jenny. *Roads to Rome: The Antebellum Protestant Encounter with Catholicism*. Berkeley: University of California Press, 1994.

Frank, Gillian. "'The Civil Rights of Parents': Race and Conservative Politics in Anita Bryant's Campaign against Gay Rights in 1970s Florida," *Journal of the History of Sexuality* 22:1 (January 2013): 126–160.

Freudenthal, Gad, ed., *AIDS in Jewish Thought and Law*. Hoboken, NJ: KTAV Publishing House, Inc., 1998.

Fumento, Michael. *The Myth of Heterosexual AIDS*. New York: Basic Books, 1990.

Gallup, George, and Jim Castelli. *The American Catholic People*. Garden City, NY: Doubleday, 1987.

Gardner, Christine J. *Making Chastity Sexy: The Rhetoric of Evangelical Abstinence Campaigns*. Berkeley: University of California Press, 2011.

Gasaway, Brantley W. *Progressive Evangelicals and the Pursuit of Social Justice*. Chapel Hill: University of North Carolina, 2014.

Gerber, Lynne. "The Opposite of Gay: Nature, Creation, and Queerish Ex-gay Experiments," *Novo Religio* 11:4 (May 2008): 8–30.

———. *Seeking the Straight and Narrow*. Chicago: University of Chicago Press, 2011.

Gerbert, Barbara, and Bryan Maguire. "Public Acceptance of the Surgeon General's Brochure on AIDS." *U.S. Department of Health and Human Services; Public Health Reports* 104 (April 1989): 130–133.

Gilbert, Dorie J., and Ednita M. Wright. *African American Women and HIV/AIDS: Critical Responses*. Westport, CT: Praeger, 2003.

Goldberg, Michelle. *Kingdom Coming: The Rise of Christian Nationalism*. New York: W. W. Norton & Co., 2007.

Golway, Terry. *Full of Grace: An Oral Biography of John Cardinal O'Connor*. New York: Pocket Books, 2001.

Good, Byron. *Medicine, Rationality, Experience*. Cambridge: Cambridge University Press, 1994.

Goss, Robert. *Jesus Acted Up: A Gay and Lesbian Manifesto*. San Francisco: Harper SanFrancisco, 1993.

Gould, Deborah B. *Moving Politics: Emotion and ACT UP's Fight against AIDS*. Chicago: University of Chicago Press, 2009.

Gramick, Jeannine. *Homosexuality and the Catholic Church*. Chicago: Thomas More Press, 1983.

Gramick, Jeannine, and Pat Furey. *The Vatican and Homosexuality: Reactions to the "Letter to the Bishops of the Catholic Church on the Pastoral Care of Homosexual Persons."* New York: Crossroad, 1988.

Gramick, Jeannine and Robert Nugent. *Voices of Hope: A Collection of Positive Catholic Writings on Gay & Lesbian Issues*. Mount Rainier, MD: New Ways Ministry, 1995.

Griffin, Leslie. "American Catholic Sexual Ethics, 1789–1989," in Charles Curran and Richard McCormack, eds., *Dialogue about Catholic Sexual Teaching (Readings in Moral Theology, vol. 8)*. New York: Paulist Press, 1993: 453–484.

Griffith, R. Marie. *God's Daughters: Evangelical Women and the Power of Submission*. Berkeley: University of California Press, 1997.

———. *Born Again Bodies: Flesh and Spirit in American Christianity*. Berkeley: University of California Press, 2004.

————. "The Religious Encounters of Alfred Kinsey," *Journal of American History* 95:2 (Sept. 2008): 349–377.

Grmek, Mirko D. *History of AIDS: Emergence and Origin of a Modern Epidemic.* Princeton, NJ: Princeton University Press, 1993.

Haggerty, George E. *Gay Histories and Cultures: An Encyclopedia.* New York and London: Taylor & Francis, 2000.

Hall, David D. *Lived Religion in America: Toward A History of Practice.* Princeton, NJ: Princeton University Press, 1997.

Hall, Jyl, World Vision, et al. *A Guide to Acting on AIDS: Understanding the Global AIDS Pandemic and Responding Through Faith and Action.* Tyrone, GA: Authentic, in partnership with World Vision Resources, 2006.

Hankins, Barry. *Francis Schaeffer and the Shaping of Evangelical America.* Grand Rapids, MI: Wm. B. Eerdmans Publishing Company, 2008.

Hannaway, Caroline, Victoria Angela Harden, and John Parascandola. *AIDS and the Public Debate.* Washington, D.C.: IOS Press, 1995.

Harding, Susan Friend. "Representing Fundamentalism: The Problem of the Repugnant Culture Other," *Social Research* 58:2 (Summer 1991): 373–393.

————. *The Book of Jerry Falwell: Fundamentalist Language and Politics.* Princeton, NJ: Princeton University Press, 2001.

————. "American Protestant Moralism and the Secular Imagination: From Temperance to the Moral Majority," *Social Research* 76:4 (Winter 2009): 1277–1306.

Harris, Angelique. *AIDS, Sexuality, and the Black Church: Making the Wounded Whole.* New York: Peter Lang International Publishers, 2010.

Hart, D. G. and John R. Muether, *Seeking a Better Country: 300 Years of American Presbyterianism.* Phillipsburg, NJ: P&R Publishing, 2007.

————. *Calvinism: A History.* New Haven, CT: Yale University Press, 2013.

Hay, Louise L. *The AIDS Book: Creating a Positive Approach.* Santa Monica, CA: Hay House Press, 1988.

Health and Human Services. *Understanding AIDS,* Publication No. (CDC) HHS-88–8404. U.S. Government Printing Office, 1988.

Hedstrom, Matthew. *The Rise of Liberal Religion: Book Culture and American Spirituality in the Twentieth Century.* New York: Oxford University Press, 2013.

Hentoff, Nat. *John Cardinal O'Connor: At the Storm Center of a Changing American Catholic Church.* New York: Scribner, 1988.

Herberg, Will. *Protestant, Catholic, Jew: An Essay in American Religious Sociology.* Chicago: University of Chicago Press, 1955.

Herman, Didi. *The Antigay Agenda.* Chicago: University of Chicago Press, 1998.

Herzog, Dagmar. *Sex in Crisis: The New Sexual Revolution and the Future of American Politics.* New York: Basic Books, 2008.

Higginbotham, Evelyn Brooks. "African-American Women's History and the Metalanguage of Race," *Signs* 17:2 (Winter 1992): 251–274.

Hilferty, Robert, Bub Huff, Altar Ego Productions, P. D. R. Productions, and Frameline. *Stop the Church* [video recording]. New York: PDR Productions, 1990.

Hodes, Martha. *White Women, Black Men: Illicit Sex in the Nineteenth-Century South.* New Haven, CT: Yale University Press, 1997.

Holifield, E. Brooks. *A History of Pastoral Care in America: From Salvation to Self-Realization.* Eugene, OR: Wipf & Stock Publishers, 2003.

Hollinger, David A. *After Cloven Tongues of Fire: Protestant Liberalism in Modern American History.* Princeton, NJ: Princeton University Press, 2013.

Hughes, Joseph. *Homosexuality: A Positive Catholic Perspective.* Baltimore: Archdiocesan Gay/Lesbian Outreach, 1985.

Humber, James M., and Robert F. Almeder. *AIDS and Ethics.* Clifton, NJ: Humana Press, 1989.

Hume, David. "Of Superstition and Enthusiasm," in Eugene F. Miller, ed., *Essays, Moral, Political, and Literary.* Indianapolis, IN: Liberty Fund, Inc., 1987.

Hunter, James Davison. *American Evangelicalism: Conservative Religion and the Quandary of Modernity.* New Brunswick, NJ: Rutgers University Press, 1983.

Hunter, James Davison. *Culture Wars: The Struggle to Define America.* New York: BasicBooks, 1991.

Hunter, James Davison, and Alan Wolfe. *Is There a Culture War?: A Dialogue on Values and American Public Life.* Washington, D.C.: Brookings Institution Press, 2006.

Hunter, Susan. *AIDS in America.* New York: Palgrave, 2006.

Hutchison, William. *The Modernist Impulse in American Protestantism.* Durham, NC: Duke University Press, 1992.

Inrig, Stephen J. *North Carolina and the Problem of AIDS.* Chapel Hill: University of North Carolina Press, 2012.

Irvine, Janice M. *Talk About Sex: The Battles over Sex Education in the United States.* Berkeley: University of California Press, 2004.

Jakobsen, Janet R., and Ann Pellegrini. *Love the Sin: Sexual Regulation and the Limits of Religious Tolerance.* New York: NYU Press, 2003.

——. "Introduction: Times Like These," *Secularisms.* Durham, NC: Duke University Press, 2008: 1–38.

Jameson, Fredric. "Postmodernism and Consumer Society," in Hal Foster, ed. *The Anti-Aesthetic: Essays on Postmodern Culture.* Port Townsend, WA: Bay Press, 1983.

Jenkins, Philip. *The New Anti-Catholicism: The Last Acceptable Prejudice.* New York: Oxford University Press, 2004.

Jonsen, Albert R. and Jeff Stryker, eds. "Religion and Religious Groups," *The Social Impact of AIDS in the United States,* Report of the Committee on AIDS Research and Behavior, Social, and Statistical Sciences, National Research Council. Washington, D.C.: National Academy Press, 1993.

Jordan, Mark D. *The Invention of Sodomy in Christian Theology.* Chicago: University of Chicago Press, 1997.

————. *The Ethics of Sex*. Oxford, UK, and Malden, MA: Wiley-Blackwell, 2002.

————. *The Silence of Sodom*. Chicago: University of Chicago Press, 2002.

————. *Recruiting Young Love: How Christians Talk about Homosexuality*. Chicago: University of Chicago Press, 2011.

Jorstad, Erling. *The Politics of Moralism: The New Christian Right in American Life*. Minneapolis: Augsburg Publishing House, 1981.

Jung, Patricia Beattie, and Thomas A. Shannon, eds. *Abortion and Catholicism: The American Debate*. New York: Crossroad, 1988.

Kalbian, Aline H. *Sexing the Church: Gender, Power, and Ethics in Contemporary Catholicism*. Bloomington: Indiana University Press, 2005.

Kaoma, Kapya. *Globalizing the Culture Wars: U.S. Conservatives, African Churches, and Homophobia*. Somerville, MA: Political Research Associates, 2009.

Kaplan, Esther. *With God on Their Side: George W. Bush and the Christian Right*. New York: New Press, 2005.

Kari, Camilla J. *Public Witness: The Pastoral Letters of the American Catholic Bishops*. Collegeville, MN: Liturgical Press, 2004.

Katz, Jonathan. *The Invention of Heterosexuality*. Chicago: University of Chicago Press, 2007.

Kauffman, Christopher. *Meaning and Ministry: A Religious History of Catholic Health-care in the United States*. New York: Crossroad, 1995.

Kavar, Louis F. *Pastoral Ministry in the AIDS Era: Focus on Families and Friends of Persons with AIDS*. Wayzata, MN: Woodland Pub Co., 1988.

Keane, Philip S. *Sexual Morality: A Catholic Perspective*. New York: Paulist Press, 1977.

————. *Catholicism and Health-Care Justice: Problems, Potential, and Solutions*. New York: Paulist Press, 2001.

Keenan, James F. *A History of Catholic Moral Theology in the Twentieth Century: From Confessing Sins to Liberating Consciences*. London and New York: Continuum, 2010.

Keenan, James F., Jon D. Fuller, and Lisa Sowle Cahill, eds. *Catholic Ethicists on HIV/AIDS Prevention*. New York: Continuum, 2000.

Kelly, Kevin. *New Directions in Sexual Ethics: Moral Theology and the Challenge of AIDS*. London: Chapman, 1999.

Kinsella, James. *Covering the Plague: AIDS and the American Media*. New Brunswick, NJ: Rutgers University Press, 1992.

Klassen, Pamela. *Spirits of Protestantism: Medicine, Healing, and Liberal Christianity*. Berkeley: University of California Press, 2011.

Kleinman, Arthur. *The Illness Narratives: Suffering, Healing, and the Human Condition*. New York: Basic Books, 1988.

Koop, C. Everett. *The Right to Live: The Right to Die*. Fort Collins: Life Cycle Books, 1981.

————. *The Memoirs of America's Family Doctor*. New York: HarperCollins, 1993 [1991].

Koop, C. Everett, with Timothy Johnson. *Let's Talk: An Honest Conversation on Critical Issues: Abortion, AIDS, Euthanasia, Health Care.* Grand Rapids, MI: Zondervan, 1992.

Kowalewski, Mark R. *All Things to All People: The Catholic Church Confronts the AIDS Crisis.* Albany: SUNY Press, 1994.

Kramer, Larry. *Reports from the Holocaust: The Story of an AIDS Activist.* New York: St. Martin's Press, 1994.

——. *The Normal Heart* and *the Destiny of Me.* New York: Grove Press, 2000.

Kymlicka, Will, and Wayne Normal. "Return of the Citizen: A Survey of Recent Work on Citizenship Theory," in Ronald Beiner, ed. *Theorizing Citizenship.* Albany: SUNY Press, 1995: 283–322.

LaHaye, Tim. *The Unhappy Gays.* Wheaton, IL: Tyndale House, 1978.

—— and Beverly LaHaye. *The Act of Marriage: The Beauty of Sexual Love.* Grand Rapids, MI: Zondervan, 1976.

Lantzer, Jason S. *Mainline Christianity: The Past and Future of America's Majority Faith.* New York: NYU Press, 2012.

Lawler, Ronald David, Joseph M. Boyle, and William E. May. *Catholic Sexual Ethics.* Huntington, IN: Our Sunday Visitor Publishing, 1998.

Lemke, Thomas. *Biopolitics: An Advanced Introduction,* trans. Eric Frederick Trump. New York: NYU Press, 2011.

Levenson, Jacob. *The Secret Epidemic: The Story of AIDS and Black America.* New York: Pantheon, 2004.

Lierman, Ashley Ruth. "The Plague Wars: Encounters between Gay and Lesbian Activism and the Christian Right in the Age of AIDS." Ph.D. Dissertation. United States—New Jersey: Drew University, 2009.

Lindsay, D. Michael. *Faith in the Halls of Power: How Evangelicals Joined the American Elite.* New York: Oxford University Press, 2008.

Link, William A. *Righteous Warrior: Jesse Helms and the Rise of Modern Conservatism.* New York: St. Martin's Press, 2008.

Lofton, Kathryn. "Queering Fundamentalism: John Balcom Shaw and the Sexuality of a Protestant Orthodoxy," *Journal of the History of Sexuality* 17:3 (September 2008): 439–468.

——. *Oprah: The Gospel of an Icon.* Berkeley: University of California Press, 2011.

Long, Thomas L. *AIDS and American Apocalypticism: The Cultural Semiotics of an Epidemic.* Albany: State University of New York Press, 2005.

Long, Ronald E., J. Michael Clark, and Michael J. North, *AIDS, God, and Faith: Continuing the Dialogue on Constructive Gay Theology.* Las Colinas, TX: Monument Press, 1992.

Long, Scott and Julie Dorf, "ACT UP," in George E. Haggerty, ed., *Gay Histories and Cultures: An Encyclopedia.* New York and London: Taylor & Francis, 2000.

Longfield, Bradley J. *Presbyterians and American Culture: A History.* Louisville, KY: Westminster John Knox Press, 2013.

Lord, Alexandra M. *Condom Nation: The U.S. Government's Sex Education Campaign from World War I to the Internet.* Baltimore: Johns Hopkins, 2009.

Lune, Howard. *Urban Action Networks: HIV/AIDS and Community Organizing in New York City.* Lanham, MD: Rowman & Littlefield Publishers, Inc., 2006.

Lynch, Joseph H. *Early Christianity: A Brief History.* New York: Oxford University Press, 2010.

Mahmood, Saba. *Politics of Piety: The Islamic Revival and the Feminist Subject.* Princeton, NJ: Princeton University Press, 2005.

———. "Secularism, Hermeneutics, and Empire: The Politics of Islamic Reformation," *Public Culture* 18: 2 (2006): 323–347.

Marcus, Eric. *Making Gay History: The Half-Century Fight for Lesbian and Gay Equal Rights.* New York: Harper Paperbacks, 2002.

Marina, Joseph George. "From the Heart of the Storm: The Response of Catholic Colleges and Universities to the HIV/AIDS Epidemic." Ph.D. Dissertation. United States—New York: Fordham University, 1999.

Marsden, George. *Understanding Fundamentalism and Evangelicalism.* Grand Rapids, MI: Wm. B. Eerdmans Publishing Co, 1991.

Martin, William C. *With God on Our Side: The Rise of the Religious Right in America.* New York: Broadway Books, 1996.

Mass, Lawrence D. *We Must Love One Another Or Die: The Life and Legacies of Larry Kramer.* New York: St. Martin's, 1997.

Massa, Mark S. *Anti-Catholicism in America: The Last Acceptable Prejudice.* New York: Crossroad, 2005.

Mauss, Marcel. "Techniques of the Body," *Economy and Society* 2: 1 (1973 [1935]): 70–88.

McAlister, Melani. "What Is Your Heart For?: Affect and Internationalism in the Evangelical Public Sphere," *American Literary History* 20: 4 (2008): 878–879.

McBride, David. *From TB to AIDS: Epidemics among Urban Blacks since 1900.* Albany: SUNY Press, 1991.

McBride, Duane C., Clyde B. McCoy, Dale D. Chitwood, James A. Inciardi, Edwin L. Hernandez, and Patricia M. Mutch. "Religious Institutions as Sources of AIDS Information for Street Injection Drug Users," *Review of Religious Research* 35, no. 4 (June 1994): 324–334.

McCauley, Bernadette. *Who Shall Take Care of Our Sick?: Roman Catholic Sisters and the Development of Catholic Hospitals in New York City.* Baltimore: Johns Hopkins University Press, 2005.

McCune, Jr. Jeffrey Q. *Sexual Discretion: Black Masculinity and the Politics of Passing.* Chicago: University of Chicago Press, 2014.

McIlhenny, Chuck, and Donna McIlhenny. *When the Wicked Seize a City,* written with Frank York. Lafayette, LA: Huntington House, 1993.

McGirr, Lisa. *Suburban Warriors: The Origins of the New American Right.* Princeton, NJ: Princeton University Press, 2001.

McGreevy, John T. *Catholicism and American Freedom: A History.* New York: W. W. Norton & Company, 2003.

McKay, Richard A. "'Patient Zero': The Absence of a Patient's View of the Early North American AIDS Epidemic," *Bull. Hist. Med.* 88, no. 1 (Spring 2014): 161–194.

McKeown, Elizabeth. "Drawing Lines," *U.S. Catholic Historian* 21, no. 4 (Fall 2003): 45–61.

McNeill, John J. *The Church and the Homosexual.* Boston: Beacon Press, 1993 [1976].

Melton, J. Gordon. *The Churches Speak on AIDS: Official Statements from Religious Bodies and Ecumenical Organizations.* Detroit, MI: Gale Research, 1989.

Merry, Sally Engle. *Colonizing Hawai'i: The Cultural Power of Law.* Princeton, NJ: Princeton University Press, 2000.

Metzl, Jonathan M., and Anna Kirkland, eds., *Against Health: How Health Became the New Morality.* New York: NYU Press, 2010.

Miller, Patricia. *Good Catholics: The Battle over Abortion in the Catholic Church.* Berkeley: University of California Press, 2014.

Monette, Paul. *Borrowed Time: An AIDS Memoir.* San Diego: Harcourt Brace, 1988.

———. *Becoming a Man: Half a Life Story.* New York: Harcourt Brace, 1992.

———. *Last Watch of the Night: Essays Too Personal and Otherwise.* New York: Harcourt Brace, 1993.

Moon, Dawne. *God, Sex, and Politics: Homosexuality and Everyday Theologies.* Chicago: University of Chicago Press, 2004.

Moore, Patrick. *Beyond Shame: Reclaiming the Abandoned History of Radical Gay Sexuality.* Boston: Beacon Press, 2004.

Moran, Jeffrey P. *Teaching Sex: The Shaping of Adolescence in the 20th Century.* Cambridge, MA: Harvard University Press, 2000.

Moreton, Bethany. *To Serve God and Wal-Mart: The Making of Christian Free Enterprise.* Cambridge, MA: Harvard University Press, 2009.

Morgan, Tracy. "From WHAM! to ACT UP," in Benjamin Shepard and Ronald Hayduk, eds., *From ACT UP to the WTO: Urban Protest and Community Building in the Era of Globalization.* London and New York: Verso, 2002: 141–149.

Morgan, David. *The Sacred Gaze: Religious Visual Culture in Theory and Practice.* Berkeley: University of California, 2005.

Murray, John Courtney, and J. Leon Hooper. *Religious Liberty: Catholic Struggles with Pluralism.* Louisville, KY: Westminster John Knox Press, 1993.

Murphy, Timothy. *Ethics in an Epidemic: AIDS, Morality, and Culture.* Berkeley: University of California Press, 1994.

Noebel, David A. *The Homosexual Revolution.* Tulsa, OK: American Christian College Press, 1977.

——— Wayne C. Lutton, and Paul Cameron. *AIDS: Acquired Immune Deficiency Syndrome: A Special Report.* Manitou Spring, CO: Summit Ministries Research Center, 1986.

Nugent, Robert. *A Challenge to Love: Gay and Lesbian Catholics in the Church.* New York: Crossroad, 1983.

O'Connor, John. "Cross-Cultural Interaction: An Evaluation of Some Conceptual Approaches." Ph.D. Dissertation. United States—District of Columbia: Georgetown University, 1970.

———. "From Theory to Practice in the Public-Policy Realm," in Patricia Beattie Jung and Thomas A. Shannon, eds. *Abortion and Catholicism: The American Debate.* New York: Crossroad, 1988.

O'Connor, John, and Ed Koch. *His Eminence and Hizzoner.* San Francisco: Harper-Collins Publishers, 1989.

Orsi, Robert. *Between Heaven and Earth: The Religious Worlds People Make and the Scholars Who Study Them.* Princeton, NJ: Princeton University Press, 2006.

———. "Abundant History: Marian Apparitions as Alternative Modernity," *Historically Speaking* (September/October 2008): 12–16.

———. *The Madonna of 115th Street.* New Haven, CT: Yale University Press, 3rd ed., 2010.

Overberg, Kenneth R., ed. *AIDS, Ethics, and Religion: Embracing a World of Suffering.* Maryknoll, NY: Orbis, 1994.

Palmer, Susan. *AIDS as an Apocalyptic Metaphor in North America.* Toronto: University of Toronto Press, 1997.

Patton, Cindy. *Sex and Germs: The Politics of AIDS.* Boston: South End Press, 1985.

———. *Inventing AIDS.* New York: Routledge, 1990.

———. *Fatal Advice: How Safe-Sex Education Went Wrong.* Durham, NC: Duke University Press, 1996.

———. *Globalizing AIDS.* Minneapolis: University of Minnesota Press, 2002.

Perrow, Charles, and Mauro F. Guillén. *The AIDS Disaster.* New Haven, CT: Yale University Press, 1990.

Petro, Anthony M. "Mainline Protestants and Homosexuality," in John C. Hawley, ed., *LGBTQ America Today: An Encyclopedia.* Westport, Conn: Greenwood, 2008: 943–949.

———. "Religion, Gender, and Sexuality," in Paul Harvey and Edward Blum, eds., *The Columbia Guide to Religion in American History.* New York: Columbia University Press, 2012: 188–212.

Pieters, A. Stephen. *"I'm Still Dancing!" A Gay Man's Health Experience.* Gaithersburg, MD: Chi Rho Press, 1991.

Porter, Dorothy. *Health, Civilization and the State: A History of Public Health from Ancient to Modern Times.* London: Routledge, 1999.

Porterfield, Amanda. *Healing in the History of Christianity.* New York: Oxford University Press, 2009.

Powers, Roger S., William B. Vogele, Christopher Kruegler, and Ronald M. McCarthy, eds. *Protest, Power, and Change: An Encyclopedia of Nonviolent Action from ACT-UP to Women's Suffrage.* New York and London: Garland, 1997.

Promey, Sally M. *Sensational Religion: Sensory Cultures in Material Practice.* New Haven, CT: Yale University Press, 2014.

Quimby, Ernest, and Samuel R. Friedman. "Dynamics of Black Mobilization against AIDS in New York City," *Social Problems* 36, no. 4 (October 1989): 403–415.

Quinn, John R. "Toward an Understanding of the Letter 'On the Pastoral Care of Homosexual Persons,'" in Jeannine Gramick and Pat Furey, eds. *The Vatican and Homosexuality:* New York: Crossroad, 1988.

Rauch, Jonathan. *Gay Marriage: Why It Is Good for Gays, Good for Straights, and Good for America.* New York: Holt, 2004.

Reamer, Frederic G. *AIDS & Ethics.* New York: Columbia University Press, 1991.

Robinson, Paul. *Queer Wars: The New Gay Right and Its Critics.* Chicago: University of Chicago Press, 2006.

Rodgers, Daniel. *The Age of Fracture.* Cambridge, MA: Harvard University Press, 2011.

Rofes, Eric E. *Reviving the Tribe: Regenerating Gay Men's Sexuality and Culture in the Ongoing Epidemic.* New York: Routledge, 1995.

Román, David. *Acts of Intervention: Performance, Gay Culture, and AIDS.* Bloomington: Indiana University Press, 1998.

Rosen, George. *A History of Public Health.* Baltimore: Johns Hopkins Press, 1993.

Rosenberg, Charles E. *The Cholera Years.* Chicago: University of Chicago Press, 1987.

———. *No Other Gods: On Science and American Social Thought.* Baltimore: Johns Hopkins University Press, 1997.

Royal, Robert. *American Catholics, American Culture: Tradition and Resistance.* Lanham, MD: Rowman & Littlefield Publishers, Inc., 2004.

Royles, Dan. "'Don't We Die Too': The Political Culture of African American AIDS Activism," Ph.D. Dissertation. United States—Philadelphia: Temple University, 2014.

Rubin, Gayle. "Thinking Sex: Notes for a Radical Theory of the Politics of Sexuality," in Carol S. Vance, ed. *Pleasure and Danger: Exploring Female Sexuality.* Boston: Routledge and Kegan Paul, 1984: 267–319.

Rueda, Enrique T. *The Homosexual Network: Private Lives and Public Policy.* Old Greenwich, CT: Devin-Adair Co., 1982.

Rueda, Enrique T., and Michael Schwartz. *Gays, AIDS, and You.* Old Greenwich, CT: Devin-Adair Co., 1987.

Russell, Letty M., ed. *The Church with AIDS: Renewal in the Midst of Crisis.* Louisville, KY: Westminster/John Knox Press, 1990.

Ryken, Philip Graham, ed., with Allen G. Guelzo, William S. Barker, and Paul S. Jones, *Tenth Presbyterian Church of Philadelphia: 175 Years of Thinking and Acting Biblically.* Phillipsburg, NJ: P&R Publishing, 2004.

Sager, Rebecca. *Faith, Politics, and Power: The Politics of Faith-Based Initiatives.* Oxford and New York: Oxford University Press, 2010.

Schaeffer, Francis, and C. Everett Koop. *Whatever Happened to the Human Race?* Old Tappan, NJ: F. H. Revell Co., 1979.

Schaeffer, Francis. *A Christian Manifesto*. Wheaton, IL: Crossway Books, 1981.

Schmidt, Leigh. *Restless Souls: The Making of American Spirituality*. New York: HarperCollins, 2005.

Schmidt, Leigh E. and Sally M. Promey, eds. *American Religious Liberalism*. Bloomington: Indiana University Press, 2012.

Schulman, Bruce J., and Julian E. Zelizer, eds. *Rightward Bound: Making America Conservative in the 1970s*. Cambridge, MA: Harvard University Press, 2008.

Sedgwick, Eve Kosofsky. *Epistemology of the Closet*. Berkeley: University of California Press, 1999.

Self, Robert O. *All in the Family: The Realignment of American Democracy since the 1960s*. New York: Hill and Wang, 2012.

Shelp, Earl E. and Ronald H. Sunderland. *AIDS and the Church*. Philadelphia: Westminster Press, 1987.

———. *AIDS: A Manual for Pastoral Care*. Philadelphia: Westminster Press, 1987.

———. *Handle with Care: An Outline for Care Teams Serving People with AIDS*. Nashville, TN: Abingdon Press, 1990.

Shelp, Earl E., Ronald H. Sunderland, and Peter W.A. Mansell, M.D. *AIDS: Personal Stories in Pastoral Perspective*. New York: Pilgrim Press, 1986.

Shepard, Benjamin Heim. *White Nights and Ascending Shadows: An Oral History of the San Francisco AIDS Epidemic*. London and Washington, D.C.: Cassell, 1997.

Shepard, Benjamin, and Ronald Hayduk. *From ACT UP to the WTO: Urban Protest and Community Building in the Era of Globalization*. London and New York: Verso, 2002.

Shilts, Randy. *And the Band Played On: Politics, People, and the AIDS Epidemic*. New York: St. Martin's Press, 1987.

Shokeid, Moshe. *A Gay Synagogue in New York*. Philadelphia: University of Pennsylvania Press, 2002.

Siker, Jeffrey S. *Homosexuality in the Church*. Louisville: Westminster John Knox Press, 1994.

Siplon, Patricia D. *AIDS and the Policy Struggle in the United States*. Washington, D.C.: Georgetown University Press, 2002.

Smith, Elwyn A. "The Fundamental Church-State Tradition of the Catholic Church in the United States," *Church History* 38, no. 4 (December 1969): 486–505.

Smith, Jonathan Z. "The Bare Facts of Ritual," *Imagining Religion: From Babylon to Jonestown*. Chicago: University of Chicago Press, 1982: 53–65.

Smith, Richard L. *AIDS, Gays, and the American Catholic Church*. Cleveland, OH: Pilgrim Press, 1994.

Smith, Merril D., ed., *Sex and Sexuality in Early America*. New York and London: NYU Press, 1998.

Sontag, Susan. *AIDS and Its Metaphors*. New York: Farrar, Straus, and Giroux, 1989.

Starr, Paul. *The Social Transformation of American Medicine*. New York: Basic Books, 1984.

Stein, Arlene. *The Stranger Next Door: The Story of a Small Community's Battle over Sex, Faith, and Civil Rights*. Boston: Beacon Press, 2001.

Stevens, Rosemary A. *History and Health Policy in the United States: Putting the Past Back In*. New Brunswick, NJ: Rutgers University Press, 2006.

Stockdill, Brett C. "ACT UP," in Roger S. Powers et al., eds., *Protest, Power, and Change: An Encyclopedia of Nonviolent Action from ACT-UP to Women's Suffrage*. New York and London: Taylor & Francis, 1997.

Stoller, Nancy E. *Lessons from the Damned: Queers, Whores and Junkies Respond to AIDS*. New York: Routledge, 1998.

Strub, Whitney. *Perversion for Profit: The Politics of Pornography and the Rise of the New Right*. New York: Columbia University Press, 2010.

Sullivan, Andrew. *Virtually Normal: An Argument about Homosexuality*. New York: Knopf, 1989.

Sullivan, Winnifred Fallers. *The Impossibility of Religious Freedom*. Princeton, NJ: Princeton University Press, 2005.

Swartz, David R. *Moral Minority: The Evangelical Left in an Age of Conservatism*: Philadelphia: University of Pennsylvania, 2012.

Tentler, Leslie Woodcock. *Catholics and Contraception: An American History*. Ithaca: Cornell University Press, 2004.

Thuesen, Peter J. "The Logic of Mainline Churchliness: Historical Background since the Reformation," in Robert Wuthnow and John H. Evans, eds. *The Quiet Hand of God: Faith-Based Activism and the Public Role of Mainline Protestantism*. Berkeley: University of California Press, 2002.

Tiemeyer, Phil. *Plane Queer: Labor, Sexuality, and AIDS in the History of Male Flight Attendants*. Berkeley: University of California Press, 2013.

Tomes, Nancy. *The Gospel of Germs: Men, Women, and the Microbe in American Life*. Cambridge, MA: Harvard University Press, 1998.

Tompkins, Jane. *Sensational Designs: The Cultural Work of American Fiction, 1790–1860*. New York: Oxford University Press, 1986.

Tone, Andrea. *Devices and Desires: A History of Contraceptives in America*. New York: Hill and Wang, 2002.

Treichler, Paula A. *How to Have Theory in an Epidemic: Cultural Chronicles of AIDS*. Durham, NC: Duke University Press, 1999.

Trinitapoli, Jenny. "Religious Responses to AIDS in Sub-Saharan Africa: An Examination of Religious Congregations in Rural Malawi," *Review of Religious Research* 47, no. 3 (March 2006): 253–270.

Troy, Gil. *Morning in America: How Ronald Reagan Invented the 1980's*. Princeton, NJ: Princeton University Press, 2007.

Troy, Gil, and Vincent J. Cannato, eds. *Living in the Eighties*. New York: Oxford University Press, 2009.

Turner, William B. "Mirror Images: Lesbian/Gay Civil Rights in the Carter and Reagan Administrations," in John D'Emilio, William B. Turner, and Urvashi

Vaid, eds., *Creating Change: Sexuality, Public Policy, and Civil Rights*. New York: St. Martin's Press, 2000: 3–28.

Veeder, Mary Harris. "Authorial Voice, Implied Audiences and the Drafting of the 1988 AIDS National Mailing," *Risk: Issues in Health & Safety* 4(1993): 287.

Vernon, Irene S. *Killing Us Quietly: Native Americans and HIV/AIDS*. Lincoln: University of Nebraska, 2001.

Wacker, Grant. "Billy Graham's America," *Church History* 78:3 (September 2009): 489–511.

Wald, Priscilla. *Contagious: Cultures, Carriers, and the Outbreak Narrative*. Durham, NC: Duke University Press, 2007.

Warner, Michael, ed., *Fear of a Queer Planet: Queer Politics and Social Theory*. Minneapolis: University of Minnesota Press, 1993.

———. *The Trouble with Normal: Sex, Politics, and the Ethics of Queer Life*. Cambridge, MA: Harvard University Press, 1999.

Warner, Michael S. *Changing Witness: Catholic Bishops and Public Policy, 1917–1994*. Grand Rapids, MI: Eerdmans Pub Co, 1995.

Warner, Michael S. "A New Ethic: The Social Teaching of the American Catholic Bishops, 1960–1986." Ph.D. Dissertation. United States—Illinois: The University of Chicago, 1990.

Warren, Kay. *Dangerous Surrender: What Happens When You Say Yes to God*. Grand Rapids, MI: Zondervan, 2007.

Warren, Rick. *The Purpose Driven Church: Growth Without Compromising Your Method and Mission*. Grand Rapids, MI: Zondervan, 1995.

Watney, Simon. *Policing Desire: Pornography, AIDS, and the Media*. Minneapolis: University of Minnesota Press, 1987.

Weatherford, Ronald Jeffrey, and Carole Boston Weatherford. *Somebody's Knocking on Your Door: AIDS and the African American Church*. New York: Haworth Press, 1999.

Weaver, Mary Jo. *What's Left?: Liberal American Catholics*. Bloomington: Indiana University Press, 1999.

Weaver, Mary Jo, and R. Scott Appleby. *Being Right: Conservative Catholics in America*. Bloomington: Indiana University Press, 1995.

Wenger, Tisa. *We Have a Religion: The 1920s Pueblo Indian Dance Controversy and American Religious Freedom*. Chapel Hill: University of North Carolina Press, 2009.

White, Heather. "Homosexuality, Gay Communities, and American Churches: A History of a Changing Religious Ethic, 1946—1977." Ph.D. Dissertation. United States—New Jersey: Princeton University, 2007.

———. *Reforming Sodom: Protestants and the Rise of Gay Rights*. Chapel Hill: University of North Carolina Press, forthcoming 2015.

Wilcox, Melissa. *Coming Out in Christianity: Religion, Identity, and Community*. Bloomington: Indiana University Press, 2003.

Wilcox, Clyde, and Carin Larson. *Onward Christian Soldiers: The Religious Right in American Politics*. Bloomington: Indiana University Press, 2006.

Wilentz, Sean. *The Age of Reagan: A History, 1974–2008*. New York: HarperCollins, 2008.

Wilkerson, David. *The Vision*. Old Tappan, NJ: Revell, 1974.

Williams, Daniel K. *God's Own Party: The Making of the Christian Right*. Oxford and New York: Oxford University Press, 2010.

Winston, Diane H. "Back to the Future: Religion, Politics, and the Media," *American Quarterly* 59:3 (Sept. 2007): 969–989.

———. "News Coverage of Religion, Sexuality, and AIDS," in *The Oxford Handbook of Religion and the American News Media*. New York: Oxford University Press, 2012: 377–390.

Wooding, Dan. *He Intends Victory*. Irvine, CA: Village Books, 1994.

Worthen, Molly. *Apostles of Reason: The Crisis of Authority in American Evangelicalism*. Oxford and New York: Oxford University Press, 2014.

Wuthnow, Robert. *After Heaven: Spirituality in America since the 1950s*. Berkeley: University of California Press, 1998.

———. *The Restructuring of American Religion: Society and Faith since World War II*. Princeton, NJ: Princeton University Press, 1988.

———. *Boundless Faith*. Berkeley: University of California Press, 2009.

Yamamori, Tetsunao, David Dageforde, and Tina Bruner. *The Hope Factor: Engaging the Church in the HIV/AIDS Crisis*. Waynesboro, GA: Authentic Media; Federal Way, WA: World Vision, 2003.

Yingling, Thomas. *AIDS and the National Body*. Edited by Robyn Wiegman. Durham, NC: Duke University Press, 1997.

Young, Rebecca M., and Ilan H. Meyer, "The Trouble with 'MSM' and 'WSW': Erasure of the Sexual Minority Person in Public Health Discourse," *American Journal of Public Health* 95:7 (July 2005): 1144–1149.

Zigon, Jarrett. *Morality: An Anthropological Perspective*. Oxford and New York: Berg Publishers, 2008.

———. *"HIV Is God's Blessing:" Rehabilitating Morality in Neoliberal Russia*. Berkeley: University of California Press, 2010.

Index

ABC approach, 50
   See also abstinence; condoms; sex
    education
abortion, 8–9, 21, 99, 111–112, 139,
   190
   Cuomo's stance on, 95–98, 232n17
   Koop's stance on, 55, 57–61, 64, 80,
    224n20
   O'Connor's stance on, 91–93,
    100–102, 137, 151–155
   pro-choice v. pro-life activism,
    151–167, 170–178, 184
   See also National Abortion Rights
    Action League; Operation
    Rescue; Pennsylvania Pro-
    Life Commission; Planned
    Parenthood
abstinence, 6, 9, 112, 176
   in sex education, 11, 21, 55, 111–112,
    184, 218n95
   as way to stop AIDS, 19, 43–44, 47,
    50–52, 76, 78, 83–84, 88–90,
    122, 124, 188–192, 210n4
Ad Hoc Alliance to Defend the Fourth
   Commandment, 167
Africa
   AIDS crisis in, 20–21, 47–49, 52,
    253n7
   AIDS attributed to, 3, 27, 253n8

The African American Clergy's
   Declaration of War on HIV/AIDS,
   36
African American Christian responses
   to AIDS, 36, 71, 81, 148, 216n68
African American Religious Leaders
   Summit on HIV/AIDS, 36
African Americans, 36, 166
   AIDS activism and, 36, 71, 81, 86,
    147–148
   AIDS affecting, 20, 40, 119, 132
Agudath Israel, 102
AIDS/HIV
   medical definitions of, 16, 23, 224n9
   link to HIV, 16
   moral etiology of, 6, 117, 189
   "gay cancer" and, 10, 23
   heterosexuality and, 3, 46–47
AIDS activism, 2–4, 24, 41–44, 95, 100,
   109, 135, 137–187, 191–195, 211n18,
   256n25
   biomedicine and, 130–131
   evangelical AIDS workers, 19, 21, 46,
    47, 48–52
   Koop and, 55, 71
   public health initiatives and, 12, 68,
    207n40
   race and, 36
   Reagan's AIDS policy and, 7

relation to religion, 14–16
sex education and, 79, 89–90, 93
sex positivity and, 254n10
See also individual actions,
organizations, and people
AIDS Coalition to Unleash Power (ACT
UP), 66, 195, 220n108, 229n95,
246n65, 247n82
Civil Disobedience Training Manual,
144
ethics of safe sex and, 140–146, 145,
184–185
Majority Action Committee, 148
media campaigns, 154–159, 156, 163,
169, 182, 183
religion and, 146–150, 243n31,
244n34, 251n141
Silence = Death slogan, 36, 141, 142
See also die-ins; Stop the Church
AIDS cocktail, 3, 28, 47, 200n7, 200n8
AIDS education, 100, 115, 125, 134, 149,
159, 176
Koop's version, 55, 69–76, 78, 90,
222n7
Reagan's version, 68
AIDS Healthcare Foundation (AHF),
193, 195
AIDS Project
Interfaith Council, 37
AIDS Quilt, 220n108
AIDS-Related Complex (ARC), 209n56
AIDS Task Force, 69
Alcorn, Randy, 29–30, 32, 213n41
Alfred E. Smith Memorial Dinner, 151
Allen, Jimmy, 46
Altman, Dennis, 13–14, 23, 26, 130
A.M.E. (African Methodist Episcopal)
Zion Church, 36
America, 1–2, 4, 115, 134
American Lutheran Church, 97
American Medical Association (AMA),
60, 224n20

American Public Health Association,
60
American religion, 14, 17, 147
globalization of, 255n16
sentimentality and, 48
Anderson, Carl, 72
And the Band Played On (book), 10–11,
66–67, 192, 247n82
And the Band Played On (film), 207n38
anti-Catholicism, 140, 161–171, 174, 180,
248n92
anti-Christ
as homosexual, 32
Antoninus, Archbishop Dominican, 31
Antonio, Gene, 26
apocalypse, rhetoric of, 28–34, 201n10,
211n18
Apuzzo, Virginia, 67
Aquinas, Thomas, 123, 125
Archdiocese of Military Services, 94,
124, 238n118
Archdiocese of New York, 93, 100–102,
108, 114, 123, 153
Archdiocese of San Francisco, 115
Office of Christian and Family
Development, 111
Ark of Refuge, Inc., 36
Asad, Talal, 180, 209n51
See also religious power; secularism
Asians, 144, 243n32
Augustine, 31, 149
AZT, 65, 144

Baby Doe, 63–64, 85
Baker, John, 63
The Balm in Gilead, 36
Bamforth, Nick, 38
Barbwire (blog), 194
Barnhouse, Donald, 57
Bataille, Georges, 137
bathhouses, 10–12, 44, 67–68,
208n45

Bauer, Gary, 67–69, 70, 74, 76, 81,
    87–89
Bean, Carl, 36
Bellah, Robert, 206n33
Benedict XVI, Pope
    See Ratzinger, Joseph
Bennett, William, 67, 69–70, 72, 74, 79,
    81, 87–90
Berkovitch, Sacvan, 213n39
Berkowitz, Richard, 89
Berlant, Lauren, 8–9, 186, 205n27,
    220n112
Bernardin, Joseph, 97–98, 100, 117,
    124, 126–129, 152, 239n134
Bevilacqua, Anthony, 124
Bible, 33, 42, 45, 53–54, 82, 85, 229n100
    1 Corinthians 6, 214n46
    biblical approach to AIDS, 19, 43, 45,
        50–52, 188–190
    Daniel 11:37, 32
    discussion of sodomy, 29–33, 54
    flood of Noah, 32
    Genesis 19, 31, 133, 214n46
    King James Bible, 32, 149
    Matthew, gospel of, 50, 221n116
    medicine and, 6
    New International Version, 214n47
    obligation to help the poor, 40–41
    role in evangelical Protestant
        Christianity, 15
    Romans 1, 31, 214n46
    Scofield Reference Bible, 26
Bible Belt Christians, 59, 76
Billings, Robert, 224n19
biomedicine, 2, 6, 14, 130, 135, 188,
    193–195
biopower, 5–6, 203n18, 205n21
    See also citizenship: moral
        citizenship; morality; religious
        power
bisexuality, 107, 221n120
bisexual men, 16, 41–42, 65, 84, 86, 119

Bivins, Jason, 212n23
blackness, 40, 87, 154, 166–168
    AIDS activism and, 36, 148
    See also African American Christian
        responses to AIDS; African
        Americans; National Coalition of
        Black Lesbians and Gays
Blackwell, Morton, 67
Blair, Tony, 21
blood donation, 67–68, 75, 119
blood transfusions, 24, 46, 65
Blotcher, Jay, 155
B'nai B'rith Women, 97
body
    See biopower; ritual
The Body, 35
Bono, 21
Boone, Pat, 214n44
Bosco, Anthony, 117
Bowen, Otis, 70
Bowers v. Hardwick, 7, 73, 141, 242n18
Brahmstedt, Christian, 72
Braidfoot, Larry, 81
Brandt, Edward, 66, 69
Braum, Barbara, 165
Brickner, Balfour, 102
Brier, Jennifer, 68, 74, 78, 227n68,
    229n95, 253n8
Brookins, Gary
    Surgeon General cartoon, 56, 76
Brownback, Sam, 20
Buchanan, Pat, 67
Buckalew, Judi, 67
Buckley, William F., Jr., 72
Buddhism, 14
Burger, Warren, 141
Burroughs Wellcome, 144
Bush, George W., 18–20, 188, 210n3
Bynum, Caroline Walker, 252n142

Caffarra, Carlo, 127–128
Cahill, Kevin, 108

Called to Compassion and
Responsibility, 116–117, 129–136,
149, 152
Callen, Michael, 89
Calve, John, 177–178
Cameron, Paul, 26, 73, 80
Campaign for a Smoke-Free America
by the Year 2000, 62
Campo, Rafael, 137, 186–187
Caritas Internationalis, 194
Carter, Jimmy, 59
Casanova, José, 92, 99–100, 116,
232n17
Casey, Ken, 47
Cathedral Project, 151, 176–177
Catholic Charities, 101
Catholic Coalition for Gay Civil Rights,
107
Catholic Health Association, 117
Catholic Ignatius Press, 26
Catholicism
See Roman Catholicism
Catholic New York, 4, 103–108, 110–111,
137, 161–162, 164–166, 172,
180–181, 236n80
Catholics
See Roman Catholics
Center for HIV Law and Policy, 254n16
Centers for Disease Control (CDC),
10, 23, 64, 66, 68, 74, 117, 222n5,
225n29
Central Conference of American
Rabbis, 97
The Challenge of Peace letter, 99
Chambré, Susan, 200n5
chastity, 29
as way to stop AIDS, 43, 111, 123–124,
127, 132–133, 151
Chauncey, George, 191, 196–197,
254n12
The Chicago Catholic, 126
Chilton, David, 26–27

Christian Broadcasting Network, 72
Christian Century, 4, 35, 38, 44–45
Christianity
See individual churches, denominations,
people, and publications
Christianity Today, 4, 47, 50, 60, 79,
218n95
Christian Right, 8, 13–14, 38, 40, 65, 72,
188, 252n5
AIDS as God's punishment
argument, 2, 28, 33, 54
definition of, 15
political use of AIDS, 24, 26
in Reagan era, 19
rise of, 3
views on homosexuality, 9, 21, 45,
89–90, 187, 190–191
See also Religious Right
Christians
conservative Christians, 24–25, 28–30,
32, 39, 45, 46, 73, 87, 194, 256n25
progressive Christians, 33, 42, 188
See also individual denominations and
people
citizenship, 4, 33, 105, 140, 253n8
moral citizenship, 6–9, 73, 89, 107,
179, 190–197
City of Refuge Church, 36
civil rights, 7, 37, 67–69, 78, 154, 159
civil rights for African Americans, 144
civil rights for gays and lesbians, 8–9,
14, 25, 34, 37, 71, 73, 93, 139, 161,
164–167, 171–176, 184, 187, 189,
191–192
anti-discrimination laws, 100–108,
112–114, 176
civil rights for people with AIDS, 43,
143, 157
civil rights for people with disabilities,
61, 64
civil rights for women, 60, 93, 144, 154,
157, 159, 176

Clinton, Bill, 38, 187, 210n3
Clinton, Hillary, 21
Coalition for Lesbian and Gay Rights, 102, 151, 164
Coffin, William Sloane, 28
colonialism, 202n14, 220n112
Common Threads: Stories from the Quilt, 220n108
Comstock, Anthony, 73
condoms, 11, 22–23, 43, 159, 183–184, 191–192, 194–195
    Bennett's views on, 74
    Catholic views on, 116, 122, 126–128, 131, 134, 150–152, 155, 157, 161, 175
    evangelical Christian views on, 47
    Koop's views on, 44–45, 55, 70, 72, 76, 78–79, 82–84, 88, 90, 190
    O'Connor's views on, 93, 110–112, 123–124, 135, 158–159, 162, 173
    Warrens' views on, 6, 42, 50–52
Congregation Beth Simchat Torah (CBST), 34
Congregation for the Doctrine of the Faith, 112, 128
Conservative Caucus, 67
contraception, 9, 59–60, 111, 149, 175, 232n26
    birth control pill, 194, 235n70
    See also condoms
Cooke, Terence, 94, 100–101, 108
Corrada, Alvaro, 238n120
Costello, George, 161–162
Courage, 166
criminalization of AIDS, 192–193, 254n16
Crimp, Douglas, 10, 89–90, 226n61, 230n108
Cuite, Tom, 101
culture wars, 1, 22–23, 32, 59–61, 187, 194, 248n92
    abortion's role in, 92
    challenge to binary model of, 22, 52

Koop's role in, 57, 63, 76
    Stop the Church's role in, 140, 165
Culture Wars (magazine)
    See Fidelity
Cuomo, Mario, 95–98, 100, 102, 158, 170
Curran, Charles, 151

Damian, Peter, 31
Dannemeyer, William, 68
Declaration on Certain Questions Concerning Sexual Ethics, 113
Defense of Marriage Act (DOMA), 187, 190, 192
Democrats, 21, 59–60, 95–96, 98, 100–101, 152, 187
Denver Principles, 209n57
Department of Education, 69, 74
die-ins, 138, 150, 155, 157
Dignity, 114
direct-action activism, 140–141, 143, 149, 151, 158, 177, 247n82
    See also AIDS Coalition to Unleash Power (ACT UP)
disability, 58, 61, 63–64, 95, 217n75
Dobson, James, 8
Dolores Street Southern Baptist Church, 35
Dornan, Robert, 68
Dortzbach, Deborah, 49
Douglas, Ann, 48–49
Douglas, Mary, 206n33
Douglass, Frederick, 144, 146
Dugas, Gaëtan, 10–11, 207n36
Dunagin, Ralph
    Surgeon General cartoon, 76, 77
Dunne, Richard, 141

Eagle Forum, of Schlafly, 72
Economic Justice for All letter, 99
Egan, Edward, 110–112
Elbaz, Gilbert, 147, 243n31, 243n32, 246n64

Ellis, Havelock, 30
Engel, Jonathan, 10–13, 78, 130
epidemiology, 13, 28, 224n29
Epstein, Rob
  Common Threads: Stories from the Quilt, 220n108
Erik, Servalan, 176
Estrada, Erik, 214n44
Eternal Perspective Ministries, 29
ethics, 5, 27, 58, 203n16
  sexual ethics, 17, 52, 89–90, 113, 140–146, 184, 254n15
Eucharist, 138–139, 165, 181
  See also host
Evangelical Christian Publishers Association, 213n41
evangelicals, 37, 79, 170, 194, 200n9, 214n41, 214n44, 219n108, 254n10
  in culture wars, 8
  definition, 15
  Koop and, 57–60, 72, 84–86, 90
  progressive evangelicals, 15, 37, 44–46
  views on abortion, 98
  views on AIDS as moral crisis, 3, 5–6, 19–21, 25, 30, 43–52, 81, 115, 187–190, 218n87, 220n112, 252n5
  views on homosexuality, 35, 214n47, 219n101, 221n120, 255n16
  views on witnessing, 33
Evans, Rowland, 72
Executive Order 50, 101, 233n37
Executive Task Force on AIDS, 66

Falwell, Jerry, 8, 24–25, 83, 187
family values, 8, 25, 44, 87
Fee, Elizabeth, 200n8
feminism, 8, 49, 91, 139, 144, 171, 248n92, 250n111, 254n15
Ferraro, Geraldine, 96, 100
fidelity, 19, 29, 50, 59, 78, 109
  as way to stop AIDS, 43, 47, 50–52,

74, 81, 83–84, 121–122, 132, 189, 240n148
Fidelity Magazine, 167, 249n101
First Orthodox Presbyterian Church, 82, 213n40
Flemister, Carl, 247n87
Fletcher, James, 53–54
Flunder, Yvette, 36
Flynn, Michael, 173
Focus on the Family, 8
Food and Drug Administration (FDA), 144, 193–194
Fortunato, John, 38
Foucault, Michel, 1, 5, 30, 203n16, 203n16, 203n18, 203n19, 215n49
  See also biopower; morality; religious power
Fox, Daniel M., 200n8
Francis, Pope, 253n7
Free Congress Research and Education Foundation
  Catholic Center, 26
Freud, Sigmund, 30
Friedman, Jeffrey
  Common Threads: Stories from the Quilt, 220n108
fundamentalism, 15, 24–25, 35, 186

Gagliostro, Vincent, 153–155, 159
Gallo, Robert, 135, 225n29
Garvey, J. Joseph, 167–168, 170
Gates, Bill, 21
Gates, Melinda, 21
Gay and Lesbian Alliance Against Defamation (GLAAD), 141
gay men, 35, 57, 64–65, 68–69, 110, 149, 168, 242n17, 242n18, 255n18
  care of, 39–42
  gay activists, 3, 7, 43–44, 66–67, 71, 79, 86, 87–90, 95, 109, 112, 130, 139, 141, 148– 153, 159, 161, 164–165, 171–176, 184–188, 200n5

moral AIDS rhetoric and, 2, 28–32,
45, 84, 178
race and, 36, 47, 143, 217n79
sexuality of, 9–13, 22–28, 38, 53–55,
73, 111, 119, 133, 140, 146, 177,
191–197, 207n36, 207n40
as term, 15–16
See also civil rights for gays and
lesbians; homosexuality
Gay Men's Health Crisis (GMHC), 66,
140–141, 143, 149, 158, 164, 196,
229n95, 242n17, 242n18
Gay-Related Immune Deficiency
(GRID), 23, 34
Gerald, Gil, 71
Gerber, Lynne, 5, 221n120
Gilead Sciences, 194
Gingrich, Newt, 68–69
Global PEACE Coalition, 18–19, 50
Global Summit on AIDS and the
Church, 20
Good, Byron, 1, 204n20
Goodwin, Ron, 67
Gould, Deborah, 242n18
Graham, Billy, 1, 21, 28–29, 59, 187,
199n1, 220n109
Graham, Franklin, 49
Graham, Ruth, 32
Grein, Richard F., 164
Groeschel, Benedict, 166–167, 181
Guzzardo, Paul, 178

Haitians, 9, 23, 27, 65, 253n8
Harding, Susan, 33
Harlem Week of Prayer for the Healing
of AIDS, 36
Harrington, Timothy, 238n120
Harvey, Linda, 194–195
healing, 21, 36, 38, 41
health
See public health
Health and Hospitals Corp, 60

Health and Human Services (HHS),
67–69, 75
He Intends Victory, 46
Helms, Jesse, 74
Helms Amendment, 74
hemophiliacs, 24, 65
Herberg, Will, 92
Herman, Didi, 26, 212n29
herpes, 28–29
heterosexuality, 6, 9, 31, 37, 40, 54
AIDS and, 3, 20, 22, 27, 46–47, 65,
85, 119, 194
in sex education, 71, 74, 88, 111, 152,
184, 187, 192
as way to stop AIDS, 13, 24, 42–43,
52, 69, 78, 121, 132–133, 140,
189–190, 240n148
Hickey, James, 238n120
Highly Active Antiretroviral Therapy
(HAART)
See AIDS cocktail
Hilferty, Robert
Stop the Church, 138, 245n43,
246n60
HIV/AIDS
See AIDS/HIV
HIV/AIDS Initiative (Saddleback
Church), 19–21, 48–52
HIV immigration ban, 253n8
Hollenbach, David, 134
Holy See, 94, 128–129, 135
homophobia, 25, 65, 155, 172, 174, 178,
194, 207n36
homosexuality, 3, 59, 208n47, 215n49,
215n55, 215n57, 221n120, 229n100,
255n16
Koop and, 57, 70–71, 73, 79–80,
83–87, 90
moral AIDS rhetoric and, 2–3, 13,
21–28, 37, 40–43, 45–47, 74,
116–117, 131–133, 136, 187–192,
197

homosexuality (*continued*)
  religious views on, 14, 35, 38, 51–52,
      54, 67–68, 93, 100–107, 112–115,
      126, 137, 139, 149, 151–152, 155,
      164–168, 171–174, 177, 214n44,
      214n47, 219n101
  sodomy and, 28–34, 213n39, 214n46
  as term, 15–16
  See also gay men; lesbians
host, 138, 140, 162, 166, 168, 173, 179,
      181, 245n43, 247n83, 251n139,
      252n142
  See also Eucharist
How to Have Sex in an Epidemic
      pamphlet, 89
Hubbard, Howard, 239n125
Hudson, Rock, 24, 45, 200n6
Hughes, William, 117, 125, 165
Human Rights Commission of New
      York City, 106
Human Rights Commission of San
      Francisco, 24–25
Hume, David, 169
Humm, Andrew, 102, 109, 151, 164,
      172–173, 175–176
Hunter, Dan, 176
Hunter, James Davison, 1, 22,
      206n33
Hunthausen, Raymond, 151
Hybels, Bill, 49
Hybels, Lynne, 49

Iakovos, Archbishop, 247n87
immunology, 64, 225n29
Independent Fundamental Churches of
      America, 43
Interfaith CarePartners, 217n75
International Conference on AIDS,
      194, 200n7
International Pentecostal Church of
      Christ, 43
Islam, 170, 186, 202n10

Jameson, Fredric, 212n26
Jenkins, Jerry B., 29
Jenkins, Philip, 171, 250n111
Jesuits, 1–2, 115, 134, 251n141
Jesus, 220n112
  AIDS activists and, 178, 181–184,
      252n142
  model for AIDS work, 40–41, 50, 82,
      119, 188
  object of protest, 173
Jews, 14, 34, 92, 102–103, 168, 186, 188,
      248n92
  in ACT UP, 147
  AIDS ministry and, 34–35, 37, 41
  Congregation Beth Simchat Torah
      (CBST), 34
  critique of Stop the Church, 164
  Koop's address to, 86–87, 229n100
  PEPFAR and, 19
  See also Judaism
John Paul II, Pope, 94
John Paul II Institute for Studies of
      Matrimony and Family, 127
Johnson, Earvin "Magic," 46, 200n6
Jones, E. Michael, 249n101
Jordan, Mark, 18, 26, 31–32, 213n39,
      215n49
Joseph, Steve, 173
Judaism
  Agudath Israel, 102
  Orthodox Judaism, 103
  Reform Judaism, 87, 229n100
  See also Jews

Kagame, Paul, 21
Kaplan, Helen Singer, 53
Kaposi's sarcoma, 23
Keating, John, 238n120
Keeler, William, 239n134
Keenan, James, 174–175
Kennedy, John F., 168
Kenslea, Ged, 195

Kerrison, Ray, 139
Kinsey, Alfred, 30, 84
Klein, Alvin F., 101
Klenk, John, 74
Koch, Edward, 101–102, 107, 110–112,
    150, 154, 234n62
Koop, C. Everett, 53, 62, 167, 193,
    224n20, 240n148, 249n102
    evangelical identity, 57–61, 227n68,
    229n100
    *Surgeon General's Report on Acquired
    Immune Deficiency Syndrome*,
    70–71, 82
    views on AIDS education, 44–45,
    55–56, 65–66, 69–90, 78–90,
    189–191, 222n7
    views on Baby Doe case, 63–64
    views on smoking, 61–63, 64
Kramer, Larry, 140–143, 149, 195,
    242n18
    Faggots, 242n17
    The Normal Heart, 192, 196
Krol, John, 98, 124

L'Abri, 58
Laghi, Pio, 94
LaHaye, Beverly, 29
LaHaye, Tim, 29–30, 32, 215n57
LaRouche Initiative, 37
Latinos, 36, 144, 147
    AIDS affecting, 20, 36, 40, 87, 119, 132
Lavender Hill Mob, 141, 151
Law, Bernard, 98, 124, 239n134
Lawrence v. Texas, 7, 73
Lazarus, William H., 248n87
Leclair, Danny, 193
lesbians, 10, 14, 53, 73, 155, 157, 168,
    184–185, 187–188, 191–192, 197
    lesbian activists, 3, 7, 21, 43–44,
    66–67, 86, 93, 95, 109, 140–141,
    144, 147, 171–176, 196, 251n41
    role in religion, 34, 36, 38, 57, 114

sexuality of, 9–10, 55, 88–89, 146
    as term, 15
    See also civil rights for gays and
    lesbians; homosexuality
Lessard, Raymond, 117, 239n134
Levi, Jeff, 67
liberalism, 59, 105, 160, 189
    definitions of religion and, 168–170,
    174, 180, 184
    See also religious freedom;
    secularism; sexual freedom
Lily, Frank, 109
lived religion, 210n58, 231n5, 251n139
Lively, Scott, 255n16
Lochrane, Patrick, 107
Long, Thomas, 211n18, 213n39, 214n44
Loots, Aubrey, 193
Los Angeles Times, 36, 71, 76–77
L'Osservatore Romano, 128, 239n130
Love Center Church, 36
Lowder, Jim, 35
Lutherans, 97, 173, 248n87
Luther, Martin, 252n142
Lutton, Wayne C., 26, 73
Lyons, Thomas, 238n120

Maggenti, Maria, 148
Mahmood, Saba, 203n16
Mahoney, Roger, 138, 238n120, 239n134
Malone, James, 95
Manoogian, Torkom, 248n87
Mansell, Peter, 39
Many Faces of AIDS statement, 115–136,
    152, 238n118, 238n120
Marino, Eugene, 238n120
marriage, 84, 190, 204n21, 232n26
    gay marriage, 21, 186, 187, 191–193,
    195–197, 227n73, 254n15
    as risk factor for AIDS, 256n25
    in sexual morality rhetoric, 6, 9, 29,
    69, 74, 80, 84, 90, 111, 112, 124,
    127, 134, 191–197

marriage (*continued*)
  as way to stop AIDS, 19, 43, 50,
    78, 80, 121–122, 152, 189–190,
    240n148
Marsden, George, 15
Mason, James O., 69
Mauss, Marcel, 91, 203n16
May, John, 123, 126–127
Mayberry, Eugene, 109–110
McAlister, Melani, 49
McBeath, William, 60
McGovern, Terry, 175–176, 180
McIlhenny, Chuck, 82, 213n40
McIlhenny, Donna, 213n40
McKeon, Richard D., 165
McLaughlin, Loretta, 71
Melbourne Declaration, 194
Mendolia, Victor, 153, 157, 176–177
men who have sex with men (MSMs),
    16, 255n18
methodology of book, 4
Metropolitan Community Church
    (MCC), 34–35
Meyer, Michael G., 115
Meyers, Woodrow, 109
Michelman, Henry, 81, 164
Minority AIDS Program (MAP), 36
Mission: America, 194
Monette, Paul, 186–187, 252n1
monogamy, 12–13, 140, 196, 256n25
  in sexual morality rhetoric, 6, 9, 55,
    71, 78, 111, 121, 127, 152, 184,
    196, 240n148
  as way to stop AIDS, 12–13, 19, 24,
    35, 42, 44–45, 51–52, 81, 83–84,
    88–90, 190–193
Montagnier, Luc, 225n29
Moore, Paul, Jr., 102
moralism, 13, 78, 89, 207n38, 208n46,
    227n72, 247n82
morality, 65, 67, 69, 203n16, 252n5,
    253n10

AIDS as moral epidemic, 2–6, 10–17,
    20–24, 27, 43–52, 187–188,
    190–194, 197
  biopower and, 5–6, 203n16, 203n18,
    203n19
  Catholics on, 91–100, 103, 105–107,
    111–136, 140
  critiques of, 40–42
  in culture wars, 59–60
  definition, 5, 204n21
  difference from moralism, 208n46
  gay activism and, 144, 146
  Koop and, 63–64, 70–74, 76–90
  languages of, 4–6, 9, 29–34
  moral citizenship, 6–9, 73, 89, 107,
    179, 190–197
  queerness and, 189
  racism and, 202n14
  secular and religious form of, 4–5, 14
  sexual morality, 7–8, 19, 43–45,
    52–58, 78–79, 93, 99–100,
    116–118, 127, 132, 189–190
  sodomy and, 28–34, 222n4
  Stop the Church and, 151–152, 157, 160,
    161, 162, 167, 177, 181, 184–185
  See also ethics; safe sex
Moral Majority, 8, 24–25, 67, 83, 224n19
Morrison, Kendall, 250n113
Mother Teresa, 109
Mugavero, Francis, 105, 233n37
Murphy, Patrice, 28
Murphy, Ryan
  The Normal Heart, 196
Murphy, Timothy, 11

Najman, Ronald, 173–174
National Abortion Rights Action
    League, 60
National Academy of Sciences, 121
National Association of Evangelicals
    (NAE), 81
  Statement on AIDS, 43–44

National Catholic AIDS Network, 194

National Coalition of American Nuns, 107

National Coalition of Black Lesbians and Gays, 71, 81, 86

National Conference of Catholic Bishops (NCCB), 115, 123–126, 128, 132, 134, 237n93

   See also Called to Compassion and Responsibility

National Council of Churches of Christ, 37, 81

National Gay and Lesbian Task Force, 67, 71–72

National Institutes of Health (NIH), 64, 225n29

National Organization for Women, 60

National Religious Broadcasters, 84

National School Boards, 83

Native American religion, 14, 170

Navarro-Valls, Joaquin, 128

needle exchange, 50, 131–132, 135, 151, 155

neoliberalism, 206n29, 254n14

New Age religion, 14, 38

New York City Board of Health, 108

New York Post, 139, 160, 173

New York Times, 4, 61, 96, 100, 195

   coverage of AIDS activism, 160, 179

   coverage of condom debates, 110, 123

   coverage of gay rights bill, 102–103

Noebel, David A., 26, 30, 32, 73, 215n55

The Normal Heart (film), 196

The Normal Heart (play), 192

Novak, Robert, 72

Obama, Barack, 20–21, 52, 186, 191, 255n16

O'Connor, John J., 94, 149, 151, 159–162, 164, 168–169, 173–174, 176–181

   representations of, 156, 169, 182

views on abortion, 91–92, 95–98, 152–158, 169

views on AIDS, 108–110, 123–124, 135–136

views on condoms, 93, 110–112, 116

views on gay rights, 100–105, 107

views on Stop the Church, 137–140, 150, 171

Operation Rescue, 153, 157, 170, 173, 178

Opus Dei, 167

Orange County, 37, 153

O'Reilly, Kevin, 106

Orsi, Robert, 139, 202–14

Orthodox Jews, 102–103

OutWeek, 4, 155, 171–178, 180

Pacific Islanders, 144, 243n32

Palmer, Susan, 211n18

Pastoral Care of Homosexual Persons letter, 113–115

Patient Zero, 10–11

Patton, Cindy, 13, 23, 130

Pennsylvania Pro-Life Commission, 96

Pentecostals, 34, 43

people of color, 146–148

   See also individual groups

people with AIDS (PWAs), 16–17, 34–44, 51, 79, 84, 109, 117–118, 123, 143, 157, 159, 187–188, 209n57

   as movement, 209n57

people with HIV, 7, 16, 22, 36, 41, 46, 51, 66, 108, 116–118, 129, 144, 184, 188, 194

Perry, Troy, 34

Philadelphia Baptist Church in Harlem, 148

Phillips, Howard, 67

Pieters, Stephen, 34–35

Pilarczyk, Daniel, 126

Planned Parenthood, 60

Play Fair! brochure, 89

pluralism, 97, 112, 116, 118, 120,
122–126, 130, 133–136, 170
Pneumocystis carinii (PCP), 23
Poust, Mary Ann, 164
P.O.V., 138
power
See biopower; morality; religious
power
pre-exposure prophylaxis (PrEP),
193–195, 255n18
See also Truvada
Presbyterian Church (U.S.A), 37–38, 97
Presbyterian Church in America (PCA),
57
Presbyterians, 37–38, 44, 57
*See also individual churches,
organizations, and people*
Presidential Commission on HIV, 44,
109, 149
President's Emergency Plan for AIDS
Relief (PEPFAR), 18–20, 188,
210n4
promiscuity, 54, 70, 76, 84, 87, 111, 121,
134
blamed for AIDS, 3, 9–13, 23–24,
26–29, 45, 80–82, 89, 191–196,
242n17
ethical value of, 89–90
Protestant Reformation, 31–32
Protestants, 2, 15, 22, 44, 51, 59, 102,
168–171, 200n9, 214n47
in ACT UP, 147
liberal Protestants, 3, 15, 202n14,
214n47, 229n100
mainline Protestants, 6, 35, 37–38,
188, 219n108, 252n5
relation with Catholics, 92–93,
248n92
See also evangelicals; *individual
churches*, denominations, *people,
and publications*
prostitution, 12, 16, 41, 83

See also sex workers
Public Broadcasting Station (PBS), 138
public health, 3–6, 60–62, 108,
143–144, 146, 180, 222n5
AIDS discourses in, 14–15, 23, 26,
46–47, 55–56, 65–69, 77–82,
130–131, 195
morality and, 85–90
PEPFAR and, 19
promiscuity rhetoric in, 10
sexuality initiatives, 12, 43–44, 122,
188, 190, 193, 207n40, 255n16
use by religious leaders, 33, 37, 52, 73,
93, 128, 202n12
Public Health Office (PHO), 55, 74, 88
Public Health Service, 66, 193
Pullen, Penny, 44
Pusilo, Robert, 164, 177

quarantine, 37, 70–71, 80
queer activism, 193, 211n18
See also AIDS Coalition to Unleash
Power (ACT UP)
queerness, 38, 89, 90, 146, 186, 189,
196
queer studies, 49, 221n120, 254n15
Quiñones, Nathan, 110

race, 3, 17, 59, 87, 168, 189, 205n25,
220n112
ACT UP and, 146–147, 243n32
AIDS epidemic and, 36, 46–47, 71,
86–87, 253n8
in anti-discrimination bills, 102, 104
"gay men" category and, 16, 217n79
in Many Faces of AIDS, 119
See also blackness; slavery; whiteness
racism, 45, 65, 106, 146, 202n14
See also slavery
Radclyffe, Nancy, 37
Ratzinger, Joseph, 112–115, 126,
128–129, 151, 236n80, 253n7

Rauch, Jonathan, 191
Reagan, Ronald, 78, 109, 199n1,
    232n25, 249n102
    on AIDS, 7, 13, 55, 66–69, 73–74, 141,
        253n8
    Christian Right and, 19, 59–61
    conservatism of, 8, 98, 132, 205n21
    economic policies of, 65
Reformed Presbyterian Church,
    Evangelical Synod, 57
Reform Jews, 87, 229n100
religious freedom, 15, 100, 138, 140,
    158–185, 174, 191, 251n141
    See also liberalism; secularism; sexual
        freedom
religious power, 4, 16, 146
    See also morality; Asad, Talal;
        secularism
Religious Right, 25, 70, 72, 78, 224n19
    See also Christian Right
Republicans, 20, 59–60, 68, 98
Rhoades, Nick, 193
ritual, 170, 180–185, 245n43, 251n141
Riverside Church, 28
Roach, John, 239n125
Robertson, Pat, 25
    The 700 Club and, 72–73
Rockland County Coalition of Lay
    Catholics for Life, 165
Roe v. Wade, 58, 60, 92
Roman Catholicism, 4, 59, 186,
    239n125, 240n148
    social v. public Catholicism, 92
    public Catholicism, 94–100, 116
    See also anti-Catholicism; Stop the
        Church; *individual churches,
        conferences, people, and
        publications*
Roman Catholics, 3, 72, 115–117,
    150–152, 188, 252n5
    in ACT UP, 147, 159, 251n141
    conservative Catholics, 8, 15

gay Catholics, 151
lay Catholics, 3, 15, 16, 92, 94, 97, 99,
    107, 153, 155, 165, 174–175
    political division among bishops, 98
    role in AIDS work, 35, 37, 108–110,
        193–194
    sodomy and, 32
    tensions with Protestants, 93
    views on ABC approach, 50
    views on abortion, 91–92, 94–100,
        152–155, 157–158, 231n13, 232n17
    views on AIDS as moral crisis, 6,
        117–136, 189–190
    views on homosexuality, 2, 100–103,
        105–107, 112–115, 172
    See also Holy See; Vatican
Rotello, Gabriel, 250n113
Rubin, Gayle, 186, 254n15
Rueda, Enrique, 26–27, 212n29
Russell, Bertrand, 30
Russian Orthodox Church, 203n16
Rwanda, 21
Ryan White CARE Act, 192, 225n32

Saddleback Church, 19, 21, 48, 50–51
    See also HIV/AIDS Initiative
Saddleback Civil Forum on Global
    Health, 18
safe sex, 11, 35, 43–45, 66, 187, 191,
    207n40
    Catholic views on, 111, 121–122, 126–
        127, 133, 160–161, 177, 238n120
    ethics of, 140–146
    Koop's views on, 82, 84
    medicalization of, 195
    norm in gay communities, 25, 69
    posters, 145, 156
    promiscuity and, 13, 89–90
    public funding for programs, 23
Salvation Army, 101–102
Sammons, James, 224n20
San Francisco AIDS Foundation, 25

Sanger, Margaret, 30
Schaeffer, Francis, 58–59
Schlafly, Phyllis, 72
Schlesinger, Arthur, 168
Schulman, Sarah, 154
Schwartz, Michael, 26–27
Schweiker, Richard, 60
Scully, Edward, 165
secular humanism, 15, 29–30, 174
secularism
    AIDS activism and, 41, 139, 146–147,
        165, 174, 175, 202n10
    languages of, 4, 33, 202n12, 203n17
    liberalism and, 79, 93
    morality and, 4–6, 79, 190, 252n5
    public health and, 56, 79
    reading practices of, 32–33
    religion and, 3, 14, 78–79, 168–170,
        209n51, 251n140
    religious freedom and, 168–170,
        179–185
    secular media, 4, 25, 105, 140, 162,
        168
    sexuality and, 8, 42, 55, 202n11,
        227n71, 241n11
Seele, Pernessa, 36
    See also The Balm in Gilead; Harlem
        Week of Prayer for the Healing
        of AIDS
Self, Robert, 8, 78, 84, 206n29
sentimentality, 8, 48–49, 196, 205n27,
    219n108
sex education, 2, 11, 60, 68, 70–74,
    110–111, 117, 194, 204n21, 222n6,
    253n10
    Catholic views on, 121–126, 137, 175,
        177, 184, 189, 238n120
    comprehensive, 19, 21, 40, 159
    Koop's views on, 43–45, 55–57, 61,
        78–81, 84, 86–88, 90, 190–191
sexual freedom, 140, 146, 171–172,
    179–185, 191, 195

sexually transmitted diseases (STDs),
    53, 57, 71, 81, 83, 125–126, 190,
    209n56
    See also AIDS; herpes; HIV
sexually transmitted infections (STIs),
    209n56
sex workers, 9, 12, 16, 41, 83, 85, 131,
    215n57
    See also prostitution
Shelp, Earl, 38–43, 51, 217n78, 217n79
Shilts, Randy, 130, 161
    And the Band Played On (book),
        10–11, 66–67, 192, 247n82
    And the Band Played On (film),
        207n38
Shultz, Tom, 178–179
Shuster, William, 224n19
Sider, Ron, 44–45, 187, 189, 218n97
Sinski, Robert, 107
Sisters in Gay Ministry, 107
Sisters of Perpetual Indulgence, 89
slavery, 97
SLOW approach, 50
Smith, Jonathan Z., 137
smoking, 54, 61–64, 90
social justice, 41, 44, 97, 253n7
sodomy, 55, 72, 86–87, 213n39
    biblical accounts of, 29–34, 214n44,
        214n46
    criminalization/decriminalization of,
        7, 73, 141
Somfai, Bela, 134
Sonnenberg, Bruce, 46
Southern Baptist Convention, 43, 85
    Christian Life Commission, 81–82
Southern Baptist Golden Gate
    Seminary, 35
Southern Baptists, 18, 29, 35, 38, 46,
    48, 59, 154
Spellman Center, 109
spirituality, 20–21, 35, 38–39, 48, 52,
    191, 244n35

spiritual terror, 167–168
spiritual versus religious, 147
See also New Age religion
Spottiswoode, Robert
  And the Band Played On, 207n38
Stafford, J. Francis, 125
Stahel, Thomas, 2
Stanley, Charles, 35
Steinem, Gloria, 91–93, 108, 230n1
Stephen Wise Free Synagogue, 102
Stevens, Jackie, 36
Stevens, John Paul, 63
STOP approach, 50
Stop the Church (film), 138, 245n43,
  246n60
Stop the Church (protest), 137–140,
  150–151, 153–161, 187, 191
  anti-Catholicism and, 161–171
  debates over, 171–179
  representations of, 156, 179–185
  tenth anniversary of, 241n5
Stowe, Eugene L., 53
Stowe, Harriet Beecher, 48
St. Patrick's Cathedral, 93, 102, 107–108,
  137–140, 149–153, 157, 160–161, 167,
  170–171, 175–176, 241n5
St. Paul's Episcopal Church, 37
Sullivan, Andrew, 191
Summit Ministries, 26, 72, 73, 212n25
Sunderland, Ronald, 38–43, 51, 217n78,
  217n79
Sweeney, Timothy, 164
Synagogue Council of America, 81, 164

Terry, Luther, 224n25
testing, 193
  mandatory testing, 12, 70–71, 80,
  208n40, 253n8
theology, 96, 127, 132, 134, 152, 171
  AIDS theology, 38–43, 217n74
  queer theology, 38, 252n141
  See also Christian Right; Protestants;

Roman Catholicism; Roman
  Catholics
Thomas, Kendall, 148
Titchener, Carl F., 22–23
Tompkins, Jane, 48–49
Treichler, Paula, 88
Trinity Church, 143
Truvada, 194–195
  See also pre-exposure prophylaxis
  (PrEP)
Turner, William, 67

Uganda, 255n16
Understanding AIDS pamphlet, 55, 56,
  74–76, 75, 77, 88–89, 190
Union of the American Hebrew
  Congregations, 86
Unitarian Universalist Church of
  Amherst, 22
United States Catholic Conference
  (USCC), 81, 95–96, 99, 115, 117,
  123–126, 134, 237n93
United States Conference of Catholic
  Bishops (USCCB), 237n93

Vaid, Urvashi, 71
Vallone, Peter, 101
Vatican, 127–130, 136, 151, 236n83, 253n7
  AIDS conference, 135, 157, 172
  Declaration on Certain Questions
    Concerning Sexual Ethics, 113
  L'Osservatore Romano, 128, 239n130
  Pastoral Care of Homosexual Persons
    letter, 113–115
  Second Vatican Council, 92, 98, 130,
    232n26, 237n93
  support for O'Connor, 94
  See also Holy See
Vaughan, Austin, 153
Village Voice, 155, 231n13
virology, 64, 225n29
Vitillo, Robert, 194

Wacker, Grant, 1
Wald, Priscilla, 18
Warner, Michael, 189
Warren, Kay, 6, 19–21, 48–52, 189, 193, 220n109
Warren, Rick, 6, 18–21, 48–52, 189, 193, 220n109, 221n116
Watkins, James, 110
Waxman, Henry, 60
Weinstein, Michael, 195
Welfare Reform bill (1996), 210n3
Weyrich, Paul, 212n29
White, C. Dale, 248n87
White, Heather, 214n47
White, Ryan, 65–66
whiteness, 76, 96
    AIDS activism and, 143–144, 146–148
    AIDS and, 22, 36, 43, 47, 119
    evangelicals and, 59, 86
    gay identity and, 16, 192, 217n79
Whittlesey, Faith Ryan, 67

Wilkerson, David, 214n44
Willow Creek Community Church, 49
Winston, Diane, 65
Wolfenden Report, 215n57
Women of the Episcopal Church, 97
Women's Health Action and
    Mobilization (WHAM!), 137–138, 150, 154–155, 157, 159, 184
Women's Suburban Clinic, 153
Wooding, Dan, 46
Woods, Cathi, 218n95
Woosley, John, 111
World AIDS Day, 18
World Relief, 49
World Vision, 47
World War II, 3, 59, 87, 92, 147, 248n92

Yingling, Thomas, 9
Yorba-Gray, Joan, 46

Zigon, Jarrett, 203n16